BEDSIDE ULTRASONOGRAPHY IN CLINICAL MEDICINE

Notice

BEDSIDE ULTRASONOGRAPHY IN CLINICAL MEDICINE

Alexander B. Levitov, MD, FCCM, RDCS

Professor, Department of Medicine
Eastern Virginia Medical School
Norfolk, Virginia

Apostolos P. Dallas, MD, FACP

Attending Physician, Carilion Medical Center
Assistant Professor, Department of Medicine
Virginia-Tech-Carilion School of Medicine
Roanoke, Virginia

Anthony D. Slonim, MD, DrPH

Vice President, Medical Affairs
Attending Physician, Carilion Medical Center
Professor, Departments of Basic Sciences
Internal Medicine, and Pediatrics
Virginia-Tech-Carilion School of Medicine
Roanoke, Virginia

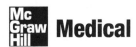

New York   Chicago   San Francisco   Lisbon   London   Madrid   Mexico City
New Delhi   San Juan   Seoul   Singapore   Sydney   Toronto

Bedside Ultrasonography in Clinical Medicine

1 2 3 4 5 6 7 8 9 0   DOW/DOW   14 13 12 11 10

Set ISBN 978-0-07-166331-1; MHID 0-07-166331-2
Book ISBN 978-0-07-166330-4; MHID 0-07-166330-4
DVD ISBN 978-0-07-166332-8; MHID 0-07-166332-0

This book was set in Cheltenham-Book by Glyph International.
The editors were James Shanahan and Karen Edmonson.
The production supervisor was Catherine Saggese.
Project management was provided by Rajni Pisharody, Glyph International.
RR Donnelley was printer and binder.

This book is printed on acid-free paper.

Library of Congress Cataloging-in-Publication Data

Bedside ultrasonography in clinical medicine / [edited by] Alexander Levitov, Apostolos P. Dallas, Anthony D. Slonim.
   p. ; cm.
   Includes bibliographical references and index.
   ISBN-13: 978-0-07-166331-1 (alk. paper)
   ISBN-10: 0-07-166331-2 (alk. paper)
   1. Diagnostic ultrasonic imaging.   2. Ultrasonics in medicine.   3. Point-of-care testing.   I. Levitov, Alexander.   II. Dallas, Apostolos P. (Apostolos Paul)   III. Slonim, Anthony D.
   [DNLM: 1. Ultrasonography—methods.   2. Point-of-Care Systems. WN 208 B413   2011]
RC78.7.U4B43 2011
616.07'543—dc22

                                                                                                    2010007596

To Irina in gratitude and to Sophia in anticipation.
Alex Levitov

*To Panagiotis and Maria for their sacrificial support and
to the Anargyroi for their continual guidance.*
Paul Dallas

To Mom and Dad with all of my love and gratitude.
Anthony Slonim

Contents

SECTION V: Ultrasound Use for the Evaluation of Organs of the Limbs and Musculoskeletal System

SECTION VI: Ultrasound Use for the Evaluation of Clinical Procedures and Special Populations

SECTION VII: Bedside Ultrasonography in Clinical Medicine: Preparing for and Achieving the Future State

Color insert is located between pages 178 and 179

Contributor List

Sameh Aziz, MD, FCCP, FACP
Assistant Professor of Medicine, University of Virginia and Edward Via Virginia College of Osteopathic Medicine, Pulmonary/Critical Care and Sleep Medicine, Virginia Tech Carilion School of Medicine, Carilion Clinic, Roanoke, Virginia

David P. Bahner, MD, RDMS
Associate Professor and Ultrasound, Director, Department of Emergency Medicine, The Ohio State University, Columbus, Ohio

Creagh T. Boulger, MD, RDMS
Clinical Instructor, Department of Emergency Medicine, The Ohio State University, Columbus, Ohio

Raoul Breitkreutz, MD, EDIC
Senior Lecturer, Department of Anesthesiology, Intensive Care Medicine and Pain Therapy, University Hospital of the Saarland and Medical Faculty of the University of the Saarland, Homburg, Saar, Germany

Christian H. Butcher, MD, FCCP
Assistant Professor of Medicine, Virginia Tech Carilion School of Medicine, Staff Pulmonary and Critical Care Physician, Carilion Clinic, Roanoke, Virginia

Gary E. Clagett, BS, RVT, RDMS
Vascular Technologist, Colorado Springs Surgical Associates, Colorado Springs, Colorado

Apostolos P. Dallas, MD, FACP
Attending Physician, Carilion Medical Center
Assistant Professor, Department of Medicine, Virginia Tech Carilion School of Medicine, Roanoke, Virginia

Roxanne Davenport, MD
Associate Professor of Surgery, Carilion Clinic, Roanoke, Virginia

Jonathan M. Dort, MD, FACS
Associate Professor, Department of Surgery, Virginia Tech Carilion School of Medicine, Roanoke, Virginia

Joseph S. Farmer, BS
Virginia Tech, Roanoke, Virginia

James E. Foster, II, MD, FACS, RPVI
Associate Professor, Department of Surgery, Virginia Tech Carilion School of Medicine and Research Institute, Medical Director, Non-Invasive Vascular Laboratory, Carilion Roanoke Memorial Hospital, Roanoke, Virginia

William R. Fry, MD, FACS, RVT, RDMS
Associate Professor, Virginia Tech Carilion School of Medicine and Research Institute, Division Chief, Trauma/Critical Care, Department of Surgery, Carilion Roanoke Memorial Hospital, Roanoke, Virginia

Christopher R. Fuller, PhD
Professor of Physics, Director Acoustics Laboratory Virginia Tech, Linchburg, Virginia

Ross Hanchett, MD
Resident OB/GYN Carilion Clinic, Roanoke, Virginia

Timothy A. Johnson, PhD
Associate Dean for Research, Professor and Chair of Basic Sciences, Virginia Tech Carilion School of Medicine and Research Institute, Roanoke, Virginia

Puneet Katyal, MD, MS
Assistant Professor, Department of Internal Medicine, Division of Critical Care Medicine, Virginia Tech Carilion School of Medicine, Roanoke, Virginia

Eduardo Lara-Torre, MD, FACOG
Assistant Professor/Associate Residency Program Director, Department of Obstetrics and Gynecology, Virginia Tech Carilion School of Medicine, Roanoke, Virginia

Alexander B. Levitov, MD, FCCM, RDCS
Professor, Department of Medicine
Eastern Virginia Medical School,
Norfolk, Virginia

Amanda B. Murchison, MD, FACOG
Assistant Professor, Virginia Tech Carilion School of Medicine, Roanoke, Virginia

Nicholas A. Perchiniak, MD
Chief Resident, 2009-2010, Department of Emergency Medicine, The Ohio State University Medical Center, Columbus, Ohio

Susanna Price, MB, BS, BSc, MRCP, EDICM, FESC, PhD
Consultant Cardiologist & Intensitivist, Royal Brompton Hospital, London, United Kingdom

Krish Ramachandran, MD
Assistant Professor, Department of Internal Medicine, Carilion Clinic Virginia Tech Carilion School of Medicine, Roanoke, Virginia, University of Virginia HSC, Charlottesville, Virginia

Sharan Ramaswamy, PhD
Assistant Professor, Department of Biomedical Engineering, Florida International University, Miami, Florida

Ashot E. Sargsyan, MD
Space Medical Operations Team, International Space Station, NASA Wyle Life Sciences, Houston, Texas

Rodney W. Savage, MD, FACP, FACC, FSCAI
Staff Cardiologist, Carilion Clinic, Roanoke, Virginia

Tarin A. Schmidt-Dalton, MD
Director, Clinical Sciences Year 1, Assistant Professor, Virginia Tech Carilion School of Medicine, Roanoke, Virginia

Yefim R. Sheynkin, MD, FACS
Associate Professor of Clinical Urology, State University of New York at Stony Brook, Stony Brook, New York

Anthony D. Slonim, MD, DrPH
Vice President, Medical Affairs, Attending Physician, Carilion Medical Center, Professor, Departments of Basic Sciences, Internal Medicine, and Pediatrics, Virginia-Tech-Carilion School of Medicine, Roanoke, Virginia

Holger Steiger, MD
Cardiology Center, Alice Hospital, Darmstadt, Germany

Santhanam Suresh, MD, FAAP
Attending Anesthesiologist Director, Pain Management Service and Research, Department of Pediatric Anesthesiology, Children's Memorial Hospital, Professor of Anesthesiology and Pediatrics, Northwestern University Feinberg School of Medicine, Chicago, Illinois

William T. Tsai, MD
Levine Children's Hospital, Carolina Medical Center, Charlotte, North Carolina

Shahana Uddin, MB, BS, FCARCS(I), EDICM
Consultant Anaesthetist and Intensive Care Medicine, Barts & The London NHS Trust, Department of Anaesthesia, London, United Kingdom

Marguerite Underwood, RN, RDCS
Echocardiography Department, The Carilion Clinic, Roanoke, Virginia

Richard C. Vari, PhD
Associate Dean for Medical Education, Professor of Physiology, Chair, Department of Interprofessionalism, Virginia Tech Carilion School of Medicine and Research Institute, Roanoke, Virginia

Gabriele Via, MD
Intensivist, Anesthesiologist, IRCCS Policilinico San Matteo Foundation, University of Pavia, Pavia, Italy

Patrice M. Weiss, MD, FACOG
Professor, Department of Obstetrics and Gynecology, Virginia Tech Carilion School of Medicine, Carilion Clinic, Roanoke, Virginia

Michael Wiid, MD, FACP
Assistant Professor of Clinical Internal Medicine, Virginia Tech Carilion School of Medicine, Roanoke, Virginia

Preface

The development of high-resolution portable ultrasonographic devices has revolutionized the practice of medicine. Portable ultrasound systems are presently available in most emergency departments, intensive care units, and anesthesia suites in the nation and have become the standard of care in these settings for diagnostic and therapeutic indications.

Bedside ultrasound assessment has also gained traction in general medical practice and is being vertically integrated into several medical school curricula. Arguably, bedside ultrasound is the most important medical tool of the present century and the only significant technological advancement to the art of physical examination since the advent of the stethoscope.

We have attempted to create a thoughtfully integrated textbook that introduces the reader to the use of diagnostic ultrasound as a part of an augmented physical examination. This book was conceptualized as a comprehensive yet concise "how to" guide to systematically incorporate ultrasound into the bedside physical examination. The inclusion of clinical algorithms fills an important void by providing direction for how to incorporate ultrasound into the clinical decision-making process, the formulation of the differential diagnosis, and the determination of therapy. Since ultrasonography is a visual specialty, the numerous anatomic and ultrasound images provide a de facto atlas and reference for more experienced learners.

We are hopeful that the book's content will provide adequate information to enable physicians to begin using ultrasound as a diagnostic aid from its first day of purchase. Further, we hope that it functions as a reference for educating medical students, residents, fellows, and practicing clinicians on how to incorporate advanced ultrasound principles into patient care.

Alexander Levitov
Apostolos Dallas
Anthony Slonim

Acknowledgments

We want to acknowledge and thank each one of our contributors who helped to bring this text from concept to completion in a very short period of time—Your expertise and guidance have allowed us to create a work that will help to advance care for scores of patients.

Special thanks to Julie Owen, MHSA for all that she did to make this project successful—We certainly could not have done it without your talent for editing, formatting, and organization.

Thanks also to the dynamic editorial team of Karen Edmonson, Jim Shanahan, and Priscilla Beer, who believed in the insanity and helped to ensure that we had what we needed to accomplish it.

BASIC PRINCIPLES OF ULTRASOUND USE

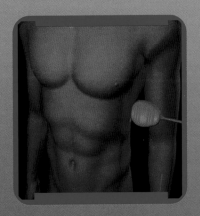

CHAPTER 1

Bedside Diagnostic Ultrasound: Potentials and Pitfalls

Joseph S. Farmer, BS and Anthony D. Slonim, MD, DrPH

INTRODUCTION

Suppose that you had access to an ultrasound unit small enough to fit around your neck or in your white-coat pocket—an easy-to-use and portable device for use at your patients' bedsides. You could generate images from these portable ultrasound systems that are so easy to operate that they walk you stepwise through image acquisition. Together with your knowledge and experience in medicine, this tool would provide you the opportunity to directly visualize a problem or realize that a problem does not exist. You could interact with your patients by having real-time conversations about the results during imaging, allaying their fears or addressing the next diagnostic or therapeutic steps.

While diagnostic bedside ultrasonography has not yet achieved mainstream application, it is likely that as available technology emerges, new and more robust clinical applications will develop. Medical students who become proficient in both the acquisition and interpretation of ultrasound images as part of their bedside clinical examinations will be prepared to fully utilize these advances over the next several decades. Physicians who already have a comfort level with ultrasound will likely drive this technology for new applications that can improve patient care.

The smaller, portable, and more user-friendly ultrasound systems have overcome the limitations of larger and more complex systems, thereby representing an area of growth for new applications of ultrasound technology. As the technology changes, it is helpful to consider the possibilities—both positive and negative—that those changes can bring.

ULTRASOUND APPLICATIONS

Figure 1.1 shows a variety of current ultrasound applications along the life cycle of the patient, from prenatal to death, categorized by specialty. While this is not an exhaustive list, it does provide a sense of the broad range of applications that are already in place, and it should also provide consideration of other potential applications for ultrasound technology.

In the life cycle of a physician (Fig. 1.1), from medical student through senior clinician, ultrasound enhances the ability to function clinically. Ultrasound availability during medical education can provide students with the ability to visualize organs and begin to formulate their three-dimensional (3D) perspective of normal and abnormal anatomy. At its foundation, medical education begins with a thorough understanding of normal structure and function, which is typically achieved at the gross and cellular level through courses such as gross anatomy, histology, and physiology. Ultrasound may provide an important adjunct to these learning experiences by giving students the opportunity to generate images, thereby building competence with ultrasound technology and informing their understanding of anatomic relationships. Once the normal structure and function of the human body are understood, the student advances toward an understanding of "abnormal" as the next step in the education process. Ultrasound provides a powerful tool for visualizing abnormalities in organs. With limited training, the difference between the image of a normal heart and one surrounded by fluid is readily apparent (Fig. 1.2 panels A and B). Similar examples exist with a healthy and diseased liver and gallbladder (Fig. 1.2 panels C–F).

After the student has a working knowledge of normal and abnormal structure and function, medical decision making can begin to take shape by understanding what to do to fix problems and diseases. Traditionally, third- and fourth-year medical students are mentored and practice their data-gathering and interpretation skills to help inform their medical decision making and treatment approaches. In these years, the student practices diagnosis and treatment skills across a variety of patient populations and builds competence in understanding the

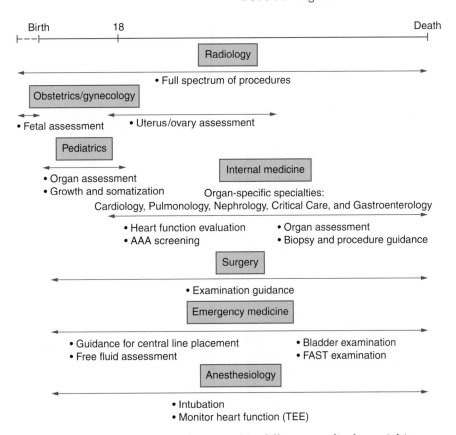

Figure 1.1. The uses for diagnostic ultrasound in different medical specialties across the lifespan of the patient.

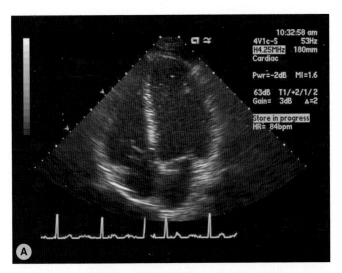

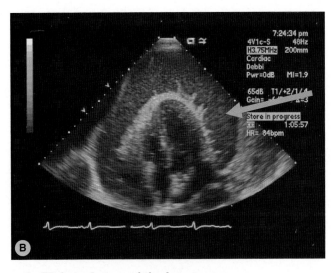

Figure 1.2. **(A)** Apical view of the heart—normal. **(B)** Apical view of the heart—cardiac tamponade highlighting the large volume of fluid (*arrow*). **(C)** Normal liver. **(D)** Diseased liver with ascites. **(E)** Normal gallbladder. **(F)** Abnormal gallbladder. *(Images A and B courtesy of Carilion Clinic. Images C and D courtesy of GE Healthcare, www.logiciqlibrary.com. Images E and F courtesy of Philips, www3.medical.philips. com/en-us/secure/images_site/index.asp?div=ultra.)*

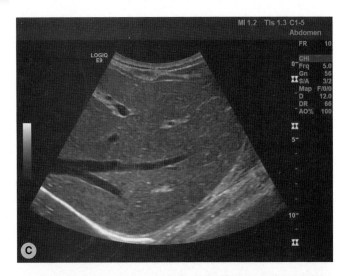

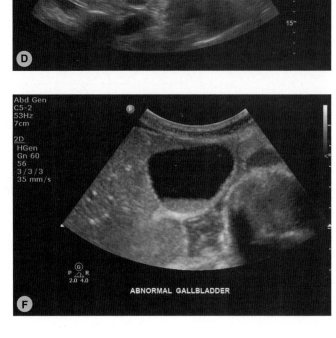

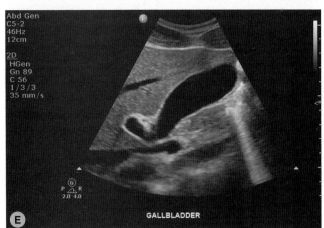

Figure 1.2. (Continued)

available treatment options and the effect these treatment options might have on disease states. When residency and fellowship begin, the focus on a specific specialty provides a deeper and more thorough understanding of a very specific content area for the trained medical student. The transition from student to practicing physician includes a dramatic increase in self-reliance and autonomy for the benefit of patients. The new attending physician has to rely on his or her skills, be confident in his or her conclusions, and know when to ask for assistance from other members of the team. Ultrasound for these clinicians is an important skill that continues to mature, as does their medical decision making.

MIGRATION OF ULTRASOUND TECHNOLOGY

As a technology, ultrasound principles are well understood, and its use as a primary diagnostic and therapeutic modality in radiology practice is well grounded.

In recent years, ultrasound technology has been evolving and now is used outside the specialty of radiology. Ultrasound use in obstetrics and cardiology is common. The application of ultrasound to other areas such as emergency medicine and the intensive care unit is growing rapidly. With this expanded use of ultrasound outside of the traditional radiology domain, device manufacturers have needed to adapt the equipment by building smaller, more portable devices that can be used at the point of care.

When compared to other imaging technologies such as computed tomography (CT) or magnetic resonance imaging (MRI), advances in ultrasound have been relatively slow; as a result, many radiologists who traditionally carried out ultrasound studies have moved toward other imaging technologies.[1] In addition, the low reimbursement rates for the expensive equipment and dedicated training that radiologists receive also contribute to the need that many radiologists feel to move to other technologies. Ultrasound utilization, however, continues to grow and is expected to reach $6 billion in equipment sales by 2012 despite the migration of radiologists toward other types of diagnostic imaging.[2] The continued overall growth of ultrasound can largely be attributed to the hand-carried ultrasound scans performed outside of radiology.

Many of the manufacturers of ultrasound equipment are predicting the continued growth of ultrasound by targeting applications in anesthesiology, emergency medicine, internal medicine, and surgery in addition to the traditional radiology market. Critical care is an area of medicine where ultrasound use is quickly becoming common for diagnosis and procedure guidance. The need for rapid action in critical care is one of the major reasons ultrasound applications are moving toward the point of care, and an understanding of the medical decision-making process provides a better understanding of how ultrasound can improve that process.

MEDICAL DECISION-MAKING PROCESS

As with any good decision-making process, medical decision making is an organized step-by-step process (Fig. 1.3). For inpatients, this commences at hospital admission, and for outpatients it begins with the clinician's first patient interaction. At the beginning of the cycle, the data-gathering step is critical to the rest of the process. Data gathering is accomplished through patient history, physical examination, and diagnostic testing. The physical examination represents an area where ultrasound has the potential to provide significant benefits (described later). The data interpretation step follows and provides an opportunity for the different data elements to be considered by the physician. Judgments as to data validity, reliability, and consistency with the patient's symptoms are made during this step. Once the clinical data are interpreted, decisions can be made. Occasionally, the data are insufficient, and the action that needs to occur is to gather more data. Mostly, the data provide enough information so that a diagnosis can be made, and a series of actions known as a treatment plan can be generated. Responses to the treatment plan are monitored as the cycle begins again with additional data-gathering steps. If the treatment actions were successful, and the patient's condition improves, the patient can be released from care, ending the cycle. If the condition does not improve with treatment, additional decisions may need to be made.

In many cases, moving a data-gathering tool such as ultrasound to the bedside can improve the speed and efficiency of the decision-making process. Portable ultrasound allows the physician who is gathering the data to interpret the data, make a decision, and take action right at the bedside. If the ultrasound were not portable, the patient would have to be moved; a technician would perform a diagnostic test and the results would be sent to a radiologist for interpretation before they could be included in the decision-making process for action to be taken.

The focused assessment with sonography in trauma (FAST) is a component of Advanced Trauma Life Support protocols and provides a rapid assessment of the trauma patient's condition with respect to internal damage. The FAST examination provides an important example of how portable ultrasound contributes to the speed of the decision-making process in the emergency department (ED) by providing quick access to vital data. With bedside ultrasound, trauma doctors are able to quickly identify free fluid in the abdomen, around the lungs, or around the heart. Quickly identifying this free fluid dictates the next steps in the treatment algorithm and is critical to patient outcome. In this and other situations, the decision-making process must move quickly; being portable, bedside ultrasonography is a tool that, when applied correctly, can have a positive impact on patient care.

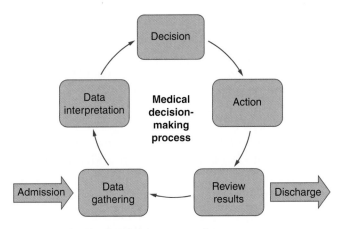

Figure 1.3. Medical decision-making process.

THE PHYSICAL EXAMINATION

The physical examination is an important part of data gathering in the decision-making process, but the time and proficiency of physicians for bedside diagnosis through physical examination have declined.[3] In addition, improvements in technology have provided additional sources for gathering data that to some extent have called into question the ultimate usefulness of the physical examination in many areas of medicine.

A 2003 study of physical examinations demonstrated that pivotal physical findings were observed in only 26% of the hospitalized patients. While these data suggest that physical examination is often poorly performed, it is also important to realize how important the physical examination is in the decision-making process. Approximately 7% of patients had physical findings that would likely have been missed by diagnostic testing alone, demonstrating the need for efficient and highly effective bedside physical examination. In addition, 19% of patients had findings that could have been addressed by physical examination alone, which might improve the speed of treatment.[4]

Laboratory testing and diagnostic images provide additional information that is helpful in understanding the abnormalities facing a patient, but they are not a replacement for a bedside assessment by the physician.[5] As part of data gathering and interpretation, the hands-on skills of a physician in inspection, palpation, percussion, and auscultation are critical to obtaining good data from a physical examination. Portable ultrasound is a tool that can enhance the physician's hands-on skills and improve the overall effectiveness of the bedside examination. Portable ultrasound technology also has the potential to allow detection of some of the subtle differences that comes only with the repetition and practice of an experienced clinician. For example, the physical examination technique for assessing the abdominal aorta through palpation is often taught during medical education. Considerations for an adequate examination include the abdominal wall thickness and the experience of the physician. Sensitivity in detecting the size of the abdominal aorta through palpation is close to 39%, compared to nearly 100% sensitivity with the use of ultrasonography.[6] Another example is the assessment for possible ascites. The physical examination technique involves rolling the patient, percussing the abdomen, and marking and listening to the movement of fluid. However, the author cautions that both these clinical signs of ascites may be misleading. Portable ultrasound offers a simple visual image of the fluid (Fig. 1.4), reducing the subjective nature of listening to wave propagation through a stethoscope. The ability of ultrasound to visualize the body's cavities,

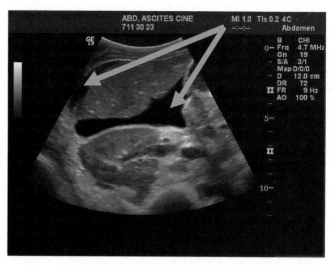

Figure 1.4. Ascites. *(Image courtesy of GE Healthcare, www.logiciqlibrary.com.)*

detecting the size and configuration of the organs and any pathology, can bring significant improvement to the bedside physical examination.

As a key element of medical decision making, the ability to gather and interpret data during a physical examination is a crucial skill, and the hands-on assessment by a physician is important to patients. The expanded use of ultrasound provides an opportunity to enhance the standard inspection, palpation, percussion, and auscultation model of the physical examination with technologic advances for visualizing anatomy while still allowing direct interaction with the patient.

A VISUAL STETHOSCOPE

The potential for hand-held ultrasound units to enhance or replace the stethoscope elicits a range of reactions, but to those who consider the possibilities, the concept is not as radical as it may first appear. In the near future physicians could see inside the body as quickly as they currently listen through the stethoscope. During a routine checkup, rather than listening for a subjective heart valve sound, an image of the heart valve itself could be viewed in just a few minutes.

Anyone who has been with an expectant mother during an ultrasound examination understands the value that ultrasound provides for allowing real-time medical conversations with patients and allaying anxiety or providing immediate answers for concerns. Ultrasound can be a very powerful tool that helps to bridge the communication gap that often exists between doctor and patient. In addition, the potential impact of moving ultrasound use from a diagnostic tool to a screening tool has attained more serious attention as technologic advances bring smaller and less expensive equipment to the bedside. While routine ultrasound use has many hurdles, it offers an amazingly simple, noninvasive way to get useful information.

Portable ultrasound represents the fastest-growing segment of ultrasonography. The growth rate of hand-carried ultrasound (HCU) units increased from $5 million to $96 million from 1999 to 2003, and as more manufacturers enter this market, growth is expected to continue.[7] Some ultrasound systems have pushed the portability envelope even further (Fig. 1.5). The Acuson P10 from Siemens weighs 1.6 pounds and is small enough to fit in a lab-coat pocket. The company's literature touts the ability to use such portable devices in screening as a component of physical examinations. There is also a new company, Signostics, Inc., that received approval from the U.S. Food and Drug Administration (FDA) in 2009 for a half-pound device called the Signos Personal Ultrasound that is marketed as a visual stethoscope. A small but powerful system from SonoSite called the NanoMaxx appears to be close to receiving FDA approval.

Another feature that the smaller systems provide is preset system settings based on the proposed scan. The operator simply needs to press a button labeled "AAA" when performing an abdominal aortic aneurysm screening, and standard settings are set for the operator, thereby greatly reducing the training for specific examinations. Some systems even provide guidance on transducer placement and angle or direct the technical aspects of image acquisition in a step-by-step manner through a FAST examination. These advances improve the usability and help reduce operator error associated with these devices.

With improved battery life, image quality, and ease of use, these systems and the systems that follow will provide dramatic improvements in clinical examinations beyond what is currently practical.

ULTRASOUND USE IN GENERAL PRACTICE: AN INTERNATIONAL STUDY

Internationally, ultrasound use by physicians in general practice is much more common than in the United States. Cost reduction measures required by nationalized

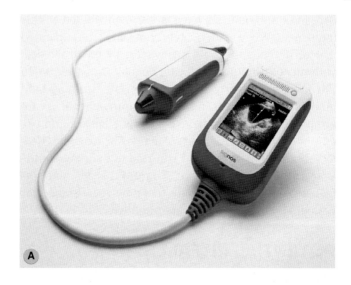

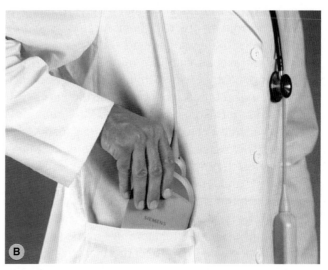

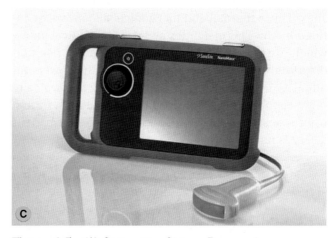

Figure 1.5. **(A)** Signostics Signos Personal Ultrasound. **(B)** Siemens Acuson P10. **(C)** SonoSite NanoMaxx.

care in other countries have largely contributed to this movement. When inadequately controlled, the expanded use of ultrasound could easily add to medical costs without contributing significant benefits; however, when introduced properly with appropriate training and guidelines, reductions in cost and improvements in care are possible and are a large reason why ultrasound use continues to expand internationally. For example, bedside abdominal ultrasound can rule out serious conditions, reduce unnecessary CT and MRI scans and specialist referrals, and provide real-time reassurance for patients by their primary care providers.[8]

POTENTIAL PITFALLS

There are certainly many pitfalls related to the expanded use of ultrasound, and proper training is one key to avoiding many of them. An understanding of the physics of ultrasound and the potential bioeffects that ultrasound can have on tissues is a critical safety component. Proper technique in image acquisition and interpretation is required for the successful application of ultrasound.

While generally considered a safe diagnostic tool, the sound waves generated by ultrasound machines, depending on their intensity and duration, can cause mechanical and thermal stress on tissues. The bone–tissue interface is an area of particular concern. The sound waves absorbed by dense bone can cause a more rapid rise in the temperature of the surrounding soft tissue. In addition to its thermal effects, ultrasound's mechanical effects on gas bubbles and the thermal stress from sound waves can also impact tissues. These thermal and mechanical effects are quantified by the Thermal Index and the Mechanical Index, which are numbers based on their relative risk and displayed on the ultrasound unit. While the power and intensity levels of hand-carried units are not typically high enough to cause significant bioeffects during brief scans, they must be understood so that patient safety is not compromised.

The American Institute of Ultrasound in Medicine has issued the following statement: "The potential benefits and risks of each examination should be considered. The As Low As Reasonably Achievable (ALARA) principle should be observed when adjusting controls that affect the acoustical output and by considering transducer dwell times."[9] The proper use of ultrasound is a skill that requires substantial training, repetition, and practice to achieve proficiency. For an untrained physician, misdiagnosis based on techniques could be common. Artifacts are typical in ultrasound, and the ability to understand and recognize them is a skill that comes with practice, so that diagnostic mistakes are not made.

Training guidelines for all levels of provider from novice to expert are included later in this text (Chapter 20). We believe that one way to improve the image acquisition and interpretation skills is to provide medical students with access to portable ultrasound devices during their rotations through anatomy, physical examination, and clinical education. Students could then become proficient in ultrasonography while they are learning 3D anatomy and in a way that does not compromise patient safety. Partnerships between device manufacturers and medical schools can assist with preparing medical students to use this important technology, not only in the medical school curriculum but also as clinicians once they graduate.

CONCLUSION

Ultrasound diagnostic imaging is continuing its migration into many areas of medicine. As medical students today become proficient in acquiring and interpreting ultrasound images in the realm of normal and abnormal anatomic structure and function, they will likely continue to drive the migration of the technology even further. For bedside physical examination, portable ultrasound is an effective tool that allows augmentation of the physical examination, enhanced doctor–patient interactions, and the reliable and objective assessment of internal structures. There will be many opportunities for medical students of today to build competence with ultrasound during their early training. The challenge is to be open-minded enough to find areas where such a tool can improve health care as it becomes easier to use, portable, and readily available.

References

1. Brice J. Ultrasound's future in play: will radiologists remain in the picture? *Diagn Imaging*. March 1, 2007.
2. Orenstein B. Ultrasound exams: bright future, but will it be in radiology? *Radiol Today*. 2009;10(6):12.
3. Bickley L, Szilagyi P. *Bates' guide to physical examination and history taking*. 9th ed. Philadelphia: Lippincott Williams & Wilkins; 2007.
4. Reilly BM. Physical examination in the care of medical inpatients: an observational study. *Lancet*. 2003;362:1100–1105.

5. Verghese A. Culture shock - patient as icon, icon as patient. *N Engl J Med.* 2008;359:26.

6. Silverstein MD, Pitts SR, Chaikof EL, Ballard DJ. Abdominal aortic aneurysm (AAA): cost-effectiveness of screening, surveillance of intermediate-sized AAA, and management of symptomatic AAA. *Proc (Bayl Univ Med Cent).* 2005;18(4):345–367.

7. Frost & Sullivan Research Service. (26 January, 2004). High-growth areas propel overall ultrasound market. Retrieved from http://www.frost.com/prod/servlet/report-brochure.pag?id=A675-01-00-00-00. Accessed on February 2, 2010.

8. Speets AM, Hoes AW, van der Graaf Y, et al. Upper abdominal ultrasound in general practice: indications, diagnostic yield, and consequences for patient management. *Fam Pract.* 2006;23:507–511.

9. Official statement of the American Institute of Ultrasound in Medicine. Retrieved from http://www.aium.org/publications/viewStatement.aspx?id=39. Accessed on February 7, 2010.

CHAPTER 2

Ultrasound Physics

Alexander B. Levitov, MD, FCCM, RDCS and Christopher Fuller, PhD

INTRODUCTION

While there certainly will be a temptation to skip over this chapter, the reader is encouraged not to do so. The physics principles presented here are fundamental to an understanding of bedside ultrasonography for the physician sonographer. Plain radiographs, computed tomography (CT), and magnetic resonance imaging (MRI) scans reflect anatomic reality. Ultrasound imaging relies on highly processed information, which makes ultrasound the least intuitive of all imaging techniques. Moreover, the physician interested in the point-of-care bedside ultrasound will also serve as an ultrasonographer. In contrast to traditional diagnostic radiology modalities, it will be the physician who will select the transducer and ultrasound system settings, obtain the images, and interpret them. All of this is impossible without a fundamental understanding of the physics of ultrasound and generation of image formation.

WAVES AND WAVE PROPAGATION

When a rock is thrown in the middle of a quiet pond, a wave will form and propagate in the poorly compressible physical medium of water. The resulting wave is a transverse one, with the predominant wave vibration occurring in a direction perpendicular to the direction of wave propagation. Sound waves created by vibrating objects are similar but are composed of the areas of increased (compression) and decreased (rarefaction) density that propagate through the medium. Although universally graphically depicted as transverse waves, sound waves are longitudinal, with the predominant vibration in the same direction as a propagating wave (Fig. 2.1). Like all waves, sound is described by the set of physical characteristics, in this case known as *acoustic parameters*.

SOUND AND ULTRASOUND: ACOUSTIC PARAMETERS

Period and Frequency

The time necessary for a sound wave to complete one cycle is termed the *period*. It is usually measured in microseconds (μsec). *Frequency* is the number of cycles per second and is the reciprocal of the period and measured in hertz (Hz). Humans can hear sound with frequencies ranging from 20 to 20,000 Hz or 20 kilohertz (20 kHz) (Fig. 2.2). Sound with frequencies less than 20 Hz is called *infrasound*, and greater than 20 kHz is termed *ultrasound* (Fig. 2.2). Neither infrasound nor ultrasound is audible by humans. Aside from these differences, ultrasound has all the characteristics of a sound wave. All sound waves reflect off large objects, forming echoes, and bend around smaller ones (diffraction). However, high-frequency ultrasound waves tend to reflect off smaller objects (relative to their wavelength), travel shorter distances, and travel in a straighter line than lower-frequency sounds. Most vibrating elastic objects produce a family of waves with frequencies that are multiples of the lower one. The lowest frequency in the family is known as the *fundamental frequency* and the multiples of the fundamental frequency are called *harmonic frequencies* or simply *harmonics* (Fig. 2.3). Diagnostic ultrasound usually utilizes sound waves with frequencies from 2 million to 20 million hertz (MHz).

Propagation Velocity

Propagation velocity is sometimes called the *speed of sound*. However, this term is technically incorrect since sound propagation is directional. Sound requires a medium to travel or propagate in and cannot travel in a vacuum. The physical nature of the medium including its density, stiffness, and temperature help to determine the propagation velocity. As a general rule, sound will propagate faster in solids than in liquids and faster in liquids than in gases. The propagation velocity for some biologic media is summarized in Table 2.1. The fact that propagation velocity is an intrinsic quality of the medium alone is far-reaching. For example, propagation velocity is independent of the movement of the sound source or the observer. In the extreme case, the velocity of the moving sound source can exceed the propagation velocity of the sound and the source can "run away" or "break the sound barrier." If the sound source or an observer is moving, the sound waves traveling in the

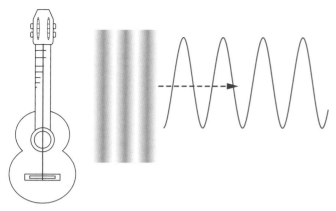

Figure 2.1. Nature of sound: A guitar string vibration is creating a longitudinal wave that is represented as a transverse wave.

Frequency of sound waves (not to scale)

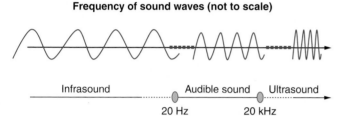

Figure 2.2. Humans can hear sound with frequencies between 20 and 20,000 Hz. Sound with frequencies less than 20 Hz (infrasound) and greater than 20,000 Hz (ultrasound) cannot be heard by most humans. However, some individuals can hear ultrasound, and most will perceive infrasound as vibration.

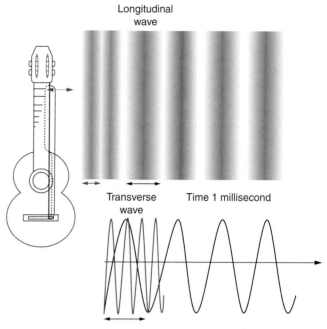

Figure 2.3. Guitar D string vibration is creating a longitudinal wave in fundamental (shades of gray) and first harmonic (shades of blue) frequencies. Longitudinal waves are represented by the transverse waves of the same frequency. The blue dotted wave is a first harmonic wave with half of the period and twice the frequency of the fundamental wave (black). The fundamental period is 2.5 milliseconds. The fundamental frequency is 400 Hz. The first harmonic frequency is 0.8 kHz. The second harmonic frequency is 1.6 kHz.

same direction have to be squeezed (acquire higher frequency), and the sound waves traveling in the opposite direction have to stretch (acquire longer frequency) to cover the same distance in the same time. This is known as the *Doppler effect* and has many applications in ultrasonography. Propagation velocity is independent of the frequency of the ultrasound wave.

Wavelength

Wavelength is the length of one cycle of the wave measured in the units of distance (usually millimeters) and depends on frequency and propagation velocity. Wavelength (mm) = propagation velocity (m/sec) × 1,000/frequency (MHz). Therefore, in soft tissue, an ultrasound wave with the frequency of 1 MHz will have a wavelength of 54 mm. The usual wavelength in diagnostic ultrasound is 0.1 mm. Shorter wavelength/higher-frequency ultrasound waves will create echo images of smaller objects, thus improving image quality (resolution), but they will decay in a shorter distance, and thus usually have less penetration.

Amplitude Power and Intensity

Sound waves can displace more or less of the medium as they propagate. The frequency will stay the same, but the motion, density, or pressure in the medium will change. The result is higher or lower "loudness" of the ultrasound, which relates to its ability to transmit more energy (power, intensity). This loudness is known as

TABLE 2.1. The Propagation Velocities for Different Biologic Media	
Biologic media	**Sound propagation velocity (m/sec)**
Lungs	300–1,000
Fat	1,400
Soft tissue	1,540
Bone	2,000–4,000

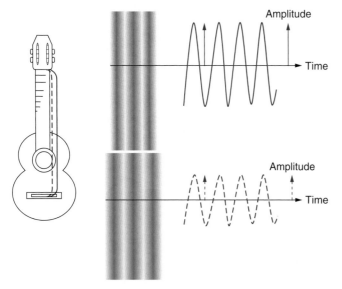

Figure 2.4. Different amplitudes of sound. **(A)** More medium displacement, higher amplitude. **(B)** Less medium displacement, lower amplitude. Power = K × Amplitude^2.

TABLE 2.2. Intensity Ratios Between Sounds A and B (Decibels)	
Sound A/sound B	*Decibels*
100:1	20
10:1	10
4:1	6
2:1	3
1:2	−3
1:10	−10

amplitude (Fig. 2.4). Because the dynamic range of the linear amplitude is huge, a logarithmic description is employed where the actual amplitude is divided by a reference value and the log taken. The ratio is measured on the logarithmic scale with the units of decibels (dB). Twenty decibels is a 10-fold increase in the amplitude of the sound, and 40 dB is a 100-fold increase. In general, however, the level of ultrasound waves is described in terms of sound intensity or power. When described sound in terms of intensity, a 10-fold increase in intensity will result in an increase of 10 dB, while a 100-fold increase will result in an increase of 20 dB. Negative decibels mean that sound B is softer or lower in amplitude or intensity than sound A (Table 2.2).

Power or the time rate of flow of energy carried and possibly released by an ultrasound wave is proportionate to the amplitude squared (where K is a coefficient, units of energy are joules, and power is measured in joule/sec or watts):

$$\text{Power} = K \times \text{Amplitude}^2$$

The amount of power delivered to a unit of surface area is called intensity and is measured in watts/cm^2. In the case of diagnostic ultrasound, where the medium is the human body, amplitude, power, and intensity are defining parameters in terms of biologic effects of the ultrasound and therefore are very important. Acoustic parameters are summarized in Table 2.3.

INTERACTIONS BETWEEN SOUND AND MEDIUM

Attenuation

An ultrasound wave propagating through the biologic medium releases some of its energy in a form of heat and tissue vibration, resulting in a decrease in the amplitude or dampening of the wave. This is known as

TABLE 2.3. Summary of Acoustic Parameters in Diagnostic Ultrasound			
Acoustic parameter	*Units*	*Determined by*	*Values in diagnostic ultrasound*
Period	μsec	Sound source	0.05–0.5 μsec
Frequency	MHz	Sound source	2–20 MHz
Amplitude	dB	Sound source	—
Power	Watts	Sound source	—
Intensity	Watts/cm^2	Sound source	0.001–100 watts/cm^2
Propagation velocity	m/sec	Medium	300–1,600 m/sec
Wavelength	mm	Sound source and medium	0.1–0.6 mm

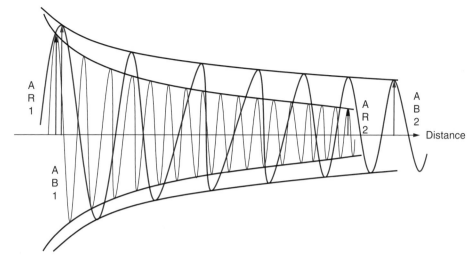

Figure 2.5. Both high-frequency black waves (R) and lower-frequency blue waves (B) attenuate (dampen) with distance. However, blue waves attenuate less. The ratio of initial amplitude A1 to final A2 illustrates the degree of attenuation and is measured in negative decibels. AB1 : AB2 > AR1 : AR2. AR1, initial amplitude of high-frequency waves; AR2, final amplitude of high-frequency waves; AB1, initial amplitude of lower-frequency waves; AB2, final amplitude of lower-frequency waves.

attenuation and is measured in decibels (Table 2.2). Attenuation does not change the wave frequency, but the magnitude of the amplitude decrease depends on the frequency of the ultrasound (Fig. 2.5). The higher the frequency of the wave, the more energy it will release and the higher will be the attenuation coefficient (decrease in amplitude per centimeter of propagation). For example, a 1-MHz-frequency wave will decrease its amplitude by 0.5 dB (–0.5 dB) per each centimeter it propagates through the tissue.

Reflection, Transmission, Acoustic Impedance, and Axial Resolution

As discussed, all sound will reflect from objects and return back to its source, in the form of an echo. In reality, it is the boundary between two layers (in the case of diagnostic ultrasound it is two tissue layers) with different physical properties that causes some of the sound energy to reflect. In order to estimate reflectivity of the boundary, a parameter known as *acoustic impedance* has been developed. The greater the difference in the acoustic impedance between the boundaries, the greater is the reflection off the boundary layer. The impedance is the product of density (kg/M^3) and propagation speed (m/sec) and is measured in rayls. The impedance of human tissue is usually between 1,250,000 and 1,750,000 rayls (25–75 Mrayls). Whatever energy is not reflected is transmitted further until another boundary with different acoustic impedance is encountered, and the

same process is repeated. Because the impedance difference between tissue layers is relatively small, only about 1% of the energy is reflected, and 99% is transmitted; this allows for the detection of multiple tissue boundaries. Both reflection and transmission are relatively predictable when the sound strikes the boundary at a 90° angle (normal incidence) (Fig. 2.6). When this is not the case, the direction and the amount of transmitted and reflected energy are difficult to predict, which will result in formation of artifacts in the resulting images. Knowing the propagation velocity

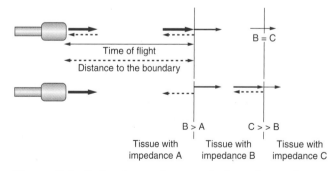

Figure 2.6. Reflection and transmission of sound at the boundaries struck at a 90° angle (normal incidence). If there is no difference in impedance between the two boundaries, no reflection will occur; the more the difference, the greater the amount of ultrasound is reflected back to the source. Distance to the boundary can be calculated from the time it takes for the ultrasound to reach the boundary and return to the source (time of flight, elapsed time).

TABLE 2.4. Elapsed Time and Position of the Boundary

Elapsed time (μsec)	Depth of the boundary on the screen (cm)
13	1
26	2
52	4
130	10

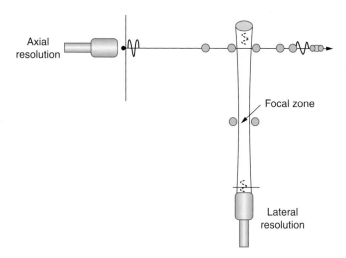

Figure 2.7. Imaging pulses are composed of two ultrasound wave cycles. Spatial length (SPL) = wavelength × 2. As two boundaries become closer in the pass of the ultrasound (axial plane), they will appear as one (limit of axial resolution). Axial resolution = SPL/2. Two objects appearing as one in the plane perpendicular to the pass of the sound is a limit of lateral resolution. Axial resolution is always better (smaller number) than lateral resolution.

and measuring the time that it takes the ultrasound impulse to reflect to the source, the ultrasound system can calculate the depth or position the boundary on the screen. For every 13 μsec of elapsed time, the boundary is positioned 1 cm deeper (Fig. 2.6, Table 2.4). In diagnostic ultrasound, this position always depends on the assumption that the propagation velocity is 1,540 m/sec, irrespective of what the actual tissue propagation velocity is (Table 2.4). If the propagation velocity differs greatly from 1,540 m/sec, the position of the boundary on the screen will not reflect the true anatomic position and is known as a *propagation velocity artifact*. As the boundaries get closer, the ability of the ultrasound system to distinguish the distance between them will diminish, until they coalesce into one image. The minimal distance when two boundaries are imaged as separate ones is known as *axial resolution* (Fig. 2.7). The shorter the wavelength, the higher the ultrasound frequency and the better the axial resolution. Typical axial resolution for the modern ultrasound system is about 0.1 mm (0.05–0.5 mm).

Scattering

If the reflective boundary is small, the sound may reflect in all directions, or *scatter*. Inconsistent scattering will deteriorate the quality of the image, but uniform scattering may provide important information about the size of the reflector. For example, red blood cells will provide a uniform scattering pattern.

Refraction

When the sound reaches the boundary with different sound propagation velocities at a non-90° angle (oblique incident angle), transmission with a change in direction, or *refraction,* will occur. The amount of deviation from the original pass of the ultrasound wave at the boundary is governed by Snell's law (Fig. 2.8).

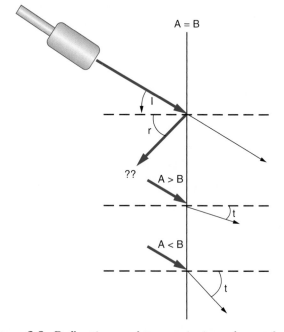

Figure 2.8. Reflection and transmission of sound at the boundaries struck at a non-90° angle (oblique incidence). Transmission and reflection are unpredictable, except for the incident angle (I) being equal to reflection angle (r). If the speed of sound in both media is equal, transmission will follow the path of the incident wave; otherwise, refraction will occur. If the speed of sound in medium A is faster than in medium B, the transmission angle will be less than the incident angle. If the speed of sound in medium A is slower than in medium B, the transmission angle will be greater than the incident angle (Snell's law).

WAVE INTERACTIONS: CONSTRUCTIVE AND DESTRUCTIVE INTERFERENCE, BEAM FORMATION, AND LATERAL RESOLUTION

Ultrasound sources emit a multitude of waves or wavelets that interact with each other. Two major forms of wave interactions are constructive and destructive interference. When two waves are in phase with each other, they combine and result in an increase in amplitude. If they are in opposition or 180° out of phase, then subtraction takes place, with a resulting wave of smaller amplitude (Fig. 2.9). Devices such as a bullhorn will maximize constructive interference in a particular direction, resulting in the formation of a beam of sound. Ultrasound systems use reflectors (ultrasound lenses) or electronically manipulate the source of ultrasound (phased array probe) to form the desired beam. This beam has a typical hourglass appearance with the narrowest point of the "waist" known as a *focal point*, or simply *focus*. Two side-by-side boundaries will appear as separate if the distance between them is greater than the width of the focal point. The ability to discriminate between two side-by-side boundaries is known as *lateral resolution* of the ultrasound system, and it is best in the focal point. High-frequency waves have a narrower focus and are associated with higher axial and lateral resolution and therefore better image quality (Fig. 2.7). Table 2.5

TABLE 2.5. High- and Low-frequency Ultrasound Waves			
	Attenuation	Image depth	Image quality
Low frequency 2–5 MHz	Low	Deep	Lower
High frequency 5–10 MHz	High	Shallow	Higher

briefly summarizes the difference between high- and low-frequency ultrasound waves used in diagnostic ultrasound.

CONTINUOUS AND PULSE ULTRASOUND

Ultrasound waves can be emitted constantly like the sound waves from a siren (continuous wave [CW]) or intermittently like the sound waves from a fog horn (pulsed wave [PW]). All imaging ultrasound is a pulsed wave. To image the object, the ultrasound system sends the pulse of ultrasound toward the reflective boundary and then listens for the echo to determine the position of the reflector. Short pulses are composed of two to four wave cycles (see earlier Period and Frequency section) and accordingly will last only 0.5 to 3 μsec. The spatial length (SPL) of the pulse will also be short—0.1 to 0 mm—depending on the wavelength and the number of cycles in the pulse. The ultrasound system listens for the returning echoes 99% to 99.9% of the time. The percentage of "talking time" is commonly referred to as a *duty factor* and is 0.1% to 1%. If the duty factor is 0%, the machine is off; if it is 100%, CW ultrasound (nonimaging) is in use. Listening times are referred to as *opened aperture time*. Short pulses are composed of high-frequency ultrasound waves and therefore improve axial resolution. In fact, axial resolution is one-half of the SPL (Fig. 2.7).

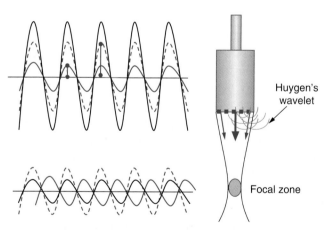

Figure 2.9. Interference and ultrasound beam formation. Constructive interference: Amplitude black = solid blue + amplitude interrupted blue. Destructive interference: Amplitude black = solid blue – amplitude interrupted blue. Constructive interference in the middle of the beam and destructive interference on the periphery of the beam form individual wavelets into the typical hourglass shape.

DOPPLER PHENOMENON

As is the case with propagation velocity, if the sound source is moving in relationship to the observer, the frequency of the sound wave changes. The same is true of the echo, if the reflective boundary is moving. If the reflector is moving toward the sound source, the frequency of the reflected sound will be higher (positive

Doppler shift) than that of the emitted one. If the reflector is moving away from the sound source, the frequency of the echo will be lower than the emitted sound (negative Doppler shift). The Doppler shift is therefore the difference between the frequency of the emitted and the reflected ultrasound wave. The frequency of the Doppler shift usually falls within the audible range, though the emitted and the reflected sound are of the ultrasonic frequency and cannot be heard. This *Doppler phenomenon* will enable the user to estimate the velocity of moving reflectors (i.e., red blood cells) (Fig. 2.10). Reflector velocity = (Doppler shift × propagation speed) / 2 × (incident frequency × cosine of the incident angle). Therefore, with a 90°

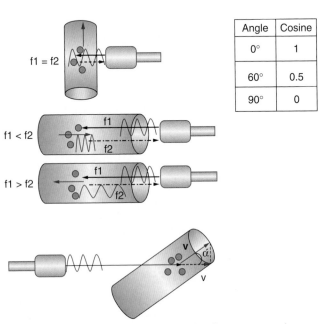

Angle	Cosine
0°	1
60°	0.5
90°	0

Doppler shift = 2 × reflector speed × incident frequency × cosine (angle ά) / propagation speed

Figure 2.10. If the blood cell is moving toward the transducer, the frequency of the reflected signal will be higher than that of the emitted or incident one (positive Doppler shift). If the blood cell is moving away, the frequency of the returning signal will be lower than the incident frequency (negative Doppler shift). Doppler shift = f1 – f2. Doppler shift depends on the angle between the reflector (red blood cell) direction and the direction of the emitted sound wave. Doppler shift = 2 × reflector speed × incident frequency × cosine (angle ×) / propagation speed. With 90° angles there is no Doppler shift, and reflector velocity calculations are impossible. Velocity calculations are most accurate with 0° incident angle. f1, incident frequency; f2, reflected frequency; ά, incident angle.

incident angle the cosine equals 0, and velocity calculations are not possible. If the incident angle is 0° (the emitted ultrasound wave is parallel to the movement of the reflector), the calculations are the most accurate.

BIOLOGIC EFFECTS OF ULTRASOUND RADIATION, THERMAL EFFECTS, AND CAVITATION AND THE ALARA PRINCIPLE

As ultrasound waves propagate through tissue, they attenuate releasing their energy. The released energy of the acoustic radiation depends on the original amplitude (power, intensity), the frequency of the ultrasound wave, focusing, and the acoustic impedance of the tissues that the sound is propagating through. The higher the amplitude of the emitted sound, the more energy is delivered; the higher the frequency, the more energy is released (higher attenuation); and the greater the difference in acoustic impedance at the boundary, the more energy is released at the boundary. A boundary between soft tissue and bone is a classic example of the release of thermal energy. Roughly half of the emitted energy is released and absorbed at such an interface. Focusing will limit energy release to a lesser extent and allow the surrounding tissues to absorb the energy. The energy of acoustic radiation is released in the form of tissue vibration and thermal energy. The latter may present itself as direct heat and in the form of cavitation. Cavitation occurs when acoustic energy is released at the boundary between soft tissue and the microscopic gas bubble and is common in such organs as the lungs. The *gaseous nuclei*, as the microbubbles are often referred to, rapidly expand and burst, injuring the neighboring cells. Tissue vibration is usually benign and has never been implicated in any adverse effects. In reality, it is used to improve the quality of the image in so-called tissue harmonic imaging. However, thermal injury and adverse effects of cavitation have been reported. Therefore, the U.S. Food and Drug Administration and the American Institute of Ultrasound in Medicine (AIUM) have set intensity limits for ultrasound radiation used in diagnostic ultrasonography. For unfocused ultrasound (see discussion on beam formation the section Wave Interaction), the limit has been set at 100 mW/cm^2, and for focused ultrasound the limit has been set at 1,000 mW/cm^2. This concern also prompted AIUM in 1988 to issue a safety statement, which is still applicable for bedside ultrasonography:

1. No study should be done without valid indications.
2. No study should be prolonged without a valid reason.
3. Minimal output power (amplitude) should be used to produce optimal images.

This set of rules is known as the *As Low As Reasonably Achievable (ALARA) principle*. However, most of the portable ultrasound systems used in bedside ultrasonography will not allow you to control the output power except in special (i.e., ophthalmologic) applications. The statement is nonetheless important to understand and follow whenever possible.

CHAPTER 3

Ultrasound Basics

Alexander B. Levitov, MD, FCCM, RDCS

ULTRASOUND TRANSDUCER STRUCTURE, FUNCTION, AND IMAGE FORMATION

In order to form images, the ultrasound signal is first transmitted into tissues, "reflects" off of interfaces of differing acoustic impedance back to the transducer, and is converted into electrical data that undergo processing to form a picture on the screen. This process is extremely complex and requires the conversion of electrical energy into mechanical (acoustic) energy, which is subsequently converted back to electrical energy. These essential tasks are performed by the ultrasound transducer, which is the most important part of the ultrasound system to understand.

Transducers can be divided into two basic types: *imaging transducers,* which produce visual representations of anatomic structures, and *Doppler transducers,* which are used to estimate the velocity of a moving reflective surface and then present it to the observer in the form of a sound, a graph, a color, or a combination of these. Either basic type can be further subdivided into several subtypes. The most common types will be discussed in this chapter, starting with the most basic single-crystal imaging transducer (Fig. 3.1).

At the core of every transducer is a piezoelectric element, also known as the active element or crystal, which is usually constructed of lead zirconium titanate (PZT) (Fig. 3.1). One property of PZT that is exploited to our advantage is that it is subject to the piezoelectric effect, which means that when mechanically deformed it will produce an electrical impulse (direct piezoelectric effect). When a positive voltage is applied to the element, it will expand, and when a negative voltage is applied, it will contract. Thus, when driven with a continuous or pulsed oscillating electrical signal, the element can be used as a source of acoustic waves. The PZT element will vibrate with the frequency of the applied electrical signal, resulting in the production of a sound wave of the same frequency. This piezoelectric property of PZT irreversibly disappears at high temperature, making it impossible to thermally sterilize (autoclave) ultrasound transducers. The higher the frequency of the electrical impulse applied to the crystal, the higher the frequency of the resulting sound wave. In the case of diagnostic ultrasound, the frequency is between 2 million and 20 million cycles per second (MHz). The PZT element is usually driven at or near its resonant frequency to maximize its output. The PZT crystal is one-half wavelength thick and is connected to wires that both deliver and carry away electrical impulses.

Imaging transducers have a dual role, acting as both the transmitter of the ultrasound wave (converting electrical impulses into the ultrasonic acoustic wave) and the receiver of the reflected ultrasound (converting the ultrasound wave into electrical impulses). Since these transducers send and receive signals, time must be allocated to the performance of each of these tasks. Therefore, all imaging transducers use what is called *pulsed ultrasound* with a dedicated "talking time," during which the ultrasound wave is generated, and "listening" is impossible. This is known as the *closed aperture time.* In addition, there is a "listening time," during which the reflected ultrasound energy is received by the PZT element and converted to electrical energy. During this interval, transmission is impossible. This is known as the *open aperture time.* Talking (transmitting) time is usually the shorter interval compared to listening time and represents 0.1% to 1% of total time.

Generally speaking, the deeper a structure, the longer it will take for an echo to return to the transducer. Since transducers can process only one signal at a time, this means that deeper structures require longer listening times and, therefore, a longer pulse repetition period, which is the combination of the transmitting and receiving times. Most machines have a depth-setting function, which can automatically adjust the listening time for the selected depth. It is possible for the transducer to emit ultrasound in the fundamental frequency but to receive echoes of the harmonic frequencies produced by tissue vibration (see also Chapter 2). This *tissue harmonic imaging* may improve image quality and reduce some artifacts. It is also possible to use higher-frequency ultrasound to interrogate shallower structures and low-frequency ultrasound for deeper structures. This is known as the *dynamic aperture.*

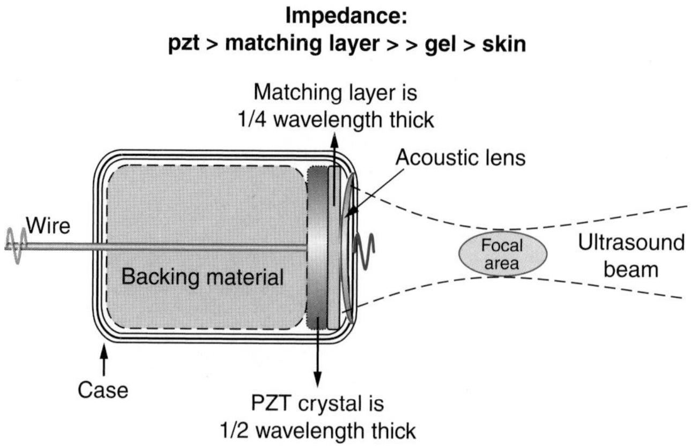

Figure 3.1. Single-crystal imaging ultrasound transducer. The imaging transducer both emits and receives signals. The lead zirconium titanate (piezoelectric) crystal converts electrical impulses from the wire into ultrasound and vice versa. The matching layer decreases internal reflections within the probe by gradually reducing acoustic impedance. The backing material reduces the length of the pulse by preventing after-ringing (dampening effect). The acoustic lens improves focusing. The case prevents electrical shock exposure for the patient and the operator. Pulse duration is the time during which the sound is emitted in each on/off cycle. It is usually 0.5 to 3 μsec and is composed of two to four cycles. The pulse repetition period is the time of the entire on/off cycle. PZT, lead zirconium titanate.

Surrounding the PZT crystal is a layer of backing or dampening material (Fig. 3.1) made of tungsten-impregnated epoxy resin. The dampening material reduces the duration of the ultrasound pulse after the electrical signal is switched off in the same way that placing a hand on a guitar string stops the vibration. In front of the active element is a matching layer, one-quarter wavelength thick, with acoustic impedance values between that of the PZT element and that of the patient's skin. This ensures a gradual change of acoustic impedance and diminishes echo formation within the transducer itself or from the skin–transducer interface. Acoustic gel is used to further reduce the impedance differences between the transducer and skin. Ultrasound gel impedance values lies between that of the skin and the matching layer, which functions to make the overall transition of acoustic impedance smoother and allows ultrasound transmission to occur without the formation of internal echoes. The gel also replaces any air between the transducer surface and the skin. The low ultrasound propagation velocity through air creates a strong impedance boundary and renders signal processing impossible, which makes the use of gel extremely important in ultrasonography.

An acoustic lens may be employed to improve the focus and lateral resolution (Fig. 3.1). The transducer is covered by a protective case that protects the operator from electric shocks and also protects the internal components of the transducer from outside elements such as water and body fluids. PZT transducers are generally driven with very high voltages. *Due to the risk of an electric shock to either the operator or the patient, one must never attempt to use a transducer with a cracked or defective housing or frayed wire.*

Single active element transducers are rarely used in ultrasound today. However, since their operation is instructive, they are briefly considered here. These transducers are capable of registering the position of the reflective surface (anatomic structure) with relationship to the transducer surface and represent the strength (energy) of the returning echoes in various shades of gray. Stronger echoes with the highest energy appear brighter (white or hyperechoic) on the screen (Fig. 3.2); the weaker ones appear darker (hypoechoic) or even black (anechoic). Typically, the image obtained with single-crystal transducers will consist of a string of dots of different shades representing the relative position of the reflective boundaries and the strength of the echo signal from each boundary. These reflective points, when plotted over time, give the standard M-mode image (Fig. 3.3). M mode is popular in echocardiography and several other applications where motion detection is essential (Fig. 3.4).

The strength of the reflected echo plotted against the distance between the reflector and the transducer will produce B-mode imaging (Fig. 3.3). Positioning a single PZT crystal on a moving head allows for "swinging" the beam across the scan plane like a spotlight, which converts dots into lines and forms a two-dimensional (2D) image (Fig. 3.5). Those so-called mechanical scanners dominated ultrasonography during the end of the last century and were still in limited use up until the late 1990s and up to 2005 (Video 3.1). Although the quality of the image achieved with mechanical transducers was acceptable, mechanical scanners had a fixed focus and were prone to failure.

TRANSDUCER TYPES, FUNCTION, AND CHOICE

Transducer Types

Currently, most imaging transducers are "array probes" that consist of multiple PZT crystals functioning in unison (Fig. 3.5). A platform of PZT crystals in an array probe is cut into multiple active elements. Each element has a separate active wire and a common

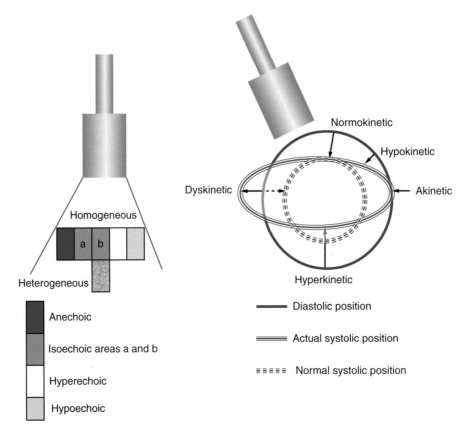

Figure 3.2. Image characteristics: static and kinetic.

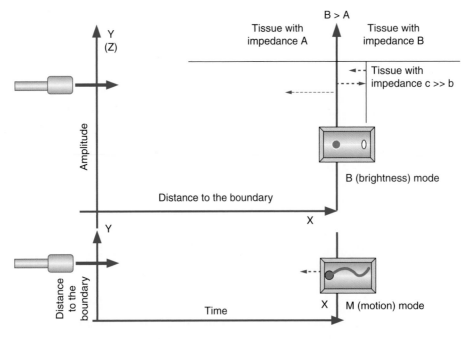

Figure 3.3. Single piezoelectric (lead zirconium titanate) transducer display modes: In B-mode parameters, the amplitude of the echo signal is represented by its brightness. The M mode displays reflector position (depth) over time.

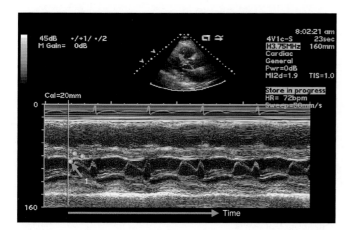

Figure 3.4. M-mode examination of the heart demonstrating the position of different cardiac structures (interventricular septum, mitral valve leaflets, and inferior wall of the left ventricle) plotted over time. Each 50 mm of the horizontal axis is 1 second. 1, Position of the anterior leaflet of the mitral valve at that time.

ground wire, which can emit and receive signals independently of its neighbor. If each crystal in the array produces the same image as the crystal positioned immediately next to it, 2D B-mode images are produced (Fig. 3.6).

Arrays are classified according to the position of the active elements into linear, curved (convex), annular, 2D, and one and one-half–dimensional ($1\frac{1}{2}$D). Linear and curved array transducers are commonly used in portable bedside ultrasound systems and will

be discussed in detail. The 2D arrays produce three-dimensional (3D) and 3D real-time (4D) images and are becoming increasingly popular in echocardiography and obstetric ultrasonography. Within the next 5 to 10 years, they probably will become commonplace for bedside applications.

The pattern of activation of the active elements further subdivides array probes into linear, curved, and phased arrays. The order of activation of crystals in linear and curved arrays is relatively simple. With linear array probes, active elements are positioned in a straight line and activated in neighboring groups of 5 to 10 at a time starting from one end of the transducer, advancing toward the other (Fig. 3.6). When the activation reaches the other end, firing starts over, and the process is repeated. The resulting image will have a typical square shape (Fig. 3.7).

Linear Arrays

Linear arrays can be activated very quickly and utilize high-frequency ultrasound waves. The images are of excellent quality, but because of attenuation, only relatively superficial structures (depth <6 cm) are amenable to visualization with linear arrays. They are therefore commonly used in vascular ultrasonography, vascular procedures, and the examination of superficial structures such as the thyroid, the eye, the testicles, and musculoskeletal structures. With the exception of ophthalmologic examinations, linear array probes may become problematic in moderately to morbidly obese patients. The other limitation of linear arrays is the fact that the size of the image can

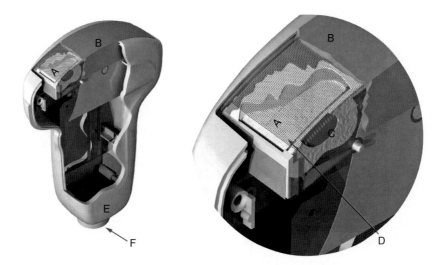

Figure 3.5. Components of an array transducer: (*A*) Piezoelectric (lead zirconium titanate) crystals: multiple crystals (active elements) can be activated separately; (*B*) matching layer; (*C*) backing material; (*D*) wires to each PZT element; (*E*) case; (*F*) cable (all wires are still separated within the cable).

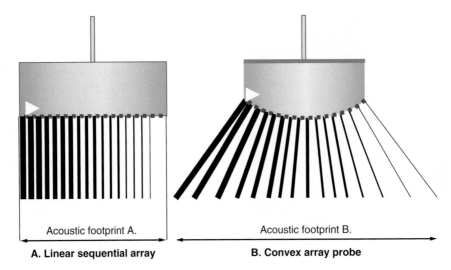

Acoustic footprint A.

A. Linear sequential array

Acoustic footprint B.

B. Convex array probe

Figure 3.6. Two-dimensional imaging. (**A**) The linear sequential array consists of multiple piezoelectric (lead zirconium titanate) crystals (elements) arranged in a line. Each one is connected to a separate wire. Elements are activated in groups from one end of the transducer to the other. (**B**) A similar arrangement is present in a convex array, but the elements are arranged in a curve, giving this type of transducer a wider view (larger footprint) in the far field. Elements in a curved array probe can be activated individually or in small groups.

be only as large as the transducer itself (Figs. 3.6 and 3.7). This "small footprint" limits the visualization of neighboring anatomy, which can be important in vascular (and other) procedures.

Curved Arrays

Curved or convex arrays are very similar to linear arrays, but PZT crystals are usually activated individually from one end of the array to the other (Fig. 3.6). They have a larger footprint and image size in both the near and far field and use lower ultrasound frequencies. Although image quality may be inferior to that of the linear array probes, curved arrays penetrate deeper into the body and provide an image of the anatomy for a large portion of the body at one time. Curved arrays are used in abdominal ultrasonography and are ideal for cavitary procedures such as paracentesis, thoracentesis, and abdominal or chest abscess or cyst drainage (Fig. 3.8). Curved probes are usually the only option in visualizing anatomic structures in morbidly obese patients.

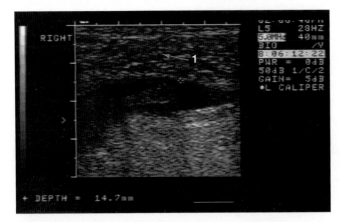

Figure 3.7. Vascular image (right common femoral vein) produced by a linear sequential array transducer. Notice the image is square and is of the same size as a vessel. The solid-looking structure (1) in the middle of the vessel is a thrombus.

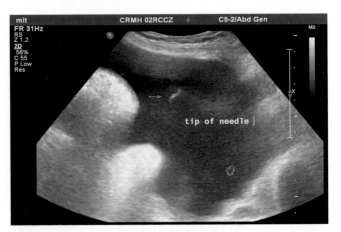

Figure 3.8. Image of the abdomen produced by the convex array transducer. Notice a large acoustic footprint in both the near and far fields.

Mechanical and phased arrays two-dimensional probes

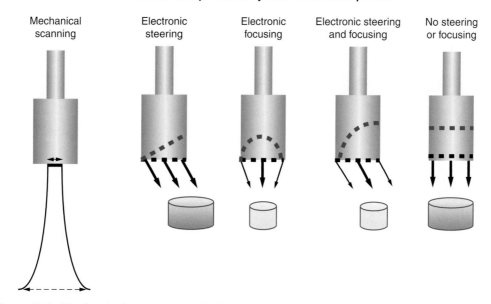

Figure 3.9. Mechanical scanning and phased array probes offer a large acoustic footprint in the far field through the small window. They are common in cardiac ultrasound, where the window is limited by intercostal spaces. In addition, phased array probes offer electronic steering (sweeping) and focusing of the ultrasound beam. The operator is capable of selecting single or multiple focal points as well as the width of the sweep. Lack of moving parts also makes phased array probes more reliable and durable.

Phased Arrays

In phased array transducers, individual PZT crystals are activated sequentially with approximately a 10-nanosecond delay. The pattern of the delay is determined by the beam former and allows for electronic steering (swinging) of the ultrasound beam, focusing, or both. A similar delay in aperture opening allows for proper echo reception and processing. Phased arrays will produce a sweeping of the ultrasound beam that is similar to that of mechanical transducers but with the advantage of an electronic focus and without moving parts. These benefits make this type of transducer particularly valuable in echocardiography, where a large organ (the heart) needs to be visualized through the small acoustic window of the intercostal space (Fig. 3.9).

Transducer Function

The signal from all of the active elements in an array produces one frame or sector of the 2D image. The next wave of the echoes will produce the next frame, and all the frames are combined into a movie clip. For the movie to be perceived as an uninterrupted continuous motion, the rate of the frames should be at least 15 frames per second. The ability of the ultrasound system to produce a movie that is perceived as smooth and uninterrupted is known as *temporal resolution.* Therefore, the minimal temporal resolution is 15 frames per second. The higher the frame rate, the better the temporal resolution of real-time 2D movies. The temporal resolution is limited by the system's time ability to generate, receive, and process signals. Since larger organs require a larger sector for visualization, it takes a longer time to interrogate them by forming a frame. Deeper structures require longer traveling times for the ultrasound to reach them and return, thereby increasing the frame formation time. Both of these situations reduce temporal resolution and the number of lines that are able to form each frame.

Line density depends on the number of active elements in the array. Additional lines (active elements) require a longer processing time and worsen the temporal resolution. A higher line density improves image quality similar to the way that the number of pixels in a digital camera improves image quality. Image quality is referred to as spatial resolution. In diagnostic ultrasonography, there exists an important trade-off between the spatial and temporal resolution in image quality (Fig. 3.10). Multifocusing improves spatial but worsens temporal resolution.

There are two methods to improve this performance: (1) find the acoustic window where the organ

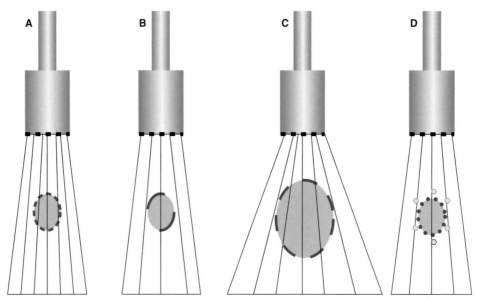

Figure 3.10. Probe A produces more ultrasound beams (lines) than probe B with resulting improvement in image quality (better spatial resolution) and deterioration of temporal resolution. Probe C produces as many lines as probe A, but a wider sector decreases line density and degrades spatial resolution. Temporal resolution is unchanged. Multifocusing requires more pulses per line and improves spatial resolution but decreases temporal resolution.

being interrogated is closer to the transducer (shallower), and (2) limit the sector size to the one necessary to evaluate the particular area of interest that provides the best possible spatial resolution (zooming). Achieving a balance between spatial and temporal resolution requires practice and experience on the part of the physician sonographer. Table 3.1 summarizes the relationships between spatial and temporal resolution of the 2D image.

DOPPLER

Doppler transducers are used to determine the velocity (speed and direction) of a moving reflector. Information derived from Doppler transducers can be presented to the operator in the acoustic (sound) or graphic (velocity over time) forms. In an acoustic form, the louder the audible, the higher is the flow volume,

and the higher the pitch, the faster is the reflector's velocity. In the graphical form, the flow direction is represented by the relationship to the baseline. When the position is above the baseline, the reflector is moving toward the transducer, and when the position is below the baseline, the reflector is moving away from the transducer. Color can also provide important guidance. When the image is red, the reflector is moving toward the transducer, and when the image is blue, the reflector is moving away from the transducer. Flow volume is represented by shades of gray and the width of the graphic. Velocity is measured by the height (or the depth) of the graphic representation. In color Doppler, velocity is presented by the color, and the color map is provided in the form of a side bar that allows the sonographer to decipher this information.

There are three basic types of Doppler transducers: continuous wave, pulsed wave, and duplex imaging.

TABLE 3.1. Factors Determining Spatial and Temporal Resolution				
Improved resolution	*Depth*	*Line density (LD)*	*Sector width*	*Focusing*
Spatial	Shallow	High	Narrow (zooming)	Multiple
Temporal	Shallow	Low	Narrow unchanged LD	Single

Continuous Wave Transducers

Continuous wave (CW) transducers have two active PZT elements, with one continuously emitting and the other receiving ultrasound waves from the moving reflector (Fig. 3.11 [see also color insert]). No backing material is necessary with a CW Doppler. By subtracting the frequency of the echo wave from the frequency of the emitted wave, Doppler shift can be calculated, and since it falls within an audible range (Chapter 2), the shift can be presented in the form of sound. The most familiar CW device is a "black box" Doppler "wand" used to obtain an audible representation of arterial flow. It is important to mention a common mistake in using this simplest ultrasound system. To obtain the best Doppler information, the wand should have an incidental angle of 0° cosine = 1 (kept parallel with the interrogated artery). A 90° angle most commonly used by operators will result in a cosine of 0 with the worst

possible Doppler shift. Doppler shift information can be converted into flow velocity information and presented graphically. As one can see from Fig. 3.11 (see also color insert), there is significant overlap between the emitted and returning beams, resulting in an inability to tell the precise location of the moving reflector. This range ambiguity is a major limitation of CW Doppler.

Pulsed Wave Doppler

If one requires the exact location of a moving reflector (i.e., valvular or stenotic vascular lesion), pulsed wave (PW) Doppler is utilized. A PW transducer structurally resembles an imaging transducer. The same PZT crystal is used to both emit and receive signals, but only echoes from the particular area (sample volume) are analyzed. The signal is emitted and received in the form of a pulse, just as with the imaging transducer, and the sample area is identified

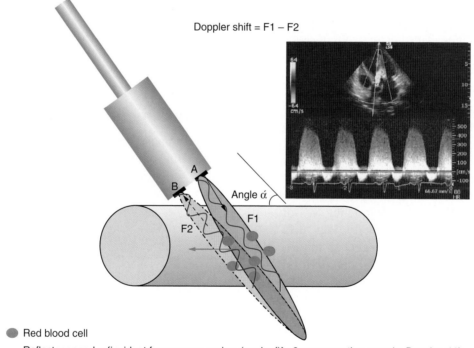

Doppler shift = F1 – F2

Angle ἁ

F1

F2

A

B

● Red blood cell

Reflector speed = {incident frequency x cosine. (angle ἁ)} : 2 × propagation speed × Doppler shift

Figure 3.11. A continuous wave (CW) Doppler transducer has two piezoelectric (lead zirconium titanate) crystals. One constantly emits, and the other receives signals. Element A transmits continuous ultrasound waves with frequency F1. Element B receives frequency F (F1 – F2 = Doppler shift). Doppler shift is in the audible frequency range and can be presented to the operator in the form of sound. Backing material is not necessary because CW signals require no dampening. The large area of overlap between the incident beam and receiver beam results in an inability to assess where the sample is located, known as range ambiguity. The CW Doppler transducer can measure very high flow velocities. Knowing Doppler shift, reflector velocity (RBC) can be calculated. Flow velocity information can be presented in graphic form. Color flow Doppler is a pulsed mode demonstrating average flow velocity (speed and direction over the sample area). The colored map in the left upper corner (see color insert) is providing reference information to the direction and speed of the moving reflectors (blood = RBCs).

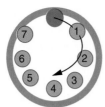 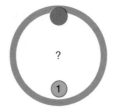 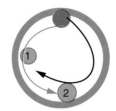

8:1 Samples per rotation: Clockwise direction is obvious.

2:1 Samples per rotation: Direction is obscure. Nyquist limit is reached.

1.5 Samples per rotation: Red dot seems to move counterclockwise (aliasing has occurred).

Figure 3.12. Nyquist limit and aliasing illustrated by sample snapshots of the ball, rotating clockwise.

by "gating," which is to limit the returning signals to a specified time interval and to ignore signals arriving earlier and later than expected. Every returning pulse is essentially a snapshot of the reflector position within the sample at the time the echo is formed. This ensures an exact knowledge of the position of the moving reflector with respect to the transducer surface, but now the frequency of sampling depends on the time of flight. This means that if a moving reflector is deep or moving fast, the sampling frequency might be insufficient for the operator to understand the velocity or direction of the flow. This is known as aliasing (Chapter 2). The sample frequency at which aliasing occurs is known as the *Nyquist limit* and is determined by pulse repetition frequency (PRF). The Nyquist limit is dependant on the frequency of the ultrasound wave, with high-frequency pulsed Doppler probes being more prone to aliasing due to the higher frequency of Doppler shift with the same reflector velocity (Figs. 3.12 and 3.13). The Nyquist limit is represented mathematically by the following equation: Nyquist limit (kHz) = PRF / 2. When aliasing occurs, there are several methods for eliminating it, including the following:

- Use a shallower sample volume (increase the PRF).
- Reduce carrier ultrasound frequency.
- Reduce the incidence angle.
- Use color wave Doppler since it is not subject to Ualiasing.

Pulsed wave Doppler information can be presented acoustically or graphically or converted into color (color flow Doppler). In this case, multiple sample volumes are analyzed simultaneously. Several pulses are delivered in one packet, and Doppler shifts are averaged to provide an average flow velocity. By convention, negative Doppler shift, where the reflector is moving away from the transducer, is represented in blue, and positive Doppler shift, where the reflector is moving toward the transducer, is represented in red. A color map is provided to assist with estimation of direction and velocity of the reflector. The distance from the center of the bar is associated with higher-flow velocity in either direction (Fig. 3.11 [see also color insert]). Colored flow Doppler is a pulsed modality and as such is subject to aliasing. The blue dots in the middle of the yellow flow in Fig. 3.11 (see also color insert) do not represent flow reversal in the sample area, but aliasing.

Duplex Imaging

Duplex imaging transducers combine the capability of producing anatomic images in shades of gray and

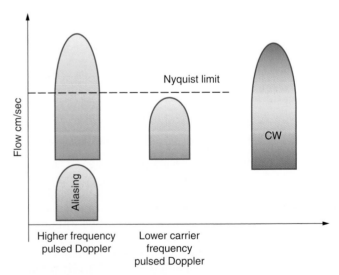

Figure 3.13. Eliminating aliasing. Aliasing can be eliminated by choosing the shallower sample (increase pulse repetition frequency), converting to continuous wave (CW) Doppler, or choosing lower-frequency pulsed wave Doppler.

colored flow Doppler information on the same screen. Arrays in duplex transducers have dedicated imaging and Doppler active elements. However, popular duplex transducers are subject to an incident angle "paradox." Anatomic images are best visualized at a 90° angle and Doppler calculations at 0°. Therefore, in extreme cases, either the anatomic image or Doppler analysis will need to be optimized. The flow velocity information can and usually is converted to a pressure gradient Δ, using a simplified Bernoulli equation: $-\Delta P = 4 \times (V_{max})^2$ where V_{max} is maximal flow velocity.

ULTRASOUND SYSTEM ANATOMY AND IMAGE PROCESSING

The seamless flow of electrical and mechanical impulses and their conversion into images are possible with ultrasonography. Increasingly sophisticated signal processing allows the development of high-quality portable ultrasound systems that can be used in bedside ultrasonography. There are six basic components of ultrasound processors; the transducer has already been discussed. The five remaining components are the master synchronizer, pulser (or beam former), receiver (processor), display (screen), and information (image) storage device, which will be discussed here.

Master Synchronizer

The master synchronizer organizes the timing of the electrical impulses into the transducer (closed aperture or talking time) and electrical impulses produced by the returning echoes in the transducer (opened aperture or listening time). Open aperture time greatly exceeds talking time, when the transducer is emitting signals into tissues.

Pulser

The pulser, or beam former, controls the sequence of activation of the active elements (PZT crystals) in the array transducers and the amplitude of the electrical impulses and, therefore, the intensity of mechanical vibration in the PZT crystals and the amount of acoustic energy released into the tissues. In most portable bedside ultrasound machines, this function is preset and is not under operator control, but in others it can be controlled by the sonographer and is referred to as an *output power*. PRF is also controlled by the pulser and can be changed by the operator through adjustment of the depth control button on the ultrasound system. The deeper the anatomy to be interrogated, the lower the PRF needs to be set.

Receiver

The receiver contains all of the elements necessary for the formation of images from the information contained in the returning echoes and, therefore, electrical impulses produced in the transducer by those returning echoes. Before these impulses can be turned into a display, they need to be amplified and undergo signal depth compensation and compression. The receiver gain control can increase the amplitude of the electrical impulses from the echo signals. Since the amplitude of the signal is presented on the display screen as brightness amplification (receiver gain), an increase will produce uniformly brighter images. Figure 3.14A illustrates proper use of the receiver gain control button. In Figure 3.14B, the gain settings are too high, obscuring anatomic details. Signal compensation refers to the process by which echo signals from the deeper (and thus more attenuated) structures will be amplified more than the less attenuated (stronger) signals from more superficial structures. This process is known as time (time of flight) gain compensation (TGC) or depth gain compensation. These terms are synonymous. The process of compensation is under operator control, and in most bedside machines, this is done through the shallow (near field)/deep (far field) gain (brightness) buttons or levers. Most portable systems will also provide an "autogain" option, in which the machine chooses the TGC settings. Figure 3.15A illustrates proper use of TGC control. In Figure 3.15B, the image is overcompensated in the near field. Figure 3.16 shows an example of the portable ultrasound system with the control marked; Video 3.2 further illustrates receiver gain and TGC use. After compensation, signal compression takes place, bringing all signals into the range of brightness visible to the human eye, followed by the rejection of the very low amplitude signals. Neither rejection nor compression is under operator control.

Image Display and Storage

After the processor, in most portable ultrasound machines, the signal is sent to a digital converter (computer chip) and is then displayed on the screen. The process is proprietary to the manufacturer. The digital image then becomes subject to postprocessing manipulations, some of which (such as electronic zooming) can be under the control of the operator or reader. The image is then passed into the system computer storage system, preferably picture archive and communication systems familiar to most physicians.

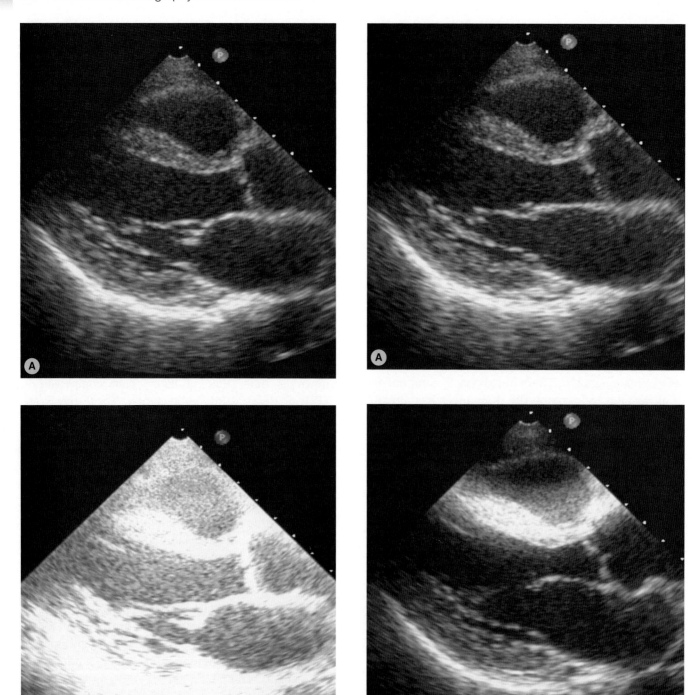

Figure 3.14. Use of the receiver gain (amplification) control button. **(A)** The image represents proper receiver gain. **(B)** The image is too bright, making detailed anatomy obscure (overgain).

Figure 3.15. Use of the time gain compensation (TGC) (depth gain compensation) control. **(A)** Image demonstrates proper use of TGC. **(B)** Image shows TCG overuse in the near field (the image is too bright, making detailed anatomy obscure).

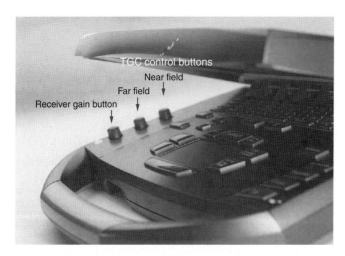

Figure 3.16. Portable ultrasound system with time gain compensation (TGC) buttons marked.

COMMON ULTRASOUND ARTIFACTS

Ultrasound image formation is a highly organized process, but it is also subject to a number of assumptions and artifacts. Artifacts by themselves are neither good nor bad and, in fact, can be utilized for diagnosis (lung ultrasound). They are always bad, however, when they are not recognized as artifacts and are assumed to be anatomic entities.

Technically, an artifact is the discrepancy between an interpreted image and the anatomic or physiologic reality present in the patient at the time of image acquisition. Artifacts include imaging errors, operator errors, and interpretation errors. One can avoid the latter two errors with a thorough knowledge of anatomy and ultrasound system operation, so we will concentrate on unavoidable imaging artifacts, which are inherent in the present diagnostic ultrasound equipment. It is important to state that, although recent technologic advances have reduced the incidence of image artifacts, they still occur frequently enough that the physician sonographer should be vigilant for their occurrence and aware of the difference from anatomic reality. This is particularly important when ultrasonography is being used to guide invasive procedures.

Acoustic Shadowing

When reaching the boundary with high acoustic impedance difference (high attenuation), an ultrasound pulse can penetrate no further, creating linear anechoic or hypoechoic "shadows" traveling in the direction of the ultrasound beam. This makes visualization of the

deeper structures impossible. As with all artifacts, the implications for acoustic shadowing are twofold. Acoustic shadowing can make some structures invisible to the ultrasound, decreasing their spatial resolution. Alternatively, acoustic shadowing can be used to improve the diagnosis for several conditions. Lesions with high acoustic impedance, such as gallstones, are diagnosed by their shadowing pattern. In chest ultrasonography, rib shadows can assist with locating a pleural line (Fig. 3.17). The dual nature of an acoustic shadowing artifact is illustrated in Figures 3.18 and 3.19.

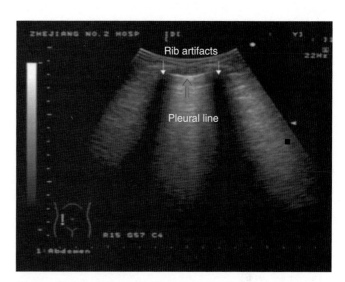

Figure 3.17. "Shadows" of the ribs (*white arrows*) assist in locating the pleural line (between visceral and parietal pleura, *blue arrow*).

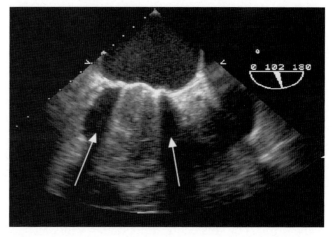

Figure 3.18. Transesophageal echo of the prosthetic mitral valve. Acoustic shadows of the prosthetic leaflets or "puppets" (*white arrows*) make underlying structures invisible and assessment of valvular function (including Doppler) difficult, if not impossible.

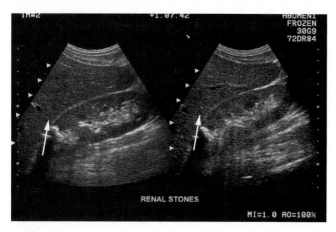

Figure 3.19. Acoustic shadow (*white arrows*) assists the operator (interpreter) in the diagnosis of a renal calculus.

Reverberations or "Ring-down" Artifacts

Ultrasound beams caught between two highly reflective layers will "bounce" between those layers, producing multiple reflections. Each of the reflections is picked up by the transducer as a separate image. The images are equally spaced and are perpendicular to the direction of the ultrasound pulse. This produces a typical "venetian blind" pattern of reverberation artifact (Fig. 3.20). As the distance between these lines diminishes, they may become confluent, resulting in production of a "comet tail" artifact. Again, the dual nature of a reverberation artifact makes it a diagnostic tool. In chest ultrasound, comet tail artifacts (also

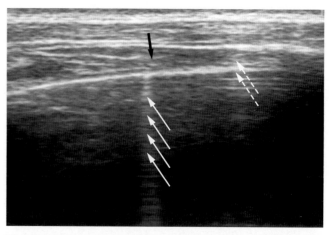

Figure 3.21. Reverberation artifacts from the pleural line including the classic pattern (*interrupted parallel arrows*) and comet tail, ring-down artifact (*solid white arrows*) assure the interpreter of the close proximity of visceral and parietal pleura and thus rule out pneumothorax.

known as *B lines*) are caused by the ultrasound pulse reverberating between the parietal and visceral pleura, which have to be in close proximity for this artifact to occur. Thus, the presence of B lines virtually excludes pneumothorax (Fig. 3.21).

Enhancement Artifacts

Just as high-attenuation structures produce shadows, low attenuation results in acoustic enhancement. An enhancement artifact is a hyperechoic band propagating in the same direction as an ultrasound. Through deteriorating spatial resolution, enhancement artifacts can assist in the differential diagnosis of cysts (low attenuation) and tumors (higher attenuation) (Fig. 3.22).

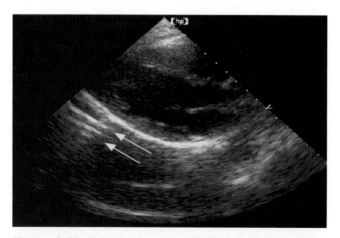

Figure 3.20. Classic reverberation artifact (*parallel white arrows*) on this echocardiogram. A venetian blind pattern causes the deterioration of image quality. It is likely caused by the ultrasound pulse being "caught" between pericardial layers and producing multiple, evenly spaced images of that one reflective boundary.

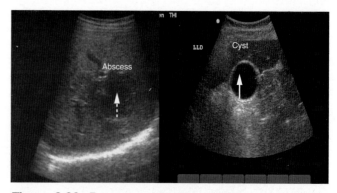

Figure 3.22. Posterior enhancement from a low-attenuation lesion (*solid white arrow*) makes it difficult to see anatomic details of the deeper structures. On the other hand, it helps to differentiate a cyst on the right from an abscess on the left, which showed no posterior enhancement (*interrupted white arrow*), because of higher ultrasound attenuation of the abscess.

Mirror-image Artifacts

Linear boundaries of very high acoustic impedance may become reflective to the ultrasound (acoustic mirror). Both direct echoes and reflected pulses will reach the transducer, resulting in image duplication. The redirected echo will always arrive later, and the ultrasound system will position it below the real image because of its longer time of flight (Fig. 3.23 [see also color insert]). The implications of this are usually benign. For example, even when a duplicate image of a carotid artery is presented, the sonographer can usually assume a single carotid artery. On some occasions, however, the artifact can be devastating (Fig. 3.23 [see also color insert]). For example, if the mirror image of the ventricle is interpreted as a pericardial effusion, pericardiocentesis may be performed when it is not indicated (Fig. 3.24). The sonographer must correlate the acquired images with the clinical condition of the patient under care.

Refraction Artifacts

If the boundary struck by the ultrasound is not at a 90° angle, refraction can occur (Chapter 2). Refraction occurs at the boundary with different propagation velocity, which may compensate for increased distance and result in similar time of flight for the ultrasound pulse. In this case, the artifact and the real image may assume any position with respect to each other, including side by side (Fig. 3.25).

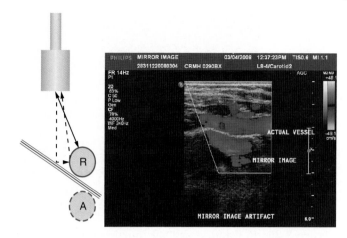

Figure 3.23. Mirror-image artifact (carotid artery duplication). The acoustic mirror (*triple black line*) reflects ultrasound toward the anatomic structure (R) (which takes longer to return to the transducer). The structure is therefore visualized twice directly (*solid black arrow*) and via the mirror reflection (*interrupted black arrow*). Since the indirect route takes longer, mirror-image artifact (A) is always positioned below the real structure. (See color insert.)

Propagation Velocity Errors

Boundary positioning on the screen is accomplished by the ultrasound system with the presumption that ultrasound propagates with a universal velocity of 1,540 m/sec. If the propagation velocity

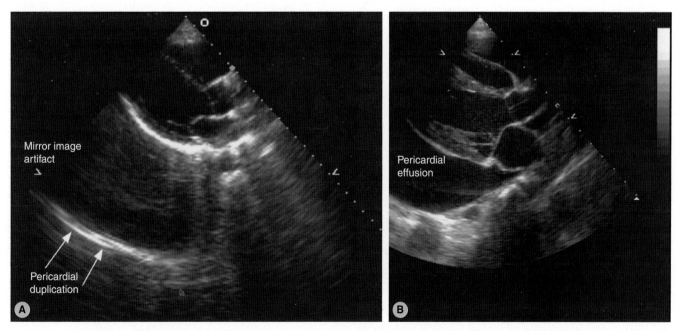

Figure 3.24. Mirror-image artifact (pericardial duplication). The mirror image of the left ventricle **(A)** may be difficult to distinguish from pericardial effusion **(B)**. The results of misinterpretation in this case may be devastating.

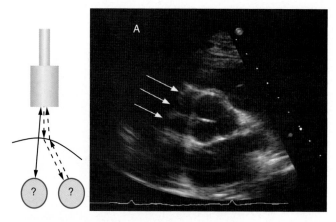

Figure 3.25. Refraction artifact (aortic duplication). The real image of the aorta on the aortic valve level is positioned side by side with the artifact.

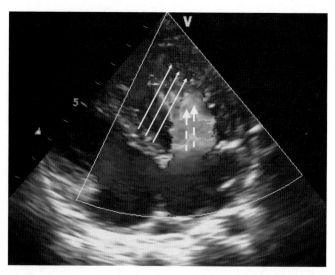

Figure 3.27. An apical four-chamber view of a non-compacted left ventricle with color flow into the noncompacted areas (*solid white arrows*). The central area within the color flow Doppler is an aliasing artifact (*interrupted white arrows*). (See color insert.)

differs significantly because of the nature of the medium (e.g., silicone-filled breast prosthesis), the reflector position on the screen will be different than in the body. In silicone, the high propagation velocity makes the reflector appear shallower than it really is.

Lobes

Lobe artifacts are produced by the parts of the ultrasound beam (pulse) traveling in a direction different from the main axis. This produces a second copy of the reflector, positioned on the screen next to the reflector (Fig. 3.26). In this case, the use of tissue harmonic imaging may reduce the incidence of this type of artifact.

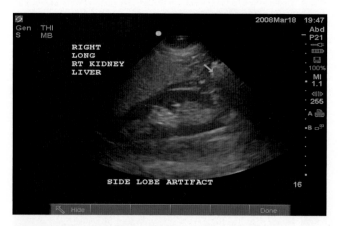

Figure 3.26. Side lobe artifact. Peripheral parts of the ultrasound beam treated by the ultrasound system as part of the main beam with the resulting partial image of the renal pelvis (*white arrow*) next to the image of the right kidney.

Doppler Artifacts

Aliasing is the most common artifact of pulsed wave and colored Doppler (Fig. 3.27 [see also color insert]); fortunately, it is relatively easy to recognize. Other Doppler artifacts include ghosting and cross-talk. Ghosting is a movement artifact where a Doppler shift is produced by the motion of a structure or material different from the one being evaluated (e.g., ventricular wall motion instead of blood flow in the ventricle). Ghosting can be eliminated by the use of a "wall filter," which rejects competing low-level Doppler shifts. Alternatively, myocardial tissue movements may be a primary target of investigation (tissue Doppler). In this case ghosting alone is evaluated, which blurs the line between what is artifact and what is useful information. Cross-talk is a mirror-image Doppler artifact (Fig. 3.28 [see also color insert]), which may occur with Doppler incidence angles close to 90° or high receiver gain settings. Therefore, this artifact can usually be eliminated by reducing either the incident angle or the receiver gain.

The recognition of artifacts is the key to correct interpretation of ultrasound images. Artifacts may provide significant diagnostic value if recognized or may result in devastating errors, depending on the operator's ability to identify them. Artifacts are usually seen in only a single view; visualization of the same structure from different transducer positions eliminates artifacts. Adequate training and expertise in image interpretation is mandatory for the physician sonographer. Adequate

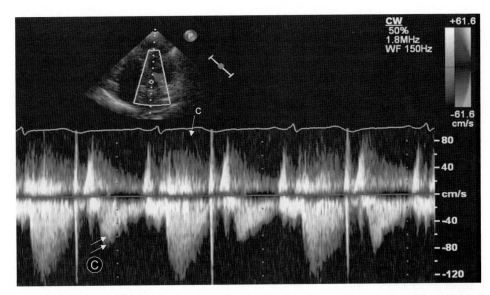

Figure 3.28. This image demonstrates the presence of cross-talk (C) artifact in a pulsed wave Doppler interrogation (see color insert). It is seen both during systole (aortic flow, *single white arrow*) and diastole (mitral flow, *two white arrows*). Please note: True aortic flow is away from the transducer and should be below the baseline, while mitral flow is directed toward the transducer and should be above the baseline. (*Image courtesy of D. Adams, RDCS.*)

knowledge for operating and maintaining the ultrasound equipment will also reduce the amount of artifacts. Finally, meticulous adherence to quality assurance recommendations will provide the patient and the operator a degree of both professional and legal protection from unrecognized artifacts.

QUALITY ASSURANCE

Although manufacturers of portable ultrasound equipment provide service contracts for machine maintenance, the primary responsibility for quality assurance rests with the operator involved in bedside ultrasonography. Routine quality assurance procedures should be adopted to ensure that patients are safe during ultrasound-guided procedures.

To ensure image quality and accuracy, simulators known as *phantoms* have been developed. These simulators have known physical characteristics including predetermined positions of reflective surfaces. The images obtained from the ultrasound system being tested are compared to the phantom information, and

any deviations are documented. If discrepancies are found, corrective measures to eliminate them are taken.

The two most commonly used and commercially available phantoms are the American Institute of Ultrasound in Medicine 100-mm test objects and tissue-equivalent phantoms (Fig. 3.29). In both of these phantoms, objects with different predetermined acoustic impedances are positioned at known distances in the medium (from the surface). The medium is constructed such that there is a propagation velocity of 1,540 m/sec. The ability of the machine to properly visualize those objects (spatial resolution) and estimate their position (calibration) is tested. Objects placed in the direction of the beam test axial resolution, and those placed perpendicular to it determine lateral resolution. Mock cysts and tumors also may be placed in phantoms to ensure the ultrasound system's ability to determine their sizes and characteristics. Doppler phantoms use either moving strings or echogenic fluid moving with known velocity in plastic tubes to test the Doppler transducer's ability to estimate the flow velocity.

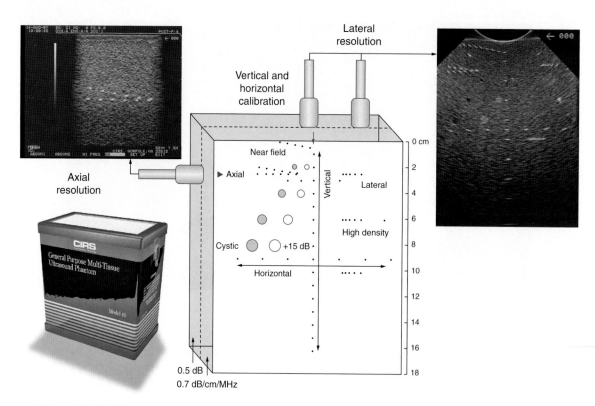

Figure 3.29. Using a tissue phantom for quality assurance to assess lateral resolution, axial resolution, and calibration.

ULTRASOUND USE FOR EVALUATION OF ORGANS OF THE HEAD AND NECK

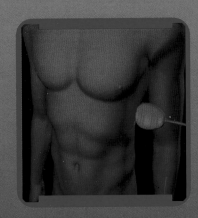

CHAPTER 4

Ultrasound of the Head and Neck

Christian Butcher, MD, FCCP

INTRODUCTION

Although uncommonly disseminated to general practitioners, the techniques and clinical applications of neck and upper respiratory ultrasonography are important to know. Physical examination of the neck provides useful clinical information that can play an integral role in diagnosing various disease states. For example, discovery of a carotid bruit alerts the provider to the presence of vascular disease; cervical lymphadenopathy in a smoker with recent weight loss and hoarseness raises the suspicion of a malignancy of the head and neck. The problem encountered in clinical practice, however, is that even proper examination of the neck often overlooks subtle abnormalities, especially in the obese population. In addition, while physical examination may identify anatomic abnormalities such as a thyroid mass, only imaging reveals whether the mass is cystic or solid, homogenous in appearance, or necrotic. Of all the imaging modalities that currently exist, only ultrasonography is amenable to being "miniaturized" into highly portable systems capable of producing high-quality images. This chapter covers some of the more uncommon clinical applications of ultrasonography—uncommon not because the clinical utility is minimal but because they are relatively unknown.

PARANASAL SINUSES

Using ultrasonography to evaluate the paranasal sinuses has been technically feasible since as early as the 1960s[1] but was not applied clinically until more recently, likely due to the development of low-cost, high-quality bedside ultrasound imaging technology. Early studies established ultrasound as a viable alternative to diagnosing maxillary sinusitis when compared to computed tomography (CT) and were instrumental in describing the typical ultrasound findings associated with sinusitis.[2,3] More recently, postural maneuvers were shown to improve the accuracy of ultrasonography to diagnose sinus disease.[4] In 2006, Vargas et al[4] investigated the role of ultrasound in performing transnasal puncture of the maxillary sinus in intubated intensive care unit patients. Patients suspected of having sinusitis first underwent ultrasound examination of the maxillary sinus followed by transnasal puncture, if the ultrasound result was positive. A total of 84 of 120 sinuses were ultrasonographically positive. Of these, 78 had positive results from transnasal puncture. The authors concluded that ultrasound evidence of sinusitis may be of value to indicate and perform transnasal puncture, thereby avoiding the overuse of CT scans and the exposure to radiation.[5]

Interestingly, there are no studies that describe an improvement in intensive care unit outcomes by using bedside ultrasonography over standard CT, even though obtaining a diagnosis by CT usually requires transport of critically ill patients to and from the radiology department. Also, one could easily imagine a significant cost savings by utilizing the bedside technique; transportation costs are eliminated, and valuable nursing time is not wasted. Although there are many benefits to the use of ultrasonography, it does not eliminate the need for CT imaging of the sinuses. Several indications for CT include any planned surgical procedure involving the sinuses, suspected sinus trauma, and suspected malignant disease. This discussion will be limited to the use of ultrasonography to evaluate paranasal sinusitis.

The importance of diagnosing sinus disease in critically ill patients has been well established. Sinusitis is a source of fever, which leads to costly workups and empiric antibiotic regimens,[6,7] many of which may be "overkill" for the most common causes of bacterial sinusitis and, thus, place the patient at unnecessary risk for antibiotic complications. Additionally, maxillary sinus disease is an independent risk factor for the development of nosocomial lung infections.[8] Although not studied in any systematic fashion, it is also conceivable that undiagnosed sinusitis may lead to significant pain and agitation, which could result in the increased use of sedatives and analgesics and impair extubation efforts.

Anatomic Review and Physical Examination Correlation With Ultrasound Anatomy and Physiology

The anatomy of the paranasal sinuses is shown in Figure 4.1 (see also color insert). The sinuses most amenable to ultrasonographic examination are the

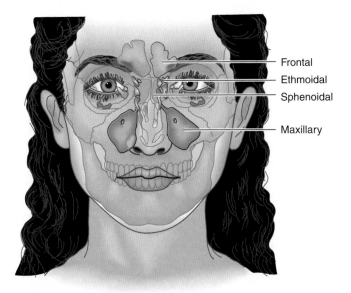

Figure 4.1. Anatomy of the paranasal sinuses. (See color insert.)

Frontal
Ethmoidal
Sphenoidal
Maxillary

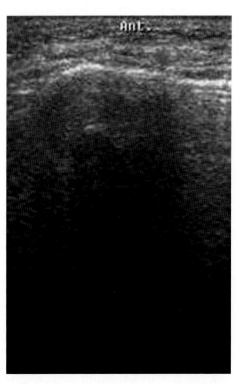

Figure 4.2. Ultrasound appearance of a normal maxillary sinus. Note that the anterior wall, including the skin and subcutaneous tissues as well as the bone, is visible at the top of the image; no other wall is visible.

maxillary and frontal sinuses; however, most studies have been performed on the maxillary sinus. The maxillary sinus is contained within the maxilla and is bordered by the orbital floor superiorly, the hard palate inferiorly, the nasal wall medially, and the zygoma laterally. In the normal state, the sinus is air filled and, thus, impairs transmission of ultrasound energy. What is seen in the normal state is the anterior wall only (Fig. 4.2). All underlying structures are obscured by air artifact; this is considered a negative study. When the sinus is filled with fluid, ultrasound waves penetrate the anterior wall, travel through the fluid, strike the posterior or lateral walls, and reflect back to the transducer, resulting in an image of the sinus cavity in its entirety (Fig. 4.3). This is known as a *sinusogram,* which is a positive study. A partial sinusogram, where only the posterior wall or a side wall is seen, occurs because of the presence of either an air-fluid level in the sinus or mucosal thickening. It is crucial to understand the effect of patient position on the behavior of fluid (if present) in the maxillary sinus, especially when attempting to ascertain the cause of a partial sinusogram. In the supine position, free fluid can "layer out" away from the anterior wall, introducing a layer of air between the anterior wall and the fluid, which causes the same acoustic shadowing seen in a completely air-filled sinus. However, when the patient is placed in a semirecumbent or upright position, the fluid (if present) will follow gravity and cover the floor of the sinus, coming in contact with the anterior wall inferiorly, which results in either a partial or complete sinusogram, depending on how much fluid is present and the transducer orientation or angulation (Fig. 4.4).

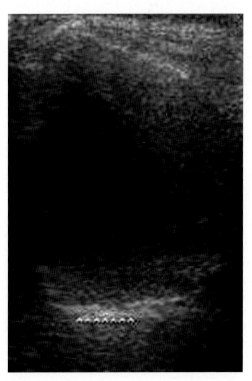

Figure 4.3. In contrast to Figure 4.2, this image clearly shows the posterior wall of the sinus cavity. This is possible because of transmission of the ultrasound energy through the sinus fluid.

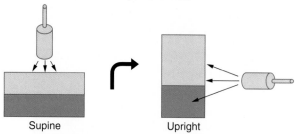

Postural maneuvers may "bring" fluid forward (against the anterior wall), enabling insonation of the posterior wall.

Supine   Upright

Figure 4.4. Effect of postural maneuvers on sinus fluid. Note that when fluid is not adjacent to the anterior wall, transmission of the ultrasound beam does not occur.

Technique

1. Most often, patients are placed in a semirecumbent position. A 6- to 13-MHz linear array probe with a small, narrow footprint is used. Proper transducer position is shown in Figure 4.5.

2. Scan in the horizontal plane first, angulating the probe cephalad (toward the orbital floor) and caudally (toward the floor of the sinus); next, turn the transducer 90°, and scan from the medial to the lateral walls.

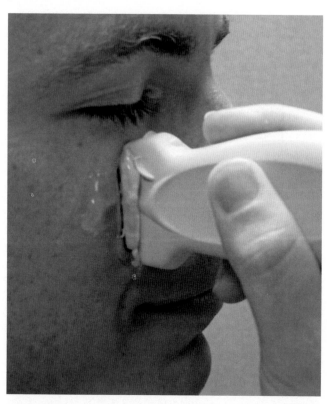

Figure 4.5. Proper position of the transducer when the maxillary sinus is being examined. The sinus can be scanned longitudinally (shown) and transversely.

3. Repeat the technique on the other side. A complete ultrasound maxillary sinus scan, in contrast to CT scanning, can be performed in less than 60 seconds. If a complete sinusogram is seen, no further evaluation is necessary; the patient should be treated for sinusitis.

4. If a partial sinusogram is obtained, postural maneuvers may help elucidate the cause: sinusitis versus mucosal thickening. Until the technique is mastered, we recommend correlating with CT scan findings unless an obvious positive result is obtained (i.e., a complete sinusogram).

Common Pitfalls

Care must be taken to scan only the maxillary sinus. Conceivably, if the probe is angled toward the orbit, or if the probe is positioned too close to the eye, retinal imaging may occur. While ocular ultrasound is routinely performed with appropriate equipment using specific ocular settings, damage to the retina may occur if inappropriate settings are used (see Chapter 5).

Another pitfall is assuming that all cases of partial, or even complete, sinusograms elicited by ultrasound are true sinusitis. Sinuses may be fluid filled for a variety of reasons. However, a sinusogram of any type in the right clinical setting (leukocytosis, fever) and in the absence of any other source of infection increases the likelihood that sinusitis is present.

LARYNX/ENDOTRACHEAL INTUBATION

Ascertaining endotracheal tube (ETT) position, both immediately after placement and on subsequent "ventilator days," uses expensive resources and exposes patients to doses of radiation that can become significant over time. In addition, waiting for "stat" portable radiographs wastes valuable time. Although the need for postintubation radiography can be debated, the reality is that many of these patients undergo confirmatory imaging.

In recent years, there have been several publications outlining the clinical application of ultrasonography to localization of the ETT in an effort to ascertain clinically important malposition events. There have also been reports of using ultrasonography to predict difficult intubation and difficult extubation, although data for these indications are limited. The majority of the following discussion, therefore, will focus on the rationale and technique underlying successful verification of ETT position.

In 1987, Raphael and Conard used B-mode two-dimensional (2D) transtracheal ultrasound to confirm

ETT placement in 24 patients already known to have successful tracheal intubations; they were not attempting to identify esophageal intubation or any other malposition. In addition to making some comments about general feasibility, they concluded that the technique could benefit certain patients, such as those who are pregnant or getting frequent chest radiographs.[9]

In 2007, a study in the emergency medicine literature showed that transtracheal 2D ultrasound could identify esophageal intubation with a sensitivity of 100%.[10] Two other studies, in both live patients and cadavers, confirmed a high sensitivity and specificity of 2D ultrasound to evaluate ETT position.[11,12] The latter of these studies demonstrated better sensitivity and specificity using a dynamic approach (visualization of the tube during placement) when compared to a static approach (confirmation of placement after the fact). Chun et al[13] in 2004 demonstrated that ETT malposition in the right mainstem bronchus could be identified with bilateral pleural ultrasound. The parietal-visceral pleural interface has a characteristic "shimmering" appearance during lung ventilation. If the ETT is positioned in a mainstem bronchus, the sliding or shimmering will be either greatly reduced or absent on the contralateral side, assuming no anatomic airway obstruction as the cause of reduced or absent pleural movement (e.g., obstructing airway tumor). Weaver et al[14] confirmed the approach, stating a sensitivity of identifying esophageal intubation of 95% to 100% and sensitivity for a right mainstem intubation versus tracheal intubation of around 70% to 75% using the sliding lung sign. Some institutions are currently investigating a combined approach of transtracheal/laryngeal ultrasonography to evaluate for *proximal malposition* of the ETT (esophageal intubation, ETT too high) and pleural ultrasound to identify *distal malposition* (mainstem intubation). Preliminary results indicate that satisfactory ETT position (in the right place without being too high or too low) can be accurately predicted using ultrasonography when compared to chest radiography; this may obviate the need for chest radiography to ascertain tube position.

There are other potential applications of upper airway ultrasonography in addition to the verification of ETT position. These include guiding the selection of ETT size by measuring the diameter of the airway in the subglottic region and predicting difficult laryngoscopy by ultrasound quantification of pretracheal soft tissue.[15–17] Unfortunately, the predictive value of this technique remains unknown. Nonetheless, it seems a worthwhile area of inquiry to predict difficult laryngoscopy, which may trigger early anesthesia consultation for suspected difficult-to-intubate patients.

Anatomic Review and Physical Examination Correlation With Ultrasound Anatomy and Physiology

The anatomy of the larynx is shown in Figure 4.6. Ultrasonographically, the posterior wall of the trachea, much like the posterior wall of an air-filled maxillary sinus, is not usually visible. This, of course, is due to the presence of air, which is a poor medium for ultrasound transmission. Therefore, only the anterior and lateral walls of the trachea are seen during the ultrasound examination. The thyroid cartilage is easily recognizable, particularly in the transverse view, due to its large size and the laryngeal prominence, which forms a characteristic anterior "point" on the ultrasound image (Fig. 4.7). Inferior to that is the cricoid cartilage, which is usually about twice as wide and twice as thick as a typical tracheal ring. Inferior to the cricoid are the tracheal rings, which can be visualized either transversely (one at a time) or longitudinally (Fig. 4.8). In the average adult, at least three tracheal rings are visible in the longitudinal view. Over the first several tracheal rings lies the isthmus of the thyroid gland; the inferior thyroid veins usually course upward from the brachiocephalic trunks on either side, running along the anterior tracheal surface to the thyroid gland. There may also be an aberrant artery in this area. The right brachiocephalic artery and left common carotid artery lie on either side of the trachea just medial and slightly posterior to the jugular veins.

A transverse ultrasonographic view of the lower cervical region is shown in Figure 4.9A and B. When intubated, the anterior wall of the ETT may be seen in either the transverse or longitudinal view as a double-walled structure just underneath the anterior wall of the trachea (Fig. 4.10). Occasionally, it may be necessary to apply gentle pressure to the trachea to promote contact of the tracheal wall with the ETT. Remember, air does not transmit ultrasound; therefore, if there is air between the ETT and the tracheal wall, the tube will not be visible. Rarely, imaging the trachea from a more lateral vantage point becomes necessary, usually after a patient is newly intubated, and the relatively stiff ETT abuts a lateral wall. The distal tip of the ETT is usually found in the proximity of the sternal notch. It may be necessary to deflate the cuff to adequately visualize the tip of the tube or to bring the tube into contact with the anterior wall of the trachea (Table 4.1). An ultrasonographic protocol that combines a translaryngeal view with bilateral pleural views to ascertain ETT position (Fig. 4.11) is currently under way.[18]

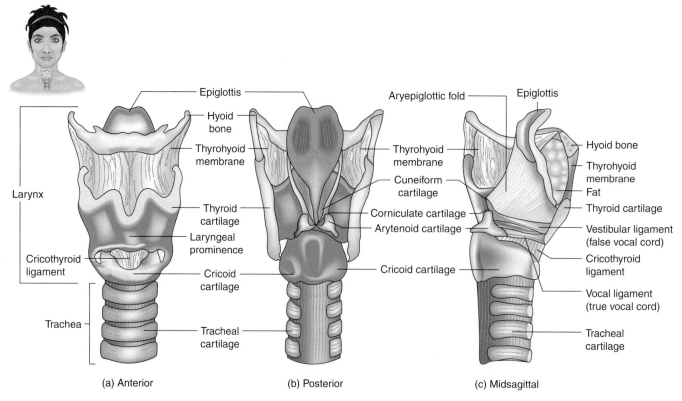

Figure 4.6. Normal anatomy of the larynx.

Technique

Two basic techniques will be discussed: translaryngeal ultrasonography, to evaluate the proximal trachea and proximal malposition, and pleural ultrasound, to evaluate for distal malposition of the ETT.

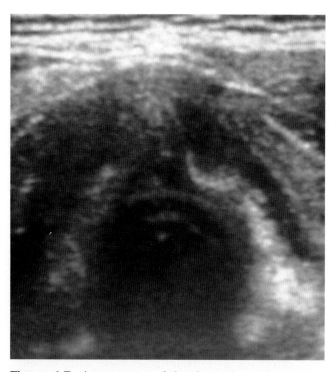

Figure 4.7. Appearance of the thyroid cartilage in cross section (transverse view). Note the typical "pointed" appearance.

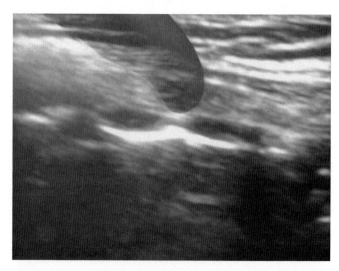

Figure 4.8. A longitudinal view of the anterior neck showing the tracheal rings as flattened, hypoechoic, oblong structures. (A super-imposed image of the thumb indicates where pressure may be applied to improve visualization of the endotracheal tube.)

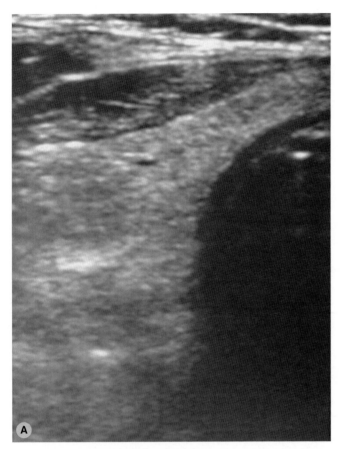 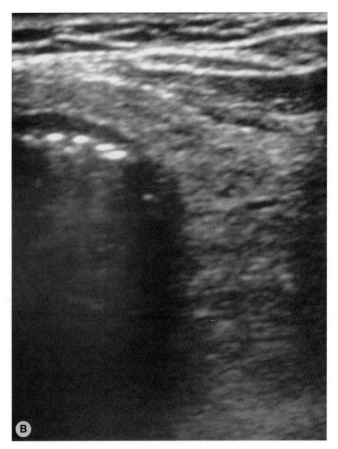

Figure 4.9. (A) Thyroid lobes draped over the anterior trachea. **(B)** Typical echotexture of the normal thyroid gland: slightly more hyperechoic than surrounding muscle and hypoechoic compared to fascial layers.

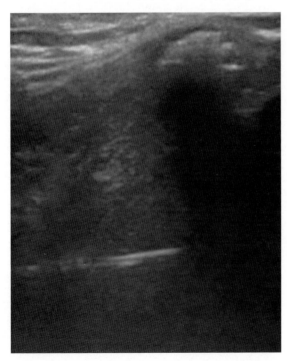

Figure 4.10. Typical appearance of an intubated trachea, with the characteristic double-wall sign.

1. A 6- to 13-MHz vascular probe works very well to image the trachea.

2. Set the depth such that the tracheal lumen, not just the anterior wall, is visualized (usually at least 3–4 cm).

3. Set the gain so that the resulting image is not too bright; this may cause reverberation artifact within the tracheal lumen and obscure the double-walled ETT.

TABLE 4.1. Maneuvers to Improve Visualization of the Endotracheal Tube (ETT)

1. Deflate the cuff.
2. Apply gentle pressure on the anterior trachea with the transducer.
3. Image from a more lateral plane.
4. Carefully advance/withdraw the ETT repeatedly while imaging.

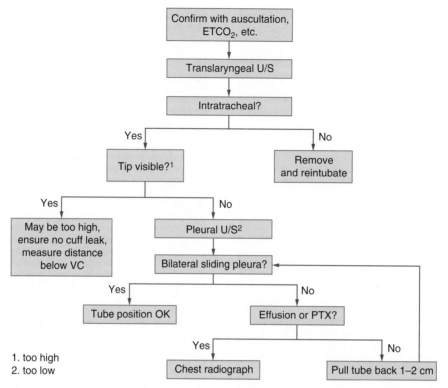

Figure 4.11. Study algorithm used to determine endotracheal tube position. ETCO$_2$, end-tidal carbon dioxide; PTX, pneumothorax; U/S, ultrasound; VC, vocal cords.

4. Image the entire trachea from the cricoid cartilage to the sternal notch, looking for the characteristic double-walled ETT.

5. Both transverse and longitudinal views should be employed.

6. It may be necessary to angle under the manubrium in an effort to locate the tip of the tube.

7. If the tube is not visible, try one or more of the following:

 a. Deflate the cuff.

 b. Apply gentle pressure on the anterior wall of the trachea with the probe; this may promote contact between the ETT and the anterior wall of the trachea.

 c. Image the trachea from a lateral probe position instead of midline (Fig. 4.12).

 d. Carefully advance and retract the ETT slightly (move the tip in and out) while imaging with a midline longitudinal view.

These maneuvers allow successful visualization of the ETT.

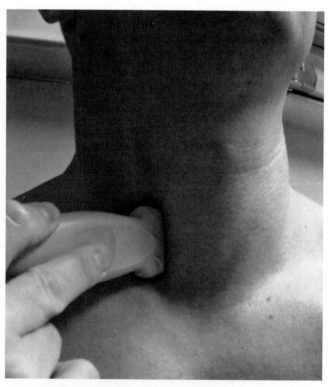

Figure 4.12. The trachea is being imaged from a more lateral position to better visualize the endotracheal tube.

Pleural ultrasonography, which is covered in Chapter 7, is an extremely useful tool to evaluate for esophageal intubation, confirm tracheal intubation, and diagnose mainstem intubation in most patients. Conveniently, the same probe used for translaryngeal ultrasonography (linear array, 6–13 MHz) can also be used to evaluate the visceral-parietal pleural interface. In cases of satisfactory tracheal intubation and in the absence of unilateral airway obstruction from tumor or foreign body, there will be bilateral and equal pleural sliding during respiration. In cases of esophageal intubation, there will be minimal pleural sliding (caused by the cardiac cycle, known as *the lung pulse*) or no pleural sliding. This is associated with decreasing oxygen saturations, a lack of auscultated breath sounds, epigastric "gurgling" with bagging, and low or undetected end-tidal CO_2 in most, but not all, cases and should prompt a repeat attempt at tracheal intubation. In cases of distal malposition, such as right mainstem intubation, there would be vigorous pleural sliding on the right side with reduced or absent sliding on the left side. There is great importance for comparing one side to the other, similar to techniques of lung auscultation learned in medical school. A combined approach of translaryngeal ultrasound to identify proximal malposition of the tube paired with pleural ultrasound to identify distal malposition may be a viable alternative to chest radiography to verify tube position. See Table 4.2 for findings seen with different types of ETT malposition.

The same basic technique used to visualize single-lumen ETTs can be applied to other situations, such as confirming proper double-lumen ETT placement.[18] Limitations of this technique include the presence of pleural fluid or air, which prevents apposition of the pleural surfaces and would not demonstrate the typical pleural sliding; prior pneumonectomy;

and significant chest wall trauma. See Chapter 7 for procedural details.

Common Pitfalls

In a substantial number of cases, the ETT is not immediately visible with only a simple transverse or midline longitudinal view. In those cases, it is imperative that the operator employ one of the several maneuvers described earlier to increase the "yield." Another very common pitfall is using inappropriate gain settings, which can cause reverberation artifact that obscures the underlying ETT. The reader is advised not to use this technique as a substitute for standard, accepted practices to ensure the intratracheal position of the ETT, such as end-tidal CO_2 and auscultation. The ultrasound technique is meant to offer additional confirmation of ETT placement, similar to the way postintubation chest radiography is used.

PERCUTANEOUS TRACHEOSTOMY

Percutaneous dilatational tracheostomy (PDT), first described in 1985,[19] has become the procedure of choice for providing long-term airway access in many institutions. Examination of the anterior neck prior to surgical tracheostomy was first described by Bertram et al 10 years later.[20] This study established the feasibility of performing a targeted ultrasound examination to identify anatomic variations that may complicate the procedure. Sustic and Zupan[21] first reported using ultrasonography for procedural guidance of percutaneous tracheostomy in 1998,[21] and the clinical utility of the technique has been confirmed in several other reports.[22–25] These studies demonstrate that ultrasonography can assist with the selection of both an insertion site and an appropriately sized tracheostomy tube,[26] in addition to allowing visualization of aberrant anatomy.

TABLE 4.2. Ultrasonographic Findings Seen in Different Types of Endotracheal Tube Malposition Events

Malposition	Translaryngeal View	Pleural Views
Esophageal	Tube not visible	Lack of sliding pleura bilaterally
Endotracheal tube too high	Tip <2.5 cm below cricoid cartilage	Bilateral sliding pleura
Mainstem intubation	Tip of tube not visible; tube extends below sternal notch	Lack of sliding pleura on contralateral side
Normal	Tip of tube >2.5 cm from cricoid cartilage OR tube extends below sternal notch	Bilateral sliding pleura

Although safe, PDT can be associated with life-threatening complications such as severe bleeding and malposition. Clinically consequential bleeding events are usually delayed (2–3 weeks after placement) and are due to erosion of the brachiocephalic artery caused by the high tracheostomy tube cuff pressures. However, bleeding can also occur at the time of tracheostomy tube placement. Muhammad et al[27] published a review of 497 cases in which bleeding occurred in 5% of patients and was usually due to an inferior thyroid vein, brachiocephalic vein, or high communicating anterior jugular vein.[27] Aberrant vascular anatomy is an important finding and should be part of the screening protocol.

Malposition is another complication of PDT. However, selecting a proper insertion site minimizes risk. Proximal malposition can cause damage to the vocal cords at the time of insertion (immediate damage) or can cause the tracheostomy tube to lie directly underneath the vocal cords and damage them over time, resulting in permanent vocal cord dysfunction and hoarseness. Distal malposition can result in the tip of the tracheostomy tube approaching the carina during neck flexion or lying in a mainstem bronchus. Contact with the carina results in cough, patient–ventilator dyssynchrony, difficult suctioning, suction trauma, and bleeding. By the use of ultrasonography, the tracheal cartilages can be counted and the appropriate site marked on the skin (usually between the second and third tracheal cartilage); this can easily eliminate proximal malposition. Sustic et al[28] demonstrated that careful ultrasound examination to identify the insertion site reduced the incidence of cranial malposition from 33% to 0%.[28] In addition, the distance from the carina to the subglottic area can be measured by bronchoscopy, providing a rough estimate of tracheal length, which minimizes the risk of distal malposition. With these two techniques, malposition of any kind can be virtually eliminated.

Another potential complication of PDT is hypercarbia. Bronchoscopic guidance is associated with hypercarbia, whereas surgical tracheostomy or tracheostomy with ultrasound guidance alone (without bronchoscopy) does not lead to elevated pCO_2 levels. In one study comparing pCO_2 levels in patients undergoing endoscopically guided PDT, ultrasound-guided PDT, or surgical tracheostomy, the pCO_2 increased up to 24 mm Hg in the bronchoscopy group, compared to 8 mm Hg in the ultrasound group and 3 mm Hg in the operative group.[29] This has potential implications for patients in whom hypercarbia is undesirable, such as patients with neurotrauma and elevated intracranial pressure or pulmonary hypertension.

Technique

1. Select an appropriately sized tracheostomy tube.

   a. Scan the pretracheal soft tissues utilizing a 6- to 13-MHz linear array probe, which allows an estimation of the distance from the skin to the anterior tracheal wall. Based on this measurement, the operator can choose either a standard tube for up to about 2.5 cm or one with a proximal long segment for longer distances. This measurement can be performed in either a longitudinal or transverse orientation but should always be performed at the proposed insertion site.

   b. Estimate the diameter of the trachea by measuring the tracheal lumen in the transverse view, also at the proposed insertion site or below. This measurement will help guide the selection of a tube with a compatible diameter.

   c. The angle of the trachea, when compared to the skin, can be measured to ensure that the standard bend of 105° will be compatible with the patient's airway. Some tracheas "dive" more deeply than others as they course inferiorly under the sternal notch. In some patients, this causes the distal tracheostomy tube opening to face the anterior wall, which then causes problems with suctioning and, occasionally, ventilation (Fig. 4.13 [see also color insert]). The caveat here is that the measurement be made when the head and neck are in a relatively neutral position (not during extension).

2. Select an insertion site by performing a midline, longitudinal view of the trachea from the cricoid cartilage to the sternal notch (Fig. 4.8). The tracheal cartilages can be counted, and the appropriate site can be marked on the skin (usually between the second and third tracheal cartilage). This requires the patient to be sedated enough that there is no movement of the head or neck between skin marking and tracheostomy insertion. If movement occurs during this window, the area needs to be rescanned to confirm that the skin mark is still appropriate.

3. After selection of an insertion site, a scan of the overlying tissues with color flow Doppler should be performed to identify any vascular structures at risk for damage during the procedure. This is performed in both a longitudinal and transverse orientation to look for "bridging" jugular veins, high brachiocephalic vessels, or thyroid veins/arteries. When examining transversely, make note of the thyroid gland, including lobes and the isthmus, as well

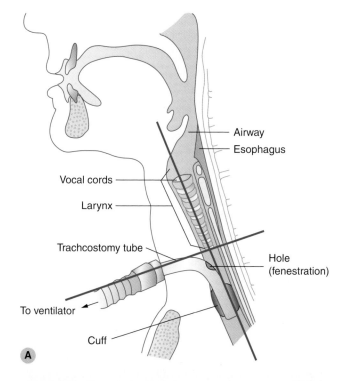

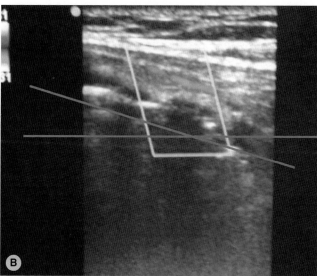

Figure 4.13. Relationship between the tracheal angle and tracheostomy tube angle. (See color insert.)

as the location of the carotid arteries and jugular veins, especially in patients with prior neck surgery.

4. Cannulation of the trachea can be visualized under dynamic guidance utilizing a longitudinal view just lateral to the midline. The cannulation needle is then applied to the skin in the midline, and the needle causes an indentation of the subcutaneous tissue, which approximates the needle tract. The

needle position can be adjusted either caudally or cranially, until this indentation overlies the desired puncture site, which is termed *longitudinal positioning*. Once the desired longitudinal position is achieved, the probe can be rotated 90° to guide the transverse position of the needle. Transverse position is less important than longitudinal position, as long as the puncture site is somewhat anterior. When the needle is in the desired position, cannulation can occur in the conventional manner. After tube placement, especially if bronchoscopy is not used to verify tube position, remember to scan the anterior chest looking for sliding pleura bilaterally; this confirms an intratracheal placement that is not too low.

Common Pitfalls

In general, ultrasound has not supplanted bronchoscopy for guidance of PDT. Bronchoscopy retains certain advantages such as direct visualization of the position of the ETT during withdrawal and visualization of the posterior tracheal wall during needle cannulation and dilation. Additionally, in cases of overzealous ETT withdrawal, one can easily reintubate the trachea over the bronchoscope.

THYROID

Ultrasound examination of the thyroid gland is commonly performed. The usual indication is to evaluate suspected thyroid nodules found either on examination or incidentally on other imaging studies (e.g., CT scan of the chest). Other indications include evaluation of suspected diffuse thyroid disease such as goiter from thyroiditis or Graves' disease. Due to the thyroid's superficial location, images with outstanding resolution can be obtained. The resolution is so good, in fact, that thyroid nodules are detected with very high sensitivity. Unfortunately, ultrasound images alone are unable to provide unequivocal diagnostic information in terms of malignancy. Although there are certain nodule characteristics that can tend to look more benign than malignant (Table 4.3), the definitive test for a thyroid nodule that might be malignant is ultrasound-guided biopsy. At present, there is no indication for routine screening of the general population for thyroid cancer. However, screening should be performed in certain high-risk populations, such as those patients with a history of familial thyroid cancer, multiple endocrine neoplasia type 2 (MEN2) syndrome, or a history of previous external beam radiation to the head or neck.

TABLE 4.3. Characteristics of Benign and Malignant Thyroid Nodules

Benign	Malignant
Multiple, small nodules	Large or dominant or solitary nodules
Cystic appearance (malignancy rarely cystic)	Solid (may also be benign)
Homogenous, hyperechoic nodule	Heterogenous isoechoic or hypoechoic nodule
Peripheral "eggshell" calcification	Punctuate "psammomatous" calcification throughout a nodule

Anatomic Review and Physical Examination Correlation With Ultrasound Anatomy and Physiology

The thyroid gland is a relatively small structure in most people, about 20 mL in volume in the adult man and 17 mL in the adult woman.[31] However, its superficial location and exposure in the neck make it ideal for ultrasonographic visualization. There are two lobes, roughly ovoid in shape, connected by the thyroid isthmus that is seen to "drape" over the proximal third of the trachea in the transverse ultrasound view (Fig. 4.9A, B). The gland is bordered anteriorly by the strap muscles, anterolaterally by the sternocleidomastoid, posterolaterally by the common carotid and internal jugular vein in the carotid sheath, and posteriorly by the trachea and the longus colli muscle. Usually, the esophagus and cervical vertebrae are not readily apparent due to air artifact from the trachea. However, on occasion, the esophagus can be seen protruding from behind the trachea at about the 4 o'clock position (posterolaterally) and can be confused with a cystic or complex-appearing thyroid nodule. Unfortunately, the normal parathyroid glands are indistinguishable from surrounding thyroid tissue. The typical echo texture is speckled but homogenous, lighter in color than surrounding muscles, but darker than fascial layers. Color Doppler reveals a richly vascularized gland that is also somewhat homogenous in distribution.

Thyroid abnormalities are varied in appearance, depending on the cause. Thyroid nodules are the most common abnormality but are quite varied in their ultrasonographic appearance in terms of size, density, and number. It becomes important, therefore, to assess the risk of malignancy in a given patient to help guide the decision of biopsy versus watchful waiting. Known risk factors for thyroid cancer are:

1. Female gender. Most thyroid cancers occur in women. However, the presence of a solitary thyroid nodule in a man is relatively unusual and requires further investigation.

2. Age between 20 and 60 years. Most thyroid cancers occur in middle age. However, solitary nodules appear to be rare in younger populations, so a nodule in a young patient should be aggressively worked up. Additionally, the development of a large, solitary thyroid nodule in advanced age (>70 years) should raise the suspicion for carcinoma.

3. Low-iodine diet.

4. Prior radiation, either in the form of medical radiation treatments or environmental radiation exposure. Childhood exposure greatly increases this risk.

5. Genetic. Medullary thyroid cancer can be familial, either alone (familial medullary thyroid cancer) or as part of the MEN2 syndrome. Patients coming from families with these disorders or who themselves are known carriers of the abnormal genes should be aggressively screened for the presence of thyroid cancer.

Malignant nodules can be associated with the following characteristics, although there is no single pathognomonic appearance:

1. Large size in conjunction with solid appearance.

2. Small areas of microcalcification spread throughout the nodule, which are associated with papillary thyroid carcinoma.

3. Irregular shape, with either very smooth borders or ill-defined boundaries if extracapsular extension occurs.

4. Presence of cervical lymphadenopathy (see next section on lymph nodes of the neck).

5. Extracapsular extension of a thyroid lesion.

Benign lesions may have the following characteristics:

1. Fluid filled (simple cyst).

2. Presence of multiple nodules.

3. Smooth edges without look of "infiltration".

4. "Warm or hot" appearance on nuclear medicine thyroid scan.

Examples of benign diseases, in addition to the benign thyroid nodule, include Graves' disease, Hashimoto thyroiditis, subacute thyroiditis, suppurative thyroiditis, and atrophic thyroiditis. Table 4.4 describes the different sonographic appearances in these disorders.

In general, suspicious lesions should be biopsied, and guidelines on this topic do exist, based largely on case reports, low-level studies, and expert opinion. A full discussion on which nodules should be biopsied can be found in the American Association of Clinical Endocrinologists/Associazione Medici Endo-crinologi guidelines published in 2006.[31] In summary, palpable thyroid nodules should prompt a thyroid-stimulating hormone (TSH) test and thyroid ultrasonography. If the TSH result is normal or low, or if the ultrasound appearance is suspicious, the lesion should be sampled with fine-needle aspiration (FNA). Or, if the lesion is cold on scintigraphy, an FNA should be performed.

Technique

Examination of the Thyroid

1. Place the patient supine, and hyperextend the neck by placing a pillow or towel roll under the shoulders (Fig. 4.14).

2. Use a high-frequency linear array transducer, such as 6 to 13 MHz.

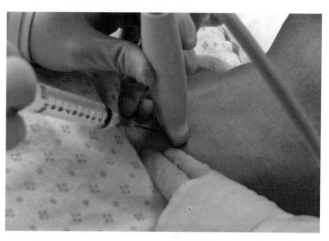

Figure 4.14. Technique of stabilizing the nodule while the operator holds both the transducer and the needle.

3. Scan the entire gland in both the transverse and longitudinal planes.

4. Calculate the thyroid size; this can be achieved in several ways. The classic technique is to measure each dimension and multiply according to the following formula: length × width × height × 0.52. Other techniques exist, however, including surface area tracing or different formulas.

Thyroid Gland Biopsy

1. Perform steps 1 through 4 of the thyroid examination.

2. Mark the position of an underlying thyroid nodule (if not palpable) on the overlying skin.

3. Prep the neck and put under sterile drape.

4. Using sterile technique, infiltrate the skin and subcutaneous tissues with lidocaine.

5. Stabilize the gland/nodule with the nonaspirating hand.

6. Perform the aspiration with a 10-mL syringe in a commercially available pistol-gripped syringe holder (or freehand) with an attached beveled needle (19 to 25 gauge). A noncutting bevel-edged needle is preferred over the standard cutting needles used for blood draws.

7. Aspiration can be statically guided (as described earlier) or dynamically guided with real-time ultrasound. If dynamic guidance is performed by the operator, an assistant may be needed to stabilize the neck and/or target nodule (Fig. 4.15).

8. Once the needle tip is thought to be in the target lesion, apply suction on the syringe plunger and gently move the needle tip in and out, which acts to shear off sheets of cells.

TABLE 4.4. Sonographic Characteristics of Diffuse Thyroid Disorders	
Disease	*Characteristics*
Graves' disease	Diffuse enlargement, may be normal in echotexture or hypoechoic, marked increased vascularity
Hashimoto thyroiditis	Diffuse, hypoechoic micronodularity, normal-to-enlarged in size, increased vascularity
Subacute (de Quervain) thyroiditis	Painful on insonation, normal-to-small size, hypoechoic or normal echogenicity, may have poorly defined hypoechoic nodules
Suppurative thyroiditis	Diffuse enlargement, focal fluid collections may be seen
Atrophic thyroiditis	Atrophic, small, hypoechoic
Adenomatous goiter	"Lumpy-bumpy" appearance due to multiple bilateral nodules of varying size and echogenicity; may have cystic areas and areas of necrosis

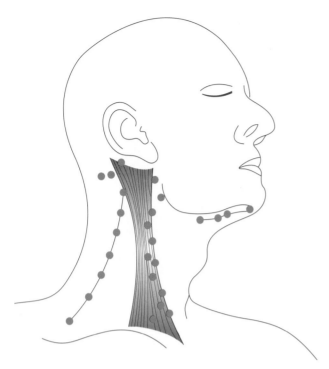

Figure 4.15. Lymph node locations in the neck region.

9. For complex cystic/solid lesions, sample the solid component before aspirating any fluid.

10. Withdraw the needle and apply gentle pressure to the needle tract.

11. Remove the needle from the syringe, aspirate a few milliliters of air into the syringe, and then replace the needle.

12. Eject the specimen, usually bloody in appearance, onto a slide and prepare in the standard fashion.

Common Pitfalls

Understanding the anatomic boundaries of the thyroid gland is essential to ensuring an adequate examination of the entire gland, to help localize abnormalities, and, in some cases, to help identify normal mimics of pathology. For example, the esophagus can occasionally be seen as a complex structure on the left, protruding from behind the trachea, but anterior to the longus colli muscle. Thyroid biopsy is often plagued by false-negative or false-positive results, but adequate tissue sampling can help alleviate this problem. Decisions regarding further testing should always be made by experienced operators in conjunction with the clinical presentation, guided by knowledge of the characteristics of benign versus malignant thyroid nodules, and based on other testing such as nuclear medicine thyroid scanning.

REGIONAL LYMPH NODES

Cervical lymphadenopathy can be caused by a staggering number of different clinical entities. The challenge to care providers is determining which cases require further diagnostic workup. Certainly history and clinical context provide guidance and reassurance in the majority of cases. However, in a small number of patients, the enlarged cervical lymph node represents malignancy and in one study represented approximately 1.1% of those presenting to primary care physicians.[32] Fortunately, ultrasound is a very effective modality for imaging the superficial lymph nodes of the neck and providing guidance for percutaneous biopsy in suspicious cases.

Anatomic Review and Physical Examination Correlation With Ultrasound Anatomy and Physiology

The nodes of the neck can be roughly divided into anterior cervical nodes, which are situated around or deep to the sternocleidomastoid muscle (SCM) and drain parts of the throat, pharynx, tonsils, and thyroid; and posterior cervical nodes, which lie posterior to the SCM in the posterior triangle of the neck and drain the scalp, back of the head, sides of the neck, some skin of the shoulder, and some parts of the nose and throat cavities. In addition, there are submandibular nodes, which drain the posterior oropharynx and floor of the mouth, and submental nodes, which largely drain the intraoral cavity. Supraclavicular nodes (lowest of the internal jugular chain) are also included in the neck examination, although they largely drain thoracic and even intra-abdominal regions, especially Virchow's node on the left.

A normal lymph node is an encapsulated ovoid-shaped structure that resembles a kidney and receives afferent lymph vessels along the outer surface, with efferent lymphatics emanating from the hilus. Lymph follicles are found in the outer cortex, while the medulla contains multiple components, such as aggregates of blood vessels, stromal components, and some cords of lymphocytes such as activated B lymphocytes.

Ultrasonographically, normal lymph nodes appear small, flattened, and much longer than they are wide (short axis–to–long axis ratio of <0.5). The echotexture is generally homogenous, with a distinct hilum and cortex. On color Doppler imaging, central hilar vessels are usually identified, and there is a paucity of peripheral vascularity.[33,34] The margins show no infiltration of surrounding tissue or vessels.

Malignant nodes, however, can be more rounded in appearance, with a short axis–to–long axis ratio of greater than 0.5, and the margins can actually appear smoother than in benign nodes. The echotexture may be more heterogeneous, depending on the type of malignancy, and there may even be cystic components present. Irregular patterns of vascularity are frequently encountered, with intense peripheral or focal vascularity (in an area other than the hilum) being particularly suspicious.[33] Calcifications, in the right clinical context, should also raise the suspicion of malignancy. Aside from the initial diagnosis of malignant nodes, ultrasonography may be clinically useful in surveillance following treatment to help establish whether or not a favorable response occurred.[35]

Although, when combined, the above characteristics can help to differentiate benign from malignant nodes, it is important to understand that the predictive value is not great enough to preclude FNA. Therefore, any strategy employed must ultimately lead to FNA of suspicious nodes or neck dissection in those patients with a known diagnosis of certain head and neck malignancies.[36,37]

Sonoelastography is a relatively new technique that helps map the elastic properties of ultrasonographically examined tissues, including lymph nodes. While used mainly as a research tool, this technique can assist with the diagnosis of breast, thyroid, and prostate cancers.[38-40] A study by Lyshchik[39] demonstrated that the technique can differentiate between benign and metastatic cervical nodes, with 92% accuracy, in patients suspected of having thyroid or hypopharyngeal cancer.

Technique

1. Position the patient appropriately; supine positioning on a flat table with the neck slightly extended over a pillow usually works best.

2. A linear array, high-frequency transducer (6 to 13 MHz) provides optimal images.

3. Perform a standard gray-scale 2D examination, locating the lymph node groups along the anterior cervical chain (internal jugular), posterior to the sternocleidomastoid, and posterior triangle (accessory chain). Also, attempt to locate the submandibular and submental nodes, but keep in mind that these nodal groups tend to be smaller than the cervical nodes. Also, evaluate the supraclavicular node.

4. Measure the nodes in three planes (length, width, and height) using electronic calipers.

5. Calculate the ratio of short axis to long axis.

6. Note the general appearance of the node, assessing for shape (round vs. oblong), echotexture, and calcification. The normal echotexture should be compared to surrounding muscle; normal lymph nodes are relatively isoechoic.

7. Note the appearance of the hilum: a normal or reactive lymph node has a distinct hyperechoic hilum, while malignant nodes may have a compressed or absent hilum.

8. Using color Doppler, interrogate the entire node for the overall pattern of vascularity. Normal lymph nodes tend to have highly vascular hila, whereas metastatic nodes tend to have notable peripheral vascularity and/or areas of focally abnormal vasculature.

9. Assess for punctuate microcalcifications.

10. Refer or perform FNA on any suspicious nodes.

Common Pitfalls

Do not base a treatment decision on ultrasonographic criteria alone. Suspicious nodes, or any nodes in certain head and neck cancers, should either be biopsied or removed during neck dissection according to standard practice and guidelines. This is particularly true for inexperienced sonographers. If ultrasound is performed, it is imperative that the sonographer track the outcome of any biopsy procedure in an effort to gain experience with the technique and to reinforce the appearance of benign versus malignant nodes.

CODING AND REIMBURSEMENT

Billing for these services requires the procedure to be in the scope of practice of the operator. In addition, images need to be permanently stored for future review if audited. The general code for ultrasonography of the head and neck is 76536. If ultrasound guidance is used during FNA or biopsy, the code 76942 can be used, but should be used only once, even if multiple biopsies were taken. Both 76536 and 76942 can be used for the same patient at the same encounter; if a suspicious node is first identified under 76536, and an FNA was then performed that required ultrasound guidance, it is acceptable to also bill 76942. Code 10022 should be used for FNA with image guidance and can be used in combination with 76942 (needle placement). The modifier -59 can be used when aspirating a different site (10022-59). If the specimen is smeared, stained, and assessed on site for adequacy, the code 88172 can be used, but the laboratory must be certified by the Clinical Laboratory Improvement

Amendments. If a follow-up ultrasound is performed to assess the stability of a node or thyroid nodule, 76970 can be used.

FUTURE DEVELOPMENTS

Ultrasonography has been used for many years and with excellent success in interventional radiology suites and endocrinologists' offices to assess the neck. In addition, clinical researchers are more clearly defining the

potential role of ultrasonography in looking at the sinuses, upper airway, and other head and neck structures. As these applications and techniques become disseminated to nonradiologist practitioners, through mediums such as this textbook, the limits of what is "standard" will change. There are currently experts in whole-body ultrasound in most emergency departments (and an increasing number of intensive care units) in the United States. However, as with any new technology or application, adequate training requirements must be established to ensure quality of care.

References

1. Abdurasulov DM, Amilova AA, Fazylov AA, et al. On the use of ultrasonics in the diagnosis of diseases of the maxillary sinuses. *Nov Med Priborostr.* 1964;24:30–33.

2. Lichtenstein D, Biderman P, Meziere G, et al. The sinusogram, a real-time ultrasound sign of maxillary sinusitis. *Intensive Care Med.* 1998;24:1057–1061.

3. Hilbert G, Vargas F, Valentino R, et al. Comparison of B-mode ultrasound and CT in the diagnosis of maxillary sinusitis in mechanically ventilated patients. *Crit Care Med.* 2001;29:1337–1342.

4. Vargas F, Boyer A, Bui HN, et al. A postural change test improves the prediction of a radiological maxillary sinusitis by ultrasonography in mechanically ventilated patients. *Intensive Care Med.* 2007;33:1474–1478.

5. Vargas F, Bui HN, Boyer A, et al. Transnasal puncture based on echographic sinusitis evidence in mechanically ventilated patients with suspicion of nosocomial maxillary sinusitis. *Intensive Care Med.* 2006;32: 858–866.

6. Holzapfel L, Chastang C, Demingeon G, et al. A randomized study assessing the systematic search for maxillary sinusitis in nasotracheally mechanically ventilated patients. *Am J Respir Crit Care Med.* 1999;159:695–670.

7. Marik PE. Fever in the ICU. *Chest.* 2000;117:855–869.

8. Rouby JJ, Laurent P, Gosnach M, et al. Risk factors and clinical relevance of nosocomial maxillary sinusitis in the critically ill. *Am J Respir Crit Care Med.* 1994;150:776–783.

9. Raphael DT, Conard FU 3rd. Ultrasound confirmation of ETT placement. *J Clin Ultrasound.* 1987;15:459–462.

10. Milling TJ, Jones M, Khan T, et al. Transtracheal 2-d ultrasound for identification of esophageal intubation. *J Emerg Med.* 2007;32:409–414.

11. Werner SL, Smith CE, Goldstein JR, et al. Pilot study to evaluate the accuracy of ultrasonography in confirming ETT placement. *Ann Emerg Med.* 2007;49:75–80.

12. Ma G, Davis DP, Schmitt J, et al. The sensitivity and specificity of transcricothyroid ultrasonography to confirm ETT placement in a cadaver model. *J Emerg Med.* 2007;32: 405–407.

13. Chun R, Kirkpatrick AW, Sirois M, et al. Where's the tube? Evaluation of hand-held ultrasound in confirming ETT placement. *Prehosp Disaster Med.* 2004;19:366–369.

14. Weaver B, Lyon M, Blaivas M. Confirmation of ETT placement after intubation using the sliding lung sign. *Acad Emerg Med.* 2006;13:239–244.

15. Lakhal K, Delplace X, Cottier JP, et al. The feasibility of ultrasound to assess subglottic diameter. *Anaesth Analg.* 2007;104:611–614.

16. Ezri T, Gewurtz G, Sessler DI, et al. Prediction of difficult laryngoscopy in obese patients by ultrasound quantification of anterior neck soft tissue. *Anaesthesia.* 2003;58: 1111–1114.

17. Komatsu R, Sengupta P, Wadhwa A. Ultrasound quantification of anterior soft tissue thickness fails to predict difficult laryngoscopy in obese patients. *Anaesth Intensive Care.* 2007;35:32–37.

18. Sustic A. Role of ultrasound in the airway management of critically ill patients. *Crit Care Med.* 2007;35:S173–S177.

19. Ciaglia P, Firsching R, Syniec C. Elective percutaneous dilatational tracheostomy. A new simple bedside procedure; preliminary report. *Chest.* Jun 1985;87(6):715–9.

20. Bertram S, Emshoff R, Norer B. Ultrasonographic anatomy of the anterior neck: implications for tracheostomy. *J Oral Maxillofac Surg.* 1995;53:1420–1424.

21. Sustic A, Zupan Z. Ultrasound guided tracheal puncture for non-surgical tracheostomy. *Intensive Care Med.* 1998; 24:92.

22. Bonde J, Norgaard N, Antonsen K, et al. Implementation of percutaneous dilation tracheotomy-value of preincisional ultrasonic examination? *Acta Anaesthesiol Scand.* 1999;43:163–166.

23. Hatfield A, Bodenham A. Portable ultrasonic scanning of the anterior neck before percutaneous dilational tracheostomy. *Anaesthesia.* 1999;54:660–663.

24. Muhammad JK, Patton DW, Evans RM, et al. Percutaneous dilational tracheostomy under ultrasound guidance. *Br J Oral Maxillofac Surg.* 1999;37:309–311.

25. Sustic A, Zupan Z, Eskinja N, et al. Ultrasonographically guided percutaneous dilational tracheostomy after anterior cervical spine fixation. *Act Anaesthesiol Scand.* 1999;43:1078–1080.

26. Muhammad JK, Major E, Patton DW. Evaluating the neck for percutaneous dilational tracheostomy. *J Craniomaxillofac Surg.* 2000;28:336–342.

27. Muhammad JK, Major E, Wood A, et al. Percutaneous tracheostomy: hemorrhagic complications and the vascular anatomy of the anterior neck. A review based on 497 cases. *Int J Oral Maxillofac Surg.* 2000;29:217–222.

28. Sustic A, Kovac D, Zgaljardic Z, et al. Ultrasound guided percutaneous dilational tracheostomy: a safe method to avoid cranial misplacement of the tracheostomy tube. *Intensive Care Med.* 2000;26:1379–1381.

29. Reilly PM, Sing RF, Giberson FA, et al. Hypercarbia during tracheostomy: a comparison of percutaneous endoscopic, percutaneous Doppler, and standard surgical tracheostomy. *Intensive Care Med.* 1997 Aug;23(8):859-64.

30. Hegedus L, Perrild H, Pulsen L, et al. The determination of thyroid volume by ultrasound and its relationship to body weight, age, and sex in normal subjects. *J Clin Endocrinol Metab.* 1983;56:260–263.

31. AACE/AME Task Force on Thyroid Nodules. American Association of Clinical Endocrinologists and Associazione Medici Endocrinologi medical guidelines for clinical practice for the diagnosis and management of thyroid nodules. *Endocr Pract.* 2006;12(1):63–102.

32. Fijten GH, Blijham GH. Unexplained lymphadenopathy in family practice. An evaluation of the probability of malignant causes and the effectiveness of physicians' workup. *J Fam Pract.* 1988;27:373–376.

33. Na DG, Lin HK, Byun HS, et al. Differential diagnosis of cervical lymphadenopathy: usefulness of color Doppler sonography. *AJR Am J Roentgenol.* 1997;168(5):1311–1316.

34. Dangore-Khasbage S, Degwekar SS, Bhowate RR, et al. Utility of color Doppler ultrasound in evaluating the status of cervical lymph nodes in oral cancer. *Oral Surg Oral Med Oral Pathol Oral Radiol Endod.* 2009;108(20):255–263.

35. Correa P, Arya S, Laskar SG, et al. Ultrasonographic changes in malignant neck nodes during radiotherapy in head and neck squamous carcinoma. *Australas Radiol.* 2005;49(2):113–118.

36. To EW, Tsang WM, Cheng J, et al. Is neck ultrasound necessary for early stage oral tongue carcinoma with clinically N0 neck? *Dentomaxillofac Radiol.* 2003;32(3):156–159.

37. De Bondt RB, Nelemans PJ, Hofman PA, et al. Detection of lymph node metastases in head and neck cancer: a meta-analysis comparing US, USgFNAC, CT, and MR imaging. *Eur J Radiol.* 2007;64(2):266–272.

38. Garra BS, Cespedes EI, Ophir J, et al. Elastography of breast lesions: initial clinical results. *Radiology.* 1997;202:79–86.

39. Lyshchik A, Higashi T, Asato R, et al. Thyroid gland tumor diagnosis at US elastography. *Radiology.* 2005;237:202–211.

40. Cochlin DL, Ganatra RH, Griffiths DF. Elastography in the detection of prostatic cancer. *Clin Radiol.* 2002;57:1014–1020.

CHAPTER 5

Ocular Ultrasound

Nicholas A. Perchiniak, MD and Dave Bahner, MD, RDMS

INTRODUCTION

The rapid evaluation and treatment of patients presenting to the primary care office or emergency department (ED) with ocular complaints is often a critical and time-sensitive endeavor since the consequences can threaten vision. The causes of ocular complaints are varied and range from infections to trauma. Approximately 2 million ocular injuries occur annually in the United States, a significant proportion of which lead to visual loss.[1] The clinician has a number of tools at his or her disposal including an appropriate history, a physical examination, and resources such as the ophthalmoscope, slit lamp, tonometer, and portable ultrasound unit to assist in the appropriate workup.

For a variety of reasons, ocular examination can be difficult to accomplish. The examination may be limited by pain, swelling, or an inability to open the eye. Advanced imaging and ophthalmologic consultation may not be immediately available or may require a prolonged delay in definitive care, thereby necessitating adequate examination by front-line providers.

Ocular ultrasonography provides a rapid and essentially noninvasive method for performing bedside evaluation to rule out acute vision-threatening emergencies. While ultrasonography has been used successfully for a number of different applications in the ED, the evaluation of ocular pathology is a relatively new approach. In 2002, the first series of ED patients presenting with ocular complaints were evaluated by bedside ultrasonography.[2] The technique was found to be highly accurate for diagnosing ocular pathology and ruling out important complications. It was also able to differentiate between emergent and vision-threatening pathology and that which could be deferred or followed on an outpatient basis.[2] Ocular ultrasonography provides guidance for the diagnosis and management of several ocular emergencies including retrobulbar hematoma, globe rupture, intraocular foreign body, lens subluxation, vitreous hemorrhage, and retinal detachment.[3]

OCULAR ANATOMY

Figures 5.1 and 5.2 depict the normal anatomy of the eye. There are three main chambers of fluid in the eye.

The anterior chamber, filled with aqueous humor, is situated between the cornea and the iris. The posterior chamber, also filled with aqueous humor, is positioned between the iris and the anterior surface of the lens. The vitreous chamber, filled with a more viscous fluid called vitreous humor, is located between the posterior surface of the lens and the retina.

The cornea is the transparent front of the eye that serves as a major refractive surface as light enters the eye. The iris is the colored part of the eye that screens out light, while the pupil adjusts the amount of light entering the eye, as determined by the sympathetic and parasympathetic innervation of the iris. The lens is a transparent, biconcave body that is suspended by the zonules behind the pupil and iris. By a process known as accommodation, these zonules contract or relax, changing the shape of the lens, and project a sharp image on the retina. The retina is neural tissue that lines the posterior vitreous cavity. It is responsible for sending the initial visual signs to the brain via the optic nerve.[4]

SCANNING TECHNIQUE

Bedside ocular ultrasonography is performed using a closed-eye approach with the patient looking straight ahead. The patient should be placed in a supine position (or reclined at 45° for potential penetrating injuries). A high-resolution 7.5- to 10.0-MHz linear array transducer is generally adequate for ocular imaging (Fig. 5.3). One can also use a dedicated high-frequency ocular transducer if available. A copious amount of standard water-soluble ultrasound transmission gel should be applied to the patient's closed eyelid (Fig. 5.4). Pressure on the globe should be avoided in the patient with any suspicion for a globe perforation; however, essentially no pressure should be required for adequate imaging, assuming that a thick layer of gel is applied.[3] The operator should stabilize the probe by resting his or her fourth and fifth fingers on either the bridge of the nose or the patient's forehead. The eye should be scanned in both sagittal and transverse planes. Depth should be adjusted so that the image of the eye fills the screen. The gain can

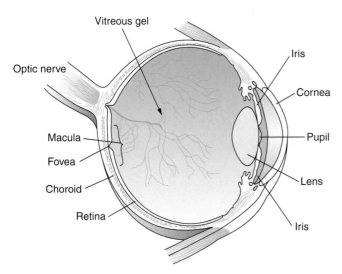

Figure 5.1. Normal ocular anatomy. *(Image source: National Eye Institute.)*

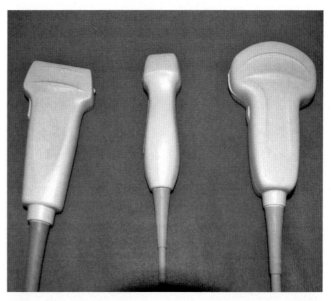

Figure 5.3. Acceptable probes for ocular ultrasound. A high-resolution linear array probe is ideal for this application.

also be adjusted to optimize acceptable imaging and reduce artifact.

NORMAL ULTRASOUND FINDINGS

Because of its fluid-filled nature, the eye provides an excellent acoustic window. The normal eye appears as a circular hypoechoic structure (Fig. 5.5). The cornea is the most anterior structure, seen as a thin hyperechoic layer parallel to the eyelid. The anterior chamber is filled with anechoic fluid, bordered by the cornea and iris anteriorly and the anterior surface of the lens posteriorly. The iris and ciliary bodies can be seen as linear structures extending from the periphery of the globe toward the lens. The lens appears as a

concave, hyperechoic reflector.[3] The vitreous chamber encompasses the majority of the image, consisting of anechoic fluid posterior to the lens. The retina is located along the posterior aspect of the vitreous chamber and cannot be differentiated from other surrounding layers on ultrasound. The optic nerve is visible posteriorly as a hypoechoic linear region radiating away from the globe.

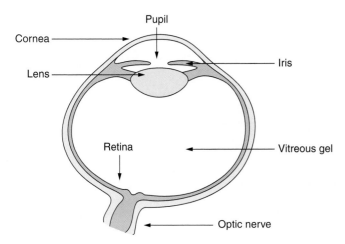

Figure 5.2. Illustration of ocular anatomy.

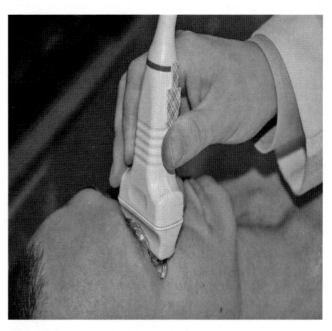

Figure 5.4. Acceptable scanning technique with minimal to no pressure applied to the eye.

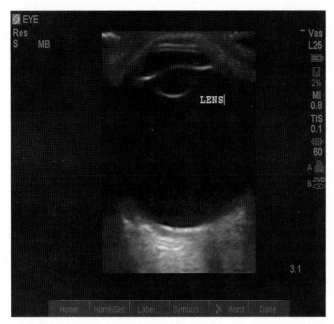

Figure 5.5. Normal ocular ultrasound image.

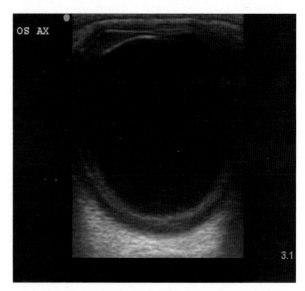

Figure 5.6. Retinal detachment.

PATHOLOGIC APPLICATIONS

Retinal Detachment

Retinal detachment is the separation of the neurosensory layer of the retina from the choroid and the underlying retinal pigment epithelium. There are three main types of retinal detachment: rhegmatogenous, exudative or serous, and tractional. Rhegmatogenous, the most common, occurs from a hole, tear, or break in the retina that allows vitreous to pass from the posterior chamber to the subretinal space. Patients typically complain of a flashing-light sensation, floaters in the affected eye, decreased visual acuity, and curtain-like visual loss.[5] Despite the fact that ophthalmologists have used ultrasound to identify retinal detachment for decades, its bedside use in the acute care setting is relatively new. However, ultrasound diagnosis of retinal detachment can be very accurate even when the operator has minimal experience.[6] The retinal detachment will appear as a hyperechoic membrane within the vitreous chamber in the posterior aspect of the globe (Fig. 5.6). This curvilinear opacity often moves in conjunction with eye movements, which assists the operator in making the diagnosis. In addition, subretinal fluid may also be visualized. When a retinal detachment becomes complete, a connection to the ora serrata is maintained anterior and posterior to the optic nerve head, accounting for the V shape in the vitreous cavity on ultrasound (Fig. 5.7).[3]

Globe Rupture

A ruptured globe is a full-thickness injury to the cornea, sclera, or both (Fig. 5.8). Penetrating ocular trauma can occur from numerous sources, including projectiles such as BB pellets, gunshot wounds, or direct penetration from a hammer or knife. Any projectile injury has the potential for penetrating the eye.[7] Clinical indicators of globe rupture include moderate to severe pain, decreased vision, hyphema, loss of anterior chamber depth, or deviation of the pupil.[5] If there is clinical suspicion for a penetrating injury, the

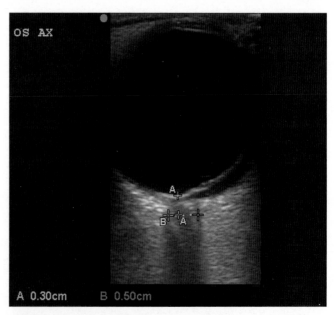

Figure 5.7. Partial retinal detachment with optic nerve sheath measured.

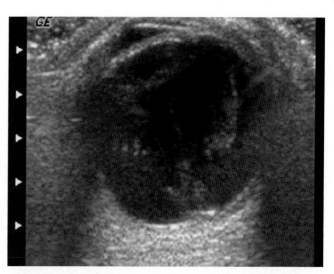

Figure 5.9. Ultrasound image of intraocular foreign body.

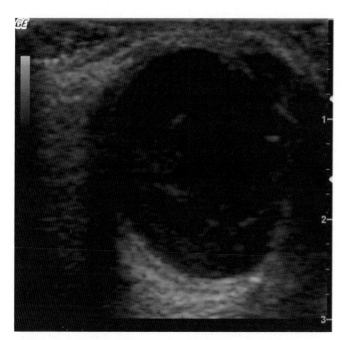

Figure 5.8. Ultrasound image of globe rupture.

Seidel test should be performed, whereby a fluorescein dye strip is applied directly to the site of injury. If a leak is present, the dye will be diluted by the aqueous, appearing as a dark stream (diluted) within a pool of bright green (concentrated dye).[8]

The use of ultrasound has clear advantages in the evaluation of possible globe rupture. Abnormalities such as hyphema or corneal edema frequently restrict the ability to directly visualize the eye on physical examination. Case reports from the military have shown that ultrasonography was able to detect penetrating injury when the Seidel test was negative.[9] Sonographically, the affected eye may appear smaller than the normal eye because of the relative reduction in globe contents. There is often evidence of anterior chamber collapse and abnormal scleral contouring or scleral buckling. The penetration site can sometimes be seen as a discontinuity of the sclera, with a hemorrhagic tract in the vitreous leading up to the rupture site. These injuries almost always require operative intervention.

Intraocular Foreign Body

Retained intraocular foreign bodies represent an important finding following ocular trauma and can often be challenging to identify clinically (Fig. 5.9).[10] The potential damage caused by an intraocular foreign body depends on several factors, including the size, shape, and momentum of the object and the point of ocular penetration. The most common causes are hammering and using power tools.

The clinical presentation is often similar to that of a patient with a ruptured globe. Ultrasound can play a useful role in the detection of intraocular foreign bodies. One study used ultrasonography for the detection of foreign bodies composed of a number of different materials.[11] They found an overall foreign body detection rate of 93%.[11] Another study used a porcine model with metallic foreign bodies of various sizes. They found a sensitivity of 87.5% and a specificity of 95.8% in the detection of these foreign bodies.[12] Intraocular foreign bodies are seen on ultrasonography by their hyperechoic acoustic profile, with either shadowing or reverberation artifacts seen in a usually echo-free vitreous (Fig. 5.9). Ultrasound patterns of shadowing and comet tails may help to differentiate between the materials of the foreign bodies.[3]

Vitreous Hemorrhage

The incidence of spontaneous vitreous hemorrhage is approximately 7 per 100,000 people.[13] Vitreous hemorrhage is the presence of extravasated blood in the posterior chamber of the globe. The three most common causes of vitreous hemorrhage are proliferative diabetic retinopathy, posterior vitreous detachment with or without retinal tear, and ocular trauma. In addition, vitreous hemorrhage may accompany subarachnoid hemorrhage and is one cause of visual loss from intracranial aneurysms.[4] Vision loss is often dramatic, with even 10 μL of blood reducing vision to hand motion. Minimal bleeding may present as new multiple floaters, visual haze, "smoke," shadows, or cobwebs. Visual acuity and slit-lamp examination should be completed, followed by ophthalmologic consultation.

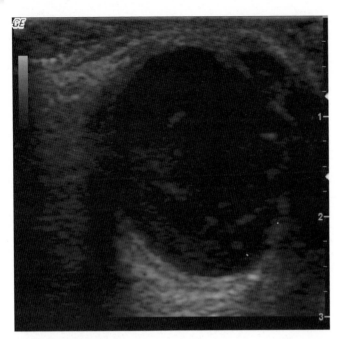

Figure 5.10. Early vitreous hemorrhage with diffuse dots of hemorrhage.

The ultrasonographic appearance of vitreous hemorrhage varies with age and severity (Figs. 5.10 and 5.11). Fresh hemorrhages produce easily detectable diffuse dots and vitreal echoes that correlate with the amount of blood present (Fig. 5.10). In older or more severe hemorrhages, the blood often organizes and forms membranes visible in the posterior chamber (Fig. 5.11). When evaluating for vitreous hemorrhage, it is important to reduce the gain to eliminate all but the densest areas of reflectivity.

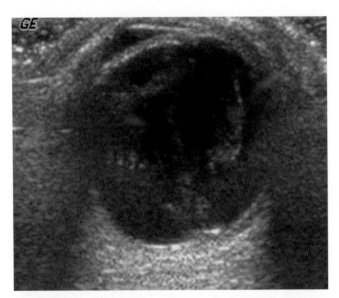

Figure 5.11. Late vitreous hemorrhage. Note the progressive layering of blood as the hemorrhage progresses.

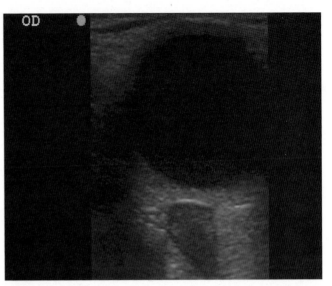

Figure 5.12. Increased optic nerve sheath diameter related to increased intracranial pressure in a patient with a cerebellar mass.

Increased Intracranial Pressure

One of the most recent advances in the use of bedside ocular ultrasonography relates to its applicability to the evaluation of increased intracranial pressure (ICP). Patients presenting with headache, altered levels of consciousness, or recent head injury may have symptoms related to elevated ICP. Physical examination is often limited for a variety of reasons, including intubation, sedation, and paralysis. Bedside ultrasonography has been useful for the diagnosis of elevated ICP via measurement of the optic nerve sheath diameter (ONSD).

The optic nerve attaches to the posterior aspect of the globe and is contiguous with the dura mater. It has an arachnoid space through which cerebrospinal fluid flows. A normal optic nerve sheath measures less than 5.0 mm in diameter. Multiple studies have confirmed that an ONSD greater than 5 mm correlates directly with clinical or radiographic evidence of elevated ICP and that this procedure is relatively easy to complete at the bedside.[14,15] The optic nerve sheath is measured 3 mm behind the posterior aspect of the globe because the ultrasound contrast is the greatest (Fig. 5.12). An initial caliper should be used to measure the distance behind the globe, while a second is used to measure the ONSD. It is important to center the nerve sheath, because an oblique measurement may be inaccurate.

SUMMARY AND KEY POINTS

Ocular ultrasonography is a rapid, noninvasive bedside procedure that can be very helpful in the evaluation of numerous ocular emergencies. It is a technique that can be easily learned and is part of the augmented physical examination of the eye. When performed, copious amounts of gel should be applied to a closed eyelid to reduce any direct pressure on the globe and the potential for contact artifacts, and the provider should scan the globe in both the sagittal and transverse planes, with clear identification of important anatomic structures. The depth and gain should be adjusted to fill the screen with the image of the eye and to reduce potential artifacts, and tissue exposure to energy should be limited to the minimal amount necessary to complete a thorough examination.

References

1. McGwin G Jr, Xie A, Owsley C. Rate of eye injury in the United States. *Arch Ophthalmol.* 2005;123:970–976.

2. Blaivas M, Theodoro D, Sierzenski PR. A study of beside ocular ultrasonography in the emergency department. *Acad Emerg Med.* 2002;9:791–799.

3. Ma O, Mateer J, Blaivas M, eds. *Emergency Ultrasound.* 2nd ed. New York, NY: McGraw-Hill; 2007.

4. Bradford C, ed. *Basic Ophthalmology.* 8th ed. San Francisco, CA: American Academy of Ophthalmology; 2004.

5. Pokhrel P, Loftus S. Ocular emergencies. *Am Fam Physician* 2007;76:829–836.

6. Shinar Z, Chan L, Orlinsky M. Use of ocular ultrasound for the evaluation of retinal detachment. *J Emerg Med.* 2009; Epub ahead of publication.

7. Tintinalli J, Kelen G, Stapczynski J, eds. *Emergency Medicine: A Comprehensive Study Guide.* 6th ed. New York, NY: McGraw-Hill; 2004.

8. Romanchuk KG. Seidel's test using 10% fluorescein. *Can J Ophthalmol.* 1979;14:253–256.

9. Sawyer N. Ultrasound imaging of penetrating ocular trauma. *J Emerg Med.* 2009;36:181–182.

10. Nair U, Aldave A, Cunningham E. Identifying intraocular foreign bodies. *Eye Net Magazine* (American Academy of Ophthalmology) 2007; October.

11. Bryden F, Pyott A, Bailey M, et al. Real time ultrasound assessment of intraocular foreign bodies. *Eye.* 1990;4: 727–731.

12. Shiver S, Lyon M, Blaivas M. Detection of metallic ocular foreign bodies with handheld sonography in a porcine model. *J Ultrasound Med.* 2005;24:1341–1346.

13. Rabinowitz R, Yagev R, Shoham A, Liftshitz T. Comparison between clinical and ultrasound findings in patients with vitreous hemorrhage. *Eye.* 2004;18:253–256.

14. Kimberly HH, Shah S, Marill K, Noble V. Correlation of optic nerve sheath diameter with direct measurement of intracranial pressure. *Acad Emerg Med.* 2008;15:201–204.

15. Blaivas M, Theodoro D, Sierzenski PR. Elevated intracranial pressure detected by bedside emergency ultrasonography of the optic nerve sheath. *Acad Emerg Med.* 2003;10:376–381.

SECTION III

ULTRASOUND USE FOR EVALUATION OF ORGANS OF THE CHEST

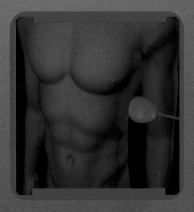

CHAPTER 6

Breast Ultrasound

Roxanne Davenport, MD

INTRODUCTION

Breast ultrasound is used primarily to evaluate palpable abnormalities, to further characterize mammographic findings, and as image guidance for percutaneous core biopsy. Because of the absence of ionizing radiation, ultrasound can be used in pregnant patients, where mammography can be of concern.

Breast ultrasound lacks the spatial resolution (detail) of mammography, and therefore is not approved by the Food and Drug Administration as a screening tool for breast cancer. Ultrasound does offer excellent contrast resolution. For this reason, a breast ultrasound can determine whether a breast lesion is cystic or solid. Doppler ultrasound techniques can be used to determine blood supply to the breast lesion.

Combining mammography with breast ultrasound for breast cancer screening continues to be an area of investigation. Certainly in a high-risk population with heterogeneously dense breast tissue, adding a single screening ultrasound to mammography increases the number of breast cancers detected, but there is also an increase in the number of patients who will require tissue biopsy because of false-positive findings of the ultrasound. Studies in this area are ongoing.

BREAST ULTRASOUND EQUIPMENT SPECIFICATIONS

The technical requirements for high-quality breast ultrasound (BUS) rely on maximizing spatial and contrast resolution. It is important that the imager be aware of the manipulations that can be made to maximize these factors.

Spatial Resolution

To optimize spatial resolution, consideration must be given to focusing in the long and short axis of the transducer and the depth of imaging (axial resolution).

Long-axis Resolution

The transducer most commonly used for breast ultrasound is the one-dimensional (1D) linear array transducer. The long-axis resolution is related to the aperture size of the transducer, element size, and the number of elements and channels. With multiple elements transmitting and receiving together in an array, the beam is electronically steered to focus along the long axis of the transducer. With this inherent fixed electronic focusing, the only manipulation made by the imager in the long axis is adjusting the depth of the focal zones once a specific area of interest is identified. It is not unusual to have to move focal zones several times during a BUS as the depth of the area of interest changes.

With the 1D linear array transducer, electronic focusing is not possible in the short axis as it is in the long axis. Short-axis focusing requires a fixed acoustic lens. The optimal focal length (depth) of the short axis in the breast is 1.5 to 2.0 cm, placing the focal length in the center of the mammary zone. Most 7- to 12-MHz linear probes have focal lengths within this range. The American Institute of Ultrasound in Medicine (AIUM) recommends a nominal center frequency of 7 MHz. Using a transducer with a frequency below 7 MHz places the focal zone within the chest wall, deep to the breast tissue in most women. This results in volume averaging, which can lead to small cystic lesions being mischaracterized as solid and to missing small cystic and solid lesions altogether as they become isoechoic with the surrounding breast tissue.

Even when using a 7- to 12-MHz probe with an appropriate short-axis focal length, small lesions that are very near the skin can be difficult to image. For lesions that are within the most superficial 1 cm of the breast, an acoustic standoff of a thick layer of gel or a standoff pad may be necessary to accurately image the lesion. The ideal standoff pad or layer of gel would be about 7 mm in thickness. Using an acoustic standoff pad that is too thick will result in placing the short-axis focal length within the standoff pad rather than within the breast, creating a greater problem than using no pad at all. If gel is being used as the standoff, use a water-soluble gel designed for ultrasound; otherwise, there could be significant air trapping in the gel, which creates artifactual shadowing.

Axial Resolution

Axial resolution is related to transducer frequency, pulse length, and bandwidth. Higher-frequency probes have better axial resolution than lower-frequency probes; this is another reason why the 7- to 12-MHz probes are superior to lower-frequency probes. For any given transducer frequency, the shorter the pulse length, the better the resolution. The pulse length varies among various ultrasound models. Lastly, wider bandwidths are preferable. Ultrasound manufacturers can provide a profile detailing these characteristics for their specific models and transducer types.

Contrast Resolution

High-quality contrast resolution is necessary to distinguish between different types of tissue in the breast and to increase the differentiation of subtle solid lesions. The single most important way to improve contrast resolution is to minimize volume averaging by improving spatial resolution. Some BUS manufacturers now offer other specialized methods to improve contrast resolution.

BREAST ULTRASOUND EXAMINATION TECHNIQUE

Performing the BUS technique correctly is just as important as having the appropriate equipment.

Patient Positioning

The positioning of the patient is influenced by the area of the breast being imaged. When imaging the medial breast, the supine position is favored. For lesions in the lateral breast, the patient is usually scanned in a contralateral posterior oblique position with the ipsilateral arm raised above the head and the hand positioned behind the head. A pillow or foam cushion can be used to support the torso if necessary. This position helps to thin the breast to the greatest degree possible, helping to ensure that a 7-MHz transducer will adequately penetrate to the chest wall.

For laterally located lesions in a very large or pendulous breast, the patient may need to be in a full contralateral lateral decubitus position to maximize tissue thinning.

Transducer Compression

Variable degrees of compression can be applied with the transducer. Compression thins the breast tissue and pushes normal tissue into a plane parallel to the transducer surface, which improves penetration and image quality.

Superficial structures, such as Cooper's ligaments, can create acoustic shadows, which prevent evaluation of deeper tissues. Moderate compression with the transducer can push an obliquely oriented Cooper's ligament into a plane that lies parallel to the transducer, eliminating acoustic shadowing.

Greater compression can be helpful when evaluating small lesions located deep in the breast tissue near the chest wall, especially when fibrous tissue lies superficial to the lesion. Too much compression can actually worsen image quality by pushing near-field shadows deeper into the breast.

EXAMINATION SPECIFICATIONS AND DOCUMENTATION

Meeting the AIUM guidelines includes evaluating an ultrasound finding in two perpendicular planes. At least one image should be obtained without calipers. The maximal dimensions of a lesion should be recorded in at least two dimensions.

The images should be labeled for laterality (right or left breast), location of the lesion (by specifying a quadrant of the breast or by using a clock-face notation), orientation of the transducer (longitudinal or transverse and radial or antiradial), and the distance from the nipple. Images of all important findings should be recorded on a retrievable and reviewable image storage format.

The sonographic features that aid in characterization of the lesion should be included in the ultrasound report. The ultrasound report should be placed in the patient's medical record.

BREAST ANATOMY

Gross Anatomy

The earliest sign of breast development occurs during the fourth week of gestation with the appearance of ectodermal thickenings known as the "milk lines." The milk line normally regresses at all sites other than the fourth intercostal space, where the breast bud begins its development by growing down into the dermis. Each primary bud gives rise to several secondary buds that develop into the lactiferous ducts.

During puberty, the lactiferous ducts give rise to approximately 15 to 20 lobes in the breast. Each lobe is made up of lobules and small branch ducts that join to form progressively larger ducts, until there is only one main central duct that drains the whole lobe.

Each major lobar duct converges in the subareolar location where each duct has a dilated portion called the lactiferous sinus, which serves as a reservoir during lactation. The ducts then course anteriorly to the apex of the nipple.

Adult female breast tissue extends between the second rib superiorly, the sixth rib inferiorly, the lateral border of the sternum medially, and the midaxillary line laterally. The breast is circular in shape with an axillary tail extending varying distances toward the axilla.

The nipple lies slightly medial and inferior to the center of the breast and is surrounded by the areola. Smooth muscle fibers in circular and longitudinal bundles erect the nipple and contract the areola in response to various stimuli. The areola contains modified sebaceous glands, known as Montgomery tubercles, which enlarge during pregnancy and secrete an oily substance that provides a protective lubricant for the areola and nipple during breast-feeding.

The fascia that lies on the anterior surface of the breast parenchyma is the premammary fascia. The premammary fascia separates the breast parenchyma from the subcutaneous fat. This fascial layer is not a smooth, continuous structure but rather is scalloped with points extending toward the skin as Cooper's ligaments. Each Cooper's ligament is made of two leaflets of closely approximated premammary fascia that separate posteriorly as they course horizontally along the anterior surface of the breast tissue. Cooper's ligaments lack the dense bundles of collagen fibers characteristic of true ligaments, but these fibrous bands do provide suspensory support to the breast, and their increasing laxity with age is believed to contribute to breast ptosis. Extensions of Cooper's ligaments cross from the anterior breast to the pectoral fascia in an unpredictable fashion, subdividing the breast parenchyma.

The fascia that lies on the posterior surface of the breast tissue, separating it from the retromammary fat, is the retromammary fascia. Between the premammary and retromammary fascia lies the mammary zone, which contains the majority of the ducts and lobules of the breast.

Histology

Breast tissue can be classified as either stromal or epithelial-myoepithelial. Stromal elements include fat and fibrous tissue. There are two types of fibrous tissue: dense interlobular and loose intralobular. The differences between the loose and dense stromal fibrous tissue are important in ultrasound because the tissues have markedly different echo textures.

The lobe, extending from the central duct out to the ductules (acini), is lined by an inner layer of epithelial cells with a more or less continuous layer of outer myoepithelial cells.

The functional unit of the breast is the terminal ductolobular unit (TDLU). Each lobule is composed of an intralobular terminal duct, individual ductules (acini), and intralobular loose fibrous tissue. Most lobules arise from peripheral ducts, but a few may arise from larger central ducts. The size of lobules varies, with most in the range of 0.5 to 2 mm in the resting adult breast.

Most breast pathology arises within the TDLUs. Most ductal carcinomas are thought to arise from within the terminal duct near its junction with the lobule.

SONOGRAPHIC BREAST ANATOMY

As in any other tissue in the body, it is most useful to use a normal structure or tissue that is near the center of the gray-scale spectrum as the standard against which other anatomic tissues and pathologic lesions are compared. In the breast, the echogenicity of normal fat serves as the standard. It is important to set up scan parameters such as total gain and time-gain curve so that fat appears to be a midlevel gray.

Zones of the Breast

The breast has three main sonographically identifiable zones from anterior to posterior: the premammary zone, the mammary zone, and the retromammary zone (Fig. 6.1).

Premammary Zone

The premammary zone lies between the skin and the premammary fascia. The premammary zone has a

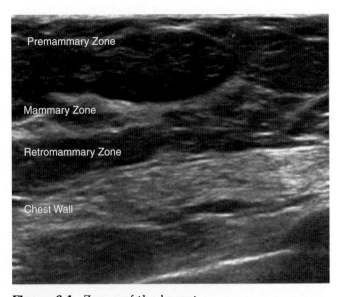

Figure 6.1. Zones of the breast.

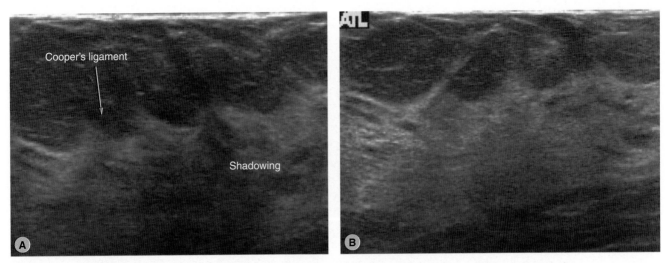

Figure 6.2. Cooper's ligaments. Split-screen images of the same scalloped Cooper's ligaments. In A, there is shadowing from ligaments perpendicular to the transducer. In B, compression eliminates shadowing.

similar appearance in all individuals: isoechoic fat with interspersed thin, echogenic scalloped Cooper's ligaments (Fig. 6.2).

Most pathologic processes that lie entirely within this region arise from the skin and subcutaneous fat. Such lesions are not specific to the breast and can occur anywhere in the body. Two common lesions in this region are lipomas and epidermal inclusion cysts (Figs. 6.3 and 6.4).

Mammary Zone

The mammary zone lies between the premammary zone and the retromammary zone and is covered anteriorly and posteriorly by mammary fascia. The sonographic appearance of the mammary zone varies greatly from individual to individual and between different areas within one breast, depending on the relative amounts and distribution of hyperechoic fibrous elements and more isoechoic fatty and epithelial-myoepithelial elements (Fig. 6.5).

Almost all of the mammary ducts and TDLUs are found within the mammary zone. Because most pathology arises in the TDLUs or ducts, the most significant breast pathology arises within the mammary zone.

Retromammary Zone

The retromammary zone lies between the retromammary fascia and the pectoralis fascia. The retromammary zone, when visible, is similar in appearance among individuals since that it is made up of fat. This zone appears to be much thinner in the anteroposterior dimension on ultrasound than on mammograms

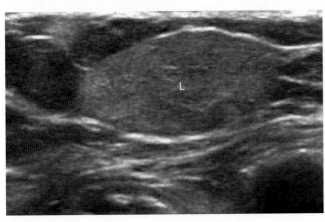

Figure 6.3. Lipoma. Well-circumscribed lipoma (L) within the premammary zone.

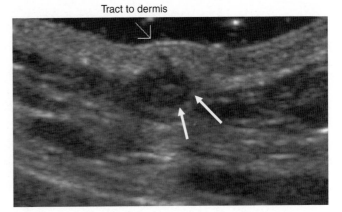

Figure 6.4. Epidermal inclusion cyst (*large white arrows*), often correlate with visual inspection of the skin.

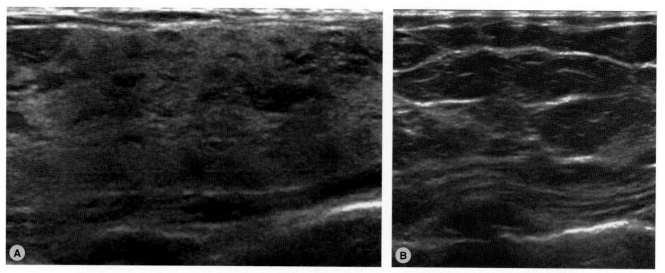

Figure 6.5. Mammary zone. This picture illustrates the variable volume and echogenicity of the mammary zone. In **A,** the mammary zone is thick and highly echogenic. In **B,** the mammary zone is composed almost entirely of fat and is comparatively hypoechoic.

or breast magnetic resonance imaging because it is compressed between the mammary zone and the chest wall during sonographic examination. This zone may be so compressed that it may not even visible on ultrasound.

Pathologic lesions that lie within the posterior half of the mammary zone can appear immediately adjacent to the pectoralis muscle. This zone contains mainly fat and few suspensory ligaments. Most of the pathologic processes in this zone arise within the mammary zone and secondarily invade the retromammary zone.

Morphology

Fat

As previously discussed, breast tissue is comprised of fat interspersed with fibrous and glandular elements. An isoechoic fat lobule can be the cause of a false-positive diagnosis. There are techniques to help distinguish fat lobules from solid breast nodules. First, per AIUM guidelines, the finding should be evaluated in more than one plane. Most fat lobules are continuous with other fat lobules, and imaging in multiple planes may show a broad sheet of fatty tissue (Fig. 6.6).

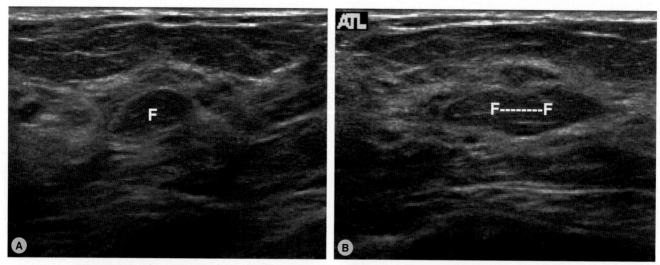

Figure 6.6. Fat lobule. Split-screen images of the same fat lobule (F). The image in **(A)** could be misinterpreted as a round mass. Imaged at a different plane **(B)**, it elongates (F--------F) as a normal fat lobule.

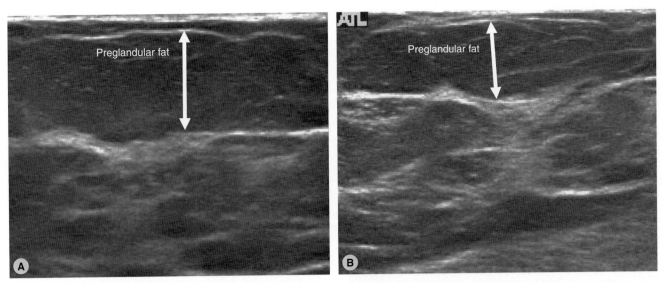

Figure 6.7. Compressibility. Split-screen images of the same premammary fat. The image in **A** is without compression. The image in **B** is with compression.

Second, fat lobules are compressible structures. Compressibility of 30% or more is strong evidence that the structure is fatty (Fig. 6.7).

Ducts

Ducts are hypoechoic-to-isoechoic linear structures extending out from the nipple in a radial fashion. The central ducts have a vertical course immediately deep to the nipple and then gradually take a more horizontal course as they move into the periphery of the breast (Fig. 6.8). The appearance of the ducts is variable depending on the amount of loose periductal

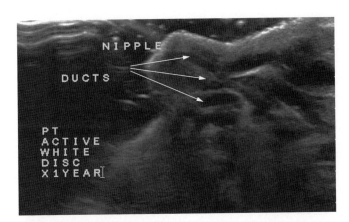

Figure 6.8. Milk ducts. Images of the nipple and subareolar ducts can be obtained by liberal gel placement and imaging with the transducer angled relative to the course of the ducts.

fibrous tissue surrounding the duct, the degree of distention of the duct by secretions, and the echogenicity of the ductal secretions.

When evaluating the central ducts, it is important to try to prevent the smooth muscle in the nipple and areola from contracting, as this can cause critical angle shadowing. Cold temperatures are one strong stimulus for contraction; therefore, the room should be warm and warm gel used when scanning. Allotting several minutes between physical examination and ultrasound examination is recommended to allow the patient to relax, as tactile stimulation will also produce contraction.

Visualization of the central ducts and the subareolar region can be enhanced by the two-handed compression technique. Placing the subareolar ductal system parallel to the transducer allows for greater visualization, and the associated pressure applied along the duct can help distinguish between echogenic secretions and a solid intraductal component.

Terminal Duct Lobular Units (TDLUs)

TDLUs are visible in a smaller percentage of individuals than are the mammary ducts. All three components of the lobule are normally isoechoic and indistinguishable from each other. The extralobular terminal duct is also isoechoic. Only when the ductules become cystically dilated, and the intralobular fibrous tissue becomes fibrotic or sclerotic and abnormally echogenic are the components of the TDLU identifiable (Fig. 6.9).

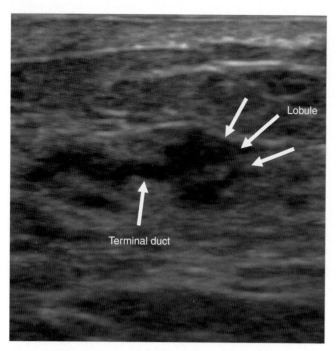

Figure 6.9. Terminal duct lobular unit (*white arrows*).

COMMON PATHOLOGY

The most common use for breast ultrasound in clinical practice is to evaluate palpable breast lesions. When evaluating a palpable abnormality with ultrasound, every attempt should be made to palpate the lesion during the scanning process. Simply demonstrating that a benign finding exists in the same area as the palpable abnormality is not sufficient; one must

be confident that the palpable lesion corresponds to the ultrasound finding.

Cysts

Ultrasound is 96% to 100% accurate in the diagnosis of a simple cyst. The strict diagnostic criteria for a simple cyst are (1) central echogenicity, (2) well-circumscribed margins, (3) completely encompassed by a thin, echogenic capsule, (4) enhanced through-transmission, and (5) thin edge shadows. All five of these criteria must be met to classify the cyst as simple. Figure 6.10 illustrates these classic features.

Simple cysts do not require aspiration, biopsy, or interval imaging follow-up. Aspiration is performed for symptomatic relief when the cysts are tender.

Complex cysts do not display the classic features of a simple cyst. They may contain internal echoes or demonstrate wall thickening or irregularity. If a cyst is not simple on ultrasound, referral to a breast center for further imaging evaluation of the lesion is recommended.

Solid Masses

Fibroadenomas are the most commonly encountered solid benign mass on ultrasound. They arise from the TDLU and are made up of variable amounts of both stromal and epithelial elements. The number of stromal and epithelial elements can be equal in some lesions, or the stromal or epithelial component can predominate.

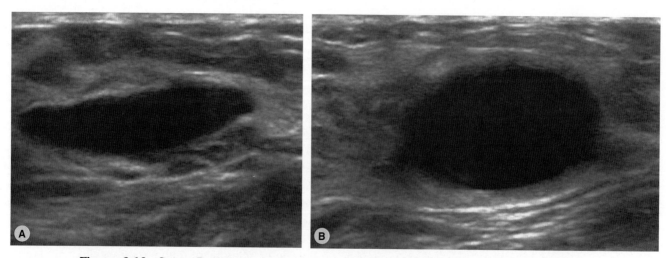

Figure 6.10. Cysts. Both cysts have classic ultrasound features. The cyst in **A** is flatter than in **B**. As fluid accumulates within a cyst it becomes rounder, and the resultant tension may result in a painful cyst.

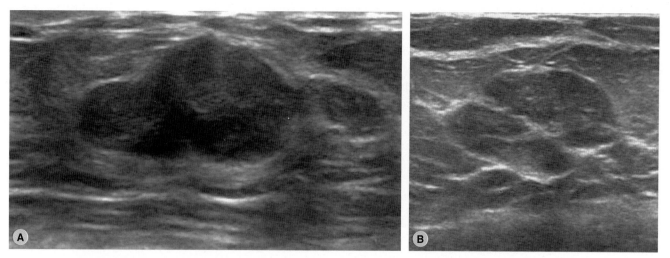

Figure 6.11. Fibroadenoma. **(A, B)** The images represent examples of two different fibroadenomas, both with classic ultrasound fibroadenoma features but each with a slightly different echo texture.

The classic findings of a fibroadenoma on ultrasound are (1) elliptical or gently lobulated shape, (2) wider than tall orientation, (3) isoechoic or mildly hypoechoic echotexture, (4) encompassed completely by a thin, echogenic capsule, (5) sound transmission that is either normal or increased in comparison to the transmission of the surrounding tissues, (6) thin edge shadows, and (7) slightly compressible. Figure 6.11 exhibits classic features. Figure 6.12 is an invasive breast cancer, which contrasts the classic findings of a fibroadenoma.

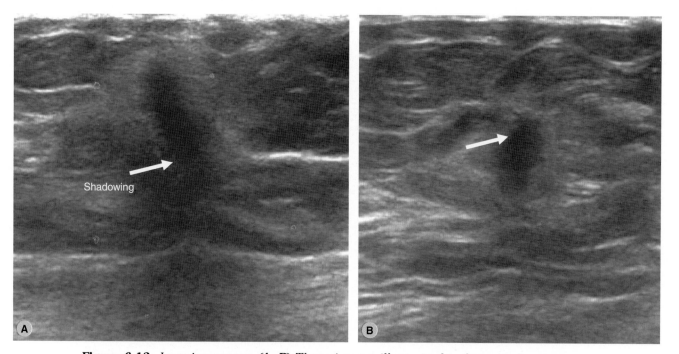

Figure 6.12. Invasive cancer. **(A, B)** These images illustrate the ultrasound appearance of invasive breast cancer. Note the poorly defined borders, thick edge, acoustic shadows (*white arrows*), and vertical growth.

Although breast ultrasound is used primarily to distinguish solid from cystic masses, imaging criteria exist that can reliably differentiate solid lesions according to benign or malignant characteristics. Discussion of those imaging characteristics is beyond the scope of this chapter. To develop a proficiency for differentiating solid benign from solid malignant lesions requires that the ultrasound operator use meticulous technique and have considerable experience. For solid lesions that do not exhibit the classic findings of a fibroadenoma, referral to a breast care center for further characterization of the lesion is recommended.

CHAPTER 7

Upper Airway and Lung Ultrasound

Sameh Aziz, MD, FCCP, FACP

INTRODUCTION

Since the development of more compact portable ultrasound units with better image quality,[1,2] ultrasound evaluation of the thorax is being utilized more consistently. The poor transmission of ultrasound waves through air in the lungs has limited ultrasound use. Interestingly, that same property has been a strength for ultrasound in the visualization of pathology, which images better than the normal lung. With the growing number of intensive care physicians trained in ultrasonography, especially lung ultrasound, and with more literature proving its effectiveness, there has been an increase in usage of portable ultrasound in the intensive care unit. In a study that compared portable chest radiography to ultrasound in critically ill patients, the use of ultrasound influenced the management of those patients 90% of the time.[3]

ULTRASOUND PHYSICS

All modalities of ultrasound—M mode, two-dimensional (2D), and Doppler assessment either through continuous, pulse wave, or color flow mapping—are useful in evaluating intrathoracic structure and pathology (see also Chapter 3).

Frequency, the number of cycles per second (Hz), can be used to advantage in lung ultrasound. Recall that ultrasound waves with low frequency have a long wavelength and are able to penetrate deeper tissue, but at the expense of good resolution. Alternatively, ultrasound waves with high frequency have a short wavelength and have the best resolution but have low tissue penetration. For an echocardiogram, a low-frequency probe would be selected because the heart is a deeper structure. In contrast, the pleural space is a superficial structure, and a high-frequency probe will offer the best resolution.[2,4]

As ultrasound waves travel through tissues, they strike a boundary between two different tissue layers, resulting in energy being reflected back to the transducer in the form of an echo. This is known as acoustic impedance and is related to certain properties of the tissue. Air

(alveolar air) has high acoustic impedance, which is responsible for almost complete reflection of the ultrasound wave at its boundary with other tissue. This property makes ultrasound evaluation of the lung parenchyma challenging.[1,2] The high acoustic impedance of the lung is responsible for the production of ultrasound artifacts (see Chapter 3), which is considered a key factor in the interpretation of lung ultrasound.[5] Refraction, attenuation, and scatter also contribute to ultrasound image acquisition and interpretation in the lung.

AIRWAY EVALUATION

Ultrasound evaluation of the upper airway is evolving (see Chapter 4). Portable ultrasound can be useful in evaluating the airway prior to intubation, in determining endotracheal tube position, and in evaluating the trachea prior to percutaneous tracheostomy (Figs. 7.1, 7.2).

A high-frequency, linear array probe is preferred for evaluating the airway. Beginning at the base of the tongue, which appears as a hypoechoic structure, one moves caudally to identify the hyoid bone, a hyperechoic structure, followed by the thyroid cartilage (see Fig. 7.13). The cricothyroid membrane and the cricoid cartilage can be identified. At this level, evaluation of the vocal cords is possible (Fig. 7.3), and in real time, the vocal cords can be seen moving. Below the cricoid, the tracheal rings can be identified and counted. For percutaneous tracheostomy, the space between the second and third tracheal rings can be confirmed.[6]

Although the trachea is filled with air, which has a high acoustic impedance, ultrasound can help to identify the position of the endotracheal tube after intubation. Visualization can be enhanced by retaining the stylet in the endotracheal tube or by increasing the echogenicity of the endotracheal tube cuff by filling it with fluid and air bubbles.

In obese patients with obstructive sleep apnea, the thickness of the lateral pharyngeal wall correlates with the apnea-hypopnea index. Ultrasound evaluation of the lateral parapharyngeal wall is possible at the level of the internal carotid artery[7] (Fig. 7.4).

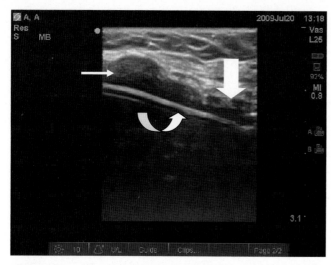

Figure 7.1. Longitudinal view of the trachea. Cricoid cartilage (*thin arrow*), tracheal rings (*thick arrow*), and endotracheal tube (*curved arrow*).

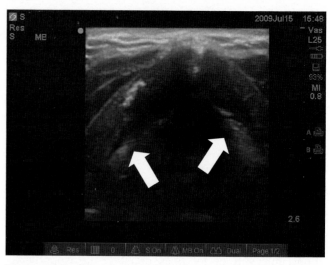

Figure 7.3. Ultrasound of the thyroid cartilage. Vocal cords can be identified (*arrows*).

ULTRASOUND OF THE DIAPHRAGM

Ultrasound is a very useful tool in evaluating the diaphragm, especially when looking for diaphragmatic paralysis. For the evaluation of the diaphragm, the ultrasound probe is placed at the midaxillary line in a longitudinal orientation, using the liver on the right side and the spleen on the left side as echo windows.

Using 2D Doppler, the diaphragm can be seen moving during respiration (Video 7.1). If the diaphragm is paralyzed, there is absence of movement ultrasonographically. Paradoxical movement can be seen with unilateral paralysis when evaluating the paralyzed side. Using M mode, the diaphragm will appear linear and hyperechoic, moving caudally during inspiration and cranially during expiration (Fig. 7.5). Absence of

movement with flat, linear artifact represents a paralyzed diaphragm.[8] Assessment of diaphragmatic movement after endotracheal intubation can confirm proper tracheal intubation, especially if combined with ultrasound evaluation looking for the endotracheal tube beneath the tracheal rings.[9]

ULTRASOUND OF THE LUNG

While any probe can be used to evaluate the lung, it is important to understand the advantages and limitations of each probe. The sector scanner is a small probe that produces a narrow view with near-field artifacts

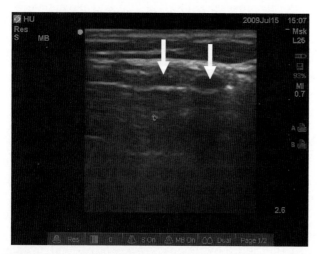

Figure 7.2. Longitudinal view of the trachea. Arrows indicate tracheal rings.

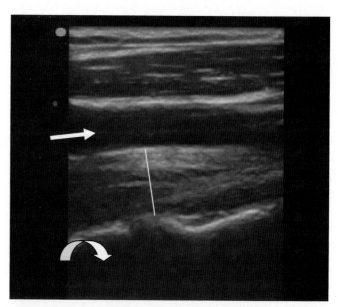

Figure 7.4. Lateral parapharyngeal wall, internal carotid artery (*straight arrow*), oropharynx (*curved arrow*), line indicates paraphyarygeal wall.

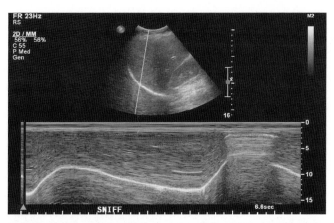

Figure 7.5. Normal movement of the diaphragm is visualized using M-mode.

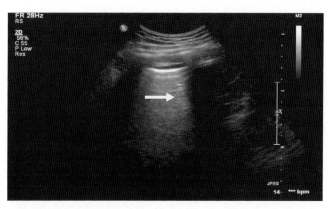

Figure 7.7. A-line artifact (*arrow*).

that may obscure the pleura, but this transducer is best suited for visualizing large pleural effusions and deeper lung structures.[5] A linear transducer provides a broad view with good visualization and evaluation of the pleura, superficial structures, and peripheral lung masses. A curved array probe provides good resolution, accesses deeper structures (low frequency), and, because of the fan-shaped image, helps to ensure visualization of appropriate landmarks.

Orientation of the ultrasound probe can be longitudinal (perpendicular to the ribs) in the long axis of the body or transverse (intercostal position). A linear transducer may be better suited for the intercostal approach. Evaluation of the thoracic structures may be performed using an intercostal approach or an abdominal approach. The abdominal approach is used mainly for visualizing the lower zones of the pleural space and the diaphragm.[5]

Normal Lung Ultrasound

In the longitudinal view, one of the most important landmarks is the ribs and the artifacts they create. These artifacts help define the location of lung pathology in

relation to the superior and inferior ribs on the ultrasound screen. In between the ribs, a hyperechoic line represents the pleural edge. The longitudinal image of the upper rib, pleural line, and lower rib resembles a flying bat with down-beating wings (Fig. 7.6).

Because of the lung–pleura interface and the high acoustic impedance of lung tissue, several artifacts can help identify normal underlying lung tissue. One such artifact is the A line presenting as a mirror image of the pleural line due to sound waves bouncing off of the smooth reflector surface of the pleura; this represents a reverberation artifact[10] (Fig. 7.7).

The lung sliding sign represents a back-and-forth movement that can be visualized under the pleural line (shimmering sign); this represents a moving lung (Video 7.2). The time motion mode (M mode), used with low depth settings, a high-frequency probe, and the intercostal approach, can enhance the physician's ability to identify moving lung. By using M mode, the parietal pleura, which is not moving, will be presented by a white hyperechoic line; the moving lung underneath will be visualized as a homogenous granular pattern producing the so-called seashore artifact[11] (Fig. 7.8, Video 7.3). Adding color Doppler will help confirm sliding lung under the pleural line.

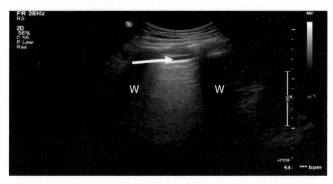

Figure 7.6. Bat sign. Pleura line (*arrow*) represents the bat's head, while the rib shadows (W) represent the bat's wings.

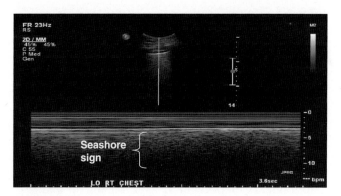

Figure 7.8. M-mode ultrasound. Seashore sign.

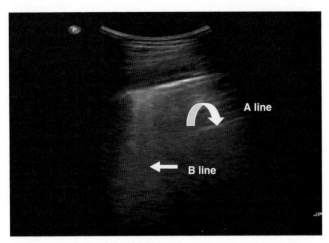

Figure 7.9. A line artifact (*curved arrow*) and B line artifact (*straight arrow*). Adding color Doppler will help confirm lung sliding under the pleural line. The combination of lung sliding, A-line, and B-line, with a positive seashore sign represents healthy underlying lung tissue.

B-line artifacts (comet tail artifact) represent the interface between the interlobular septa and the alveolar wall[12] (Fig. 7.9). In order to be classified as a B line, the artifact has to start from the pleural line, be hyperechoic, never fade throughout the field, erase A lines, and move with lung movement. The combination of lung sliding, A-line artifact, and B-line artifact with a positive seashore sign defines healthy underlying lung tissue.

The abdominal ultrasound approach may produce a mirror sign due to the reflection of ultrasound waves at the surface of the diaphragm, thus seeming as if liver appears on both sides of the diaphragm. This sign can be used as definitive evidence of air-filled lung[5] (Fig. 7.10).

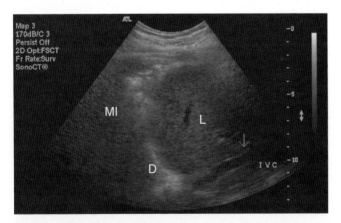

Figure 7.10. Mirror image of the liver above the diaphragm. D, diaphragm; L, liver; MI, mirror image of the liver.

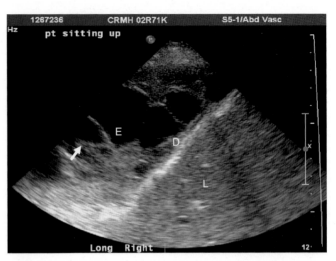

Figure 7.11. Complicated parapneumonic effusion with septation (*arrow*). E, effusion; D, diaphragm; L, liver.

Pleural Effusion

The most common indication for lung ultrasonography is evaluation for a pleural effusion. The sensitivity and specificity pf ultrasound for detecting a pleural effusion exceeds 90%.[13] Ultrasound is superior to chest radiography in imaging pleural effusions, especially in supine patients. Furthermore, ultrasound can help differentiate between pleural effusion, consolidation, and pleural thickening. While the intercostal approach can be used to image pleural effusions, smaller amounts of pleural fluid are best evaluated using an abdominal approach (subcostal).

Most transudative pleural effusions are anechoic. Exudative effusions may contain floating echogenic debris, which may scatter the ultrasound beam and produce color within the fluid, leading to the fluid color sign.[14] Pleural thickening may also accompany exudative effusions.[15] Complicated pleural effusions may demonstrate linear fibrous bands or a honeycomb appearance (Fig. 7.11). On the longitudinal view, pleural effusions are bordered by upper and lower ribs, the pleural line, and the lung line[11] (Fig. 7.12).

Dynamic findings, including diaphragmatic movement and lung floating within the pleural fluid, can be used to confirm the pleural space (Video 7.4). M mode may demonstrate a sinusoid sign, which will help confirm the presence of fluid, especially with small amounts of effusion. With the abdominal approach, an absent mirror sign due to the loss of air-filled lung above the diaphragm likewise supports the presence of an effusion. Measuring the distance between the parietal and visceral pleura, either during inspiration or expiration while the patient is supine, helps to estimate the amount of pleural fluid. A

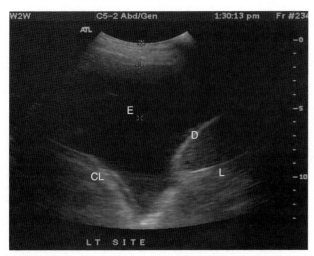

Figure 7.12. Uncomplicated pleural effusion with surrounding structures. D, diaphragm; L, liver; CL, compressed lung; E, effusion.

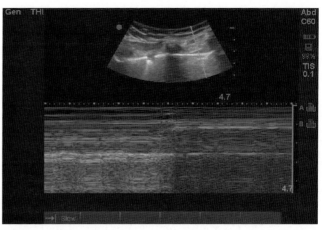

Figure 7.14. Ultrasound at the level of lung bullae. The left side represents normal lung with B-line artifact on 2-D ultrasound with seashore sign. The right side shows the absence of lung movement with the bar-code sign.

recent study showed that an interpleural distance of greater than 45 mm at the right thoracic base or 50 mm at the left thoracic base represents a pleural effusion of more than 800 mL, with a sensitivity of 94% and 100% and specificity of 76% and 67%, respectively.[16]

Pneumothorax

Ultrasound has a sensitivity of 100% and a specificity of 98%[17,18] in identifying pneumothorax. Decreasing the depth setting to magnify the pleural–lung interface improves the ability to detect pneumothorax (Fig. 7.13).

The difficulty in identifying a pneumothorax is mainly due to two factors. First, the physician is attempting to identify air, with high acoustic impedance, within the pleural space. Second, differentiating between air in the

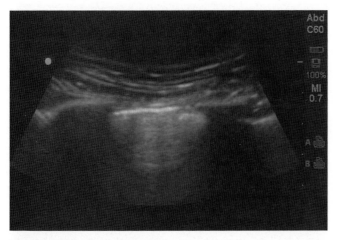

Figure 7.13. Decreasing the depth of the ultrasound beam yields greater detail of the pleura when looking for pleural pathology.

pleural space (pneumothorax) and normal lung with air-filled alveoli is a challenge. Identifying artifacts and the absence of normal looking lung helps determine whether pneumothorax is present. To confirm a normal, healthy lung, all of the following must be present: sliding lung, B-line artifact (comet tail sign), A-line artifact, and the seashore sign.[19,20]

With pneumothorax, absent lung movement produces no lung sliding on 2D mode, and on M mode the seashore sign is replaced by the stratosphere sign or bar-code sign. Absence of lung tissue under the parietal pleura will prevent the appearance of the comet tail artifact.[19] Careful evaluation of the chest at a point between normal lung and pneumothorax may identify a loculated pneumothorax with the lung point sign.[20,21] A false-positive finding of pneumothorax may occur in bullous emphysema with absence of lung sliding and a positive bar-code sign (Figs. 7.14, 7.15). Lung sliding can occur in areas with postpleurodesis pleural adhesion and in the left lung after right mainstem intubation in mechanically ventilated paralyzed patients. Also, failure to see lung sliding can be due to inappropriate technique or an inexperienced operator. False-negative findings may occur if the ultrasound examination omitted areas of localized pneumothorax. To rule out clinically significant pneumothorax, a bilateral lung examination with multiple-point interrogation must be conducted.

Multiple studies have demonstrated that ultrasound is superior to supine chest radiography in diagnosing traumatic pneumothorax.[17] Ultrasound portability makes it more effective in critically ill patients who cannot be positioned for quality chest radiographs. Ultrasonography is effective after interventional

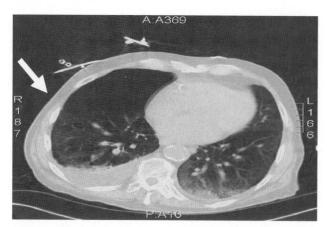

Figure 7.15. Computerized tomography of the thorax of the same patient at the same level. Transducer position (*white arrow*).

procedures[22] and central line placement to help identify complications and to confirm proper line placement at the junction between the superior vena cava and the right atrium (Figs. 7.16, 7.17).

Lung Consolidation

Pulmonary consolidation is due to the loss of lung aeration and replacement of the alveolar air with transudative fluid in pulmonary edema, exudative fluid in bronchopneumonia, and blood in lung contusion. Consolidated lung will permit the transmission of ultrasound waves through it. It will appear hypoechoic with sharply defined visceral pleural boarders.[5,23] Usually it is homogeneous in character, with complete consolidation of the lung, or heterogeneous in the partially collapsed lung. No comet tail artifact can be identified in consolidated lung. Adding Doppler to 2D ultrasound will help to

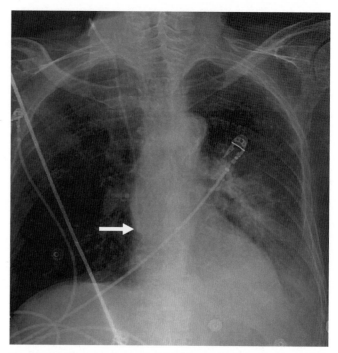

Figure 7.17. A chest X-ray of the same patient shows the appropriate position of the central line.

evaluate the vascular content of the consolidated lung and will help to differentiate between lobar pneumonia and lung cancer.[24] Air trapped inside bronchi with surrounding collapsed alveoli images as highly reflecting hyperechoic dots and lines. Even air-bronchograms may appear as echogenic branching tubular structures. Lack of pulsation, which can be confirmed using Doppler ultrasound, can differentiate between air-bronchogram and tubular pulmonary vessels.[25] Consolidated lung may act as an echo window that will permit visualization of deeper structures (Fig. 7.18).

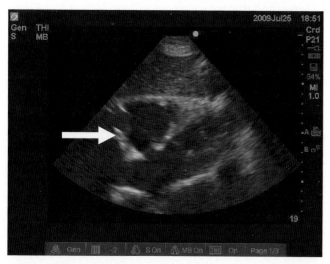

Figure 7.16. Subcostal four-chamber view of the heart. Echo artifact from the tip of the central line (*arrow*).

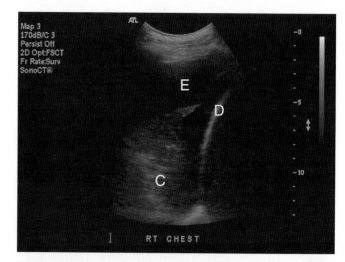

Figure 7.18. Lung consolidation due to pleural effusion. E, effusion; D, diaphragm; C, consolidated lung.

Lung Atelectasis

Loss of lung volume with lung collapse leads to atelectasis. This can occur in cases of complete bronchus obstruction, massive pleural effusion, reflexive atelectasis, or compression on the lung by tumor. Usually atelectatic lung is wedge shaped with high echogenicity. With pleural effusions, the atelectatic lung appears to move freely inside the effusion, which is one of the dynamic findings in evaluating and confirming the presence of pleural effusion.

Interstitial Lung Disease

Interstitial lung disease, due to idiopathic pulmonary fibrosis (IPF), collagen vascular disease, acute respiratory distress syndrome and other etiologies, is usually associated with thickening of the interlobular septa and a ground-glass appearance on chest computed tomography. This pattern can be identified on ultrasound by thickening of the pleura, especially in patients with IPF. Irregular borders of the pleura due to pleural traction from underlying fibrotic lung[26] and thickening of the interlobular septa represented by B lines that are 7 mm apart (B7 lines) also identify interstitial lung disease. Ground-glass areas are represented by B lines that are 3 mm apart (B3 lines).[5] In patients with pulmonary edema, the number of B3 lines correlates with the wedge pressure.[27]

DOCUMENTATION AND REIMBURSEMENT

For proper documentation, all diagnostic ultrasound images should be appropriately maintained in the patient's record. The indication for the study should be documented based on the patient's clinical history and diagnoses. In the absence of signs and symptoms, "screening" can be used as the primary indication. If any pathology is detected, it should be added to the documented diagnoses. It is the responsibility of the physician to select the appropriate code for the service. *Current Procedural Terminology* (CPT) code 76604 can be used for diagnostic ultrasound of the chest, while CPT code 76942 can be used for ultrasound-guided thoracentesis.[28]

References

1. Kendall J, Hoffenberg SR, Smith RS. History of emergency and critical care ultrasound: the evolution of a new imaging paradigm. *Crit Care Med.* 2007;35(5): S126–S129.

2. Lawrence J. Physics and instrumentation of ultrasound. *Crit Care Med.* 2007;35(8):S314–S322.

3. Yu C, Yang P, Chang D, Luh K. Diagnostic and therapeutic use of chest sonography: value in critically ill patients. *AJR Am J Roentgenol.* 1992;159:695–701.

4. Levitov A, Slonim A, Mayo P. *Critical Care Ultrasonography.* New York, NY: McGraw-Hill; 2009.

5. Rumack CM, Wilson SR, Charboneau JW. *Diagnostic Ultrasound.* 3rd ed. St. Louis, MO: Mosby; 2004.

6. Sustic A. Role of ultrasound in the airway management of critically ill patients. *Crit Care.* 2007;35:S173–S177.

7. Liu K, Chu W, To KW, et al. Sonographic measurement of lateral parapharyngeal wall thickness in patients with obstructive sleep apnea. *Sleep.* 2007;30(11):1503–1508.

8. Lloyd T, Tang YM, Benson MD, King S. Diaphragmatic paralysis: the use of M mode ultrasound for diagnosis in adults. *Spinal Cord.* 2006;44:505–508.

9. Hsieh K, Lee C, Lin C, et al. Secondary confirmation of endotracheal tube position by ultrasound image. *Crit Care.* 2004;32:S374–S377.

10. Aldrich J. Basic physics of ultrasound imaging. *Crit Care Med.* 2007;35(5):S131–S137.

11. Lichtenstein D. Ultrasound in the management of thoracic disease. *Crit Care Med.* 2007;35(5):S250–S261.

12. Lichtenstein D, Meziere G. Relevance of lung ultrasound in the diagnosis of acute respiratory failure: the BLUE protocol. *Chest.* 2008;134:117–125.

13. Lichtenstein D, Goldstein I, Mourgeon E, et al. Comparative diagnostic performances of auscultation, chest radiography and lung ultrasonography in acute respiratory distress syndrome. *Anesthesiology.* 2004;100:9–15.

14. Wu RG, Yang PC, Kuo SH, Luh KT. Fluid color sign: a useful indicator for discrimination between pleural thickening and pleural effusion. *J Ultrasound Med.* 1995;14:767–769.

15. Beckh S, Bolcskei P, Lessnau L. Real-time chest ultrasonography: a comprehensive review for the pulmonologist. *Chest.* 2002;122:1759–1773.

16. Vignon P, Chastagner C, Berkane V, et al. Quantitative assessment of pleural effusion in critically ill patients by means of ultrasonography. *Crit Care Med.* 2005;33:1757–1763.

17. Blaivas M, Lyon M, Duggal S. A prospective comparison of supine chest radiology and bedside ultrasound for diagnosis of traumatic pneumothorax. *Acad Emerg Med.* 2005;12:844–849.

18. Barofalo G, Busso M, Perotto F, De Pascale A, Fava C. Ultrasound diagnosis of pneumothorax. *Radiol Med.* 2006;111:516–525.

19. Rowan K, Kirkpatrick A, Liu D, et al. Traumatic pneumothorax detection with thoracic US: correlation with chest radiography and CT-initial experience. *Radiology.* 2002;225:210–214.

20. Lichtenstein D, Meziere G, Lascols N, et al. Ultrasound diagnosis of occult pneumothorax. *Crit Care Med.* 2005;33:1231–1238.

21. Sartori S, Tombesi P, Trevisani L, Nielsen I, Tassinari D, Abbasciano V. Accuracy of transthoracic sonography in detection of pneumothorax after sonographically guided lung biopsy: prospective comparison with chest radiography. *AJR Am J Roentgenol.* 2007;188:27–40.

22. Reibig A, Kroegel C. Accuracy of transthoracic sonography in excluding post-interventional pneumothorax and hydropneumothorax: comparison to chest radiography. *Eur J Radiol.* 2005;53:463–470.

23. Bouhemad B, Zhang M, Lu Q, Rouby J. Clinical review: bedside lung ultrasound in critical care practice. *Crit Care.* 2007;11:205–213.

24. Wernecke K. Sonographic features of pleural disease. *AJR Am J Roentgenol.* 1997;168:1061–1066.

25. Weinberg B, Diakoumakis E, Burton K, Zvi S, Zvi B. The air bronchogram: sonographic demonstration. *AJR Am J Roentgenol.* 1986;147:593–595.

26. Reibig A, Kroegel C. Transthoracic sonography of diffuse parenchymal lung disease: the role of comet tail artifacts. *J Ultrasound Med.* 2003;22:173–180.

27. Agricola E, Bove T, Oppizzi M, et al. Ultrasound comet tail images: a marker of pulmonary edema. A comparative study with wedge pressure and extravascular lung water. *Chest.* 2005;127:1690–1695.

28. CPT 2009 Professional Edition. American Medical Association, Chicago:IL.

CHAPTER 8

Cardiac Ultrasound

Rodney W. Savage, MD, FACC and Marguerite Underwood, RN, RDCS

INTRODUCTION

Echocardiography was once limited to heavy, expensive, and poorly portable machines. Now instruments are easily carried in a briefcase or even a belt harness. Appropriately trained and credentialed clinicians can employ point-of-care imaging to provide fast answers to questions that previously took hours and even days to answer. Potentially crucial in the critical care setting, valve disease, ventricular function, cardiac tamponade, shunts, and great vessel pathology can be revealed in minutes. In nonacute settings, serial studies can be performed at minimal inconvenience and cost.

This chapter serves as an instructional guide and ready reference for providers during their initial training while they are learning how to apply echocardiography as a diagnostic tool in their practice.

TWO-DIMENSIONAL WINDOWS

The four standard windows for transthoracic echocardiography are (1) left parasternal, (2) apical, (3) subxiphoid, and (4) suprasternal (Fig. 8.1A, B). Some views may be easier than others to obtain in some patients. For example, patients with severe obstructive lung disease may be best viewed from a subxiphoid approach, whereas this window may be unavailable in patients after abdominal surgery. Each of the standard windows and transducer angles is illustrated in Figures 8.2 through 8.11. The operator will know or rapidly learn that normal anatomic variation requires adjustments to optimize imaging.

M MODE

M mode provides a high-fidelity linear "ice pick" view of interrogated the structures. These "traditional" echocardiograpic images are still useful today when making measurements and when studying time relationships and associations (Fig. 8.12).

COLOR DOPPLER

Color Doppler provides a color-coded visual display of nonlaminar (turbulent) flow with standard color coding. The blue areas represent flow moving away from the transducer, while the red areas represent flow moving toward the transducer. Flow at right angles to the transducer and laminar (smooth) flow are not visualized. Accordingly, stenotic lesions, regurgitant jets, and shunts can all be seen, but several windows and views must be interrogated to avoid missing pathology. In cases of regurgitant lesions and shunts, some estimate of severity (mild, moderate, or severe) can be assessed by recognizing that turbulence is represented and not a volume or pressure change (Fig. 8.13).

PULSED DOPPLER

Pulsed Doppler presents a graphical representation of turbulent flow in a small, defined target area. To achieve spatial resolution, only limited time segments of signal transmission and reception are available in the overall imaging transmission and receiving cycle. Accordingly, high velocities or turbulent flows may exceed pulsed Doppler's capability to display (Nyquist limit). This limits the use of pulsed Doppler in the analysis of situations with low to moderate turbulence such as left and right ventricular inflow in diastole, in pulmonary vein interrogation, and in the study of lesions with mild to moderate velocity (pressure) changes (Fig. 8.14).

CONTINUOUS WAVE DOPPLER

Continuous wave (CW) Doppler enjoys constant sending and receiving of signals from red cell flow turbulence, allowing a full graphical display of high turbulence and large velocity (pressure) changes (Fig. 8.15). This advantage comes at the expense of having no visual display of interrogated structures and no spatial resolution along the beam path. For example, valvular and subvalvular left ventricular outflow tract obstructions are summed so that the operator is unaware of the respective contribution of each component. Aortic stenosis and mitral regurgitation may be confused.

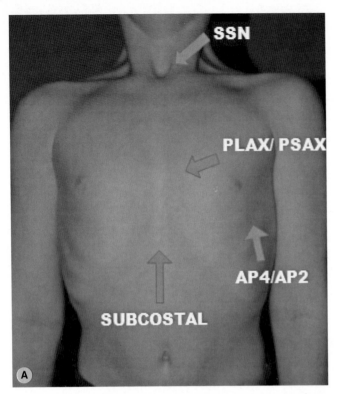

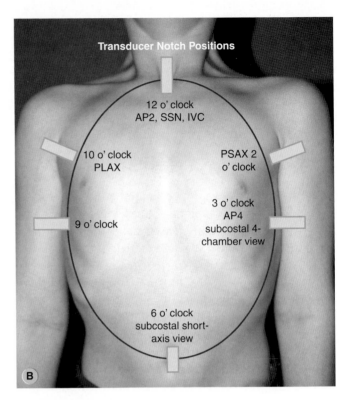

Figure 8.1. (A) Standard echocardiographic views. (*Courtesy of Jim Underwood.*) **(B)** Transducer notch position in standard echocardiographic views (long and short axis). (*Courtesy of Jim Underwood.*) AP, apical; IVC, inferior vena cava; PLAX, parasternal long axis; PSAX, parasternal short axis; SSN, suprasternal notch. AP4, Apical four-chamber view; AP2, Apical two-chamber view.

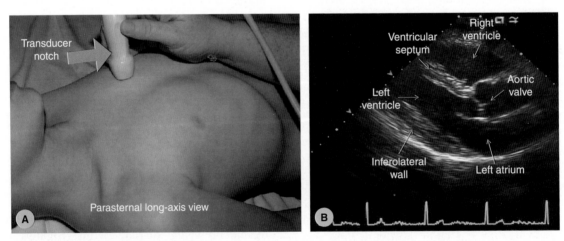

Obtaining the parasternal long axis view

• Start at the third intercostal space, move along rib space, move up and down rib spaces as needed.
• Transducer notch at approximately the 10 o'clock position.

Figure 8.2. (A) Correlation between the transducer (start at third intercostal space, move along rib space, and move up and down rib spaces as needed) and notch positions (approximately 10 o'clock) and **(B)** image obtained in parasternal long-axis view. (*Courtesy of Jim Underwood.*)

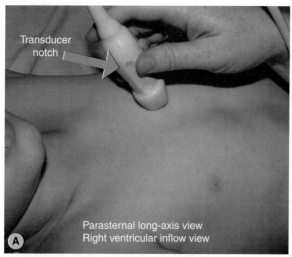

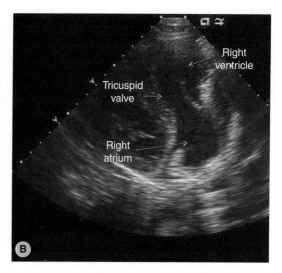

Obtaining the right ventricular inflow view

• From parasternal long axis (PLAX) view, angle inferiorly.

Figure 8.3. **(A)** Correlation between transducer (start at third intercostal space, move along rib space, move up and down rib spaces as needed, and angle inferiorly) and notch positions (approximately 10 o'clock) and **(B)** image obtained in right ventricular inflow view. (*Courtesy of Jim Underwood.*)

VALVULAR HEART DISEASE

Aortic Stenosis

Aortic stenosis may be congenital (usually bicuspid), degenerative (mostly calcific), or rheumatic. This valve is usually well seen in the left parasternal long- and short-axis views at the base. It is also well seen in the apical five- and three-chamber views. From the sub-xiphoid window, views equivalent to those available from the apical window may be obtained, but with

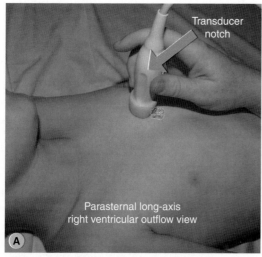

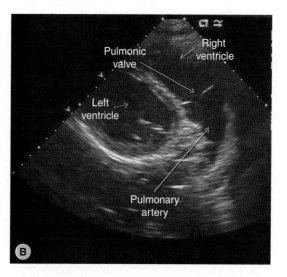

Obtaining the right ventricular inflow view

• From the parasternal long axis (PLAX) view, tilt transducer beam superiorly.
• May need to rotate the transducer notch clockwise slightly.

Figure 8.4. **(A)** Correlation between transducer (start at third intercostal space, move along rib space, move up and down rib spaces as needed, and angle inferiorly) and notch positions (approximately 10 o'clock; rotate the transducer notch clockwise slightly) and **(B)** image obtained in the right ventricular outflow view. (*Courtesy of Jim Underwood.*)

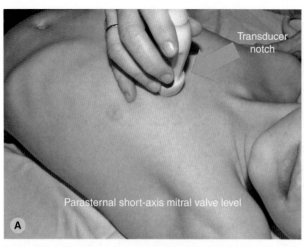

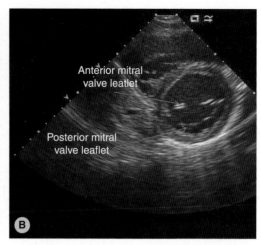

Obtaining the parasternal short-axis view (mitral valve level)
- The left ventricle should be round in appearance.
- By tilting the transducer (using superior and inferior angulation) from the patient's right shoulder to the left hip and maintaining the notch position at 2 o'clock, the operator will view the heart from apex to base.
- From the PLAX view, rotate the transducer notch clockwise to approximately 2 o'clock.

Figure 8.5. (A) Correlation between transducer (start at third intercostal space, move along rib space, and move up and down rib spaces as needed) and notch positions (approximately 2 o'clock) and **(B)** images obtained in parasternal short-axis view. Tilt the transducer superiorly and inferiorly to view the heart from apex to base. (*Courtesy of Jim Underwood.*)

more difficulty and less clarity. The left parasternal short-axis view at the base provides the most detail for valve morphology and, on occasion, can give a reasonable estimate of systolic valve area. Calcification usually makes this estimate unreliable. Color Doppler

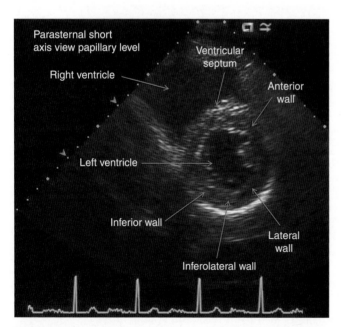

Figure 8.6. Parasternal short axis (PSAX) at papillary muscle level. Tilting the transducer superiorly and inferiorly in the PSAX position will allow viewing of the heart from apex to base. (*Courtesy of Jim Underwood.*)

shows evidence of supravalvular turbulence. CW Doppler provides an estimate of peak pressure drop using the equation: $P = 4 (V1 - V2)$, where P is the peak pressure difference across the valve in systole, V1 is the Doppler velocity just distal to the stenosis, and V2 is the velocity proximal to the stenosis (Fig. 8.16). The angle of incidence between the line of interrogation and the jet midline must be less than 30° to avoid underestimation since measured velocity differs form true velocity. Measured velocity is dependant on the angle theta and is smaller then the true one by the cosine theta (multiplication factor) (see formula in Chapter 3). The operator should interrogate several windows including apical, subxiphoid, suprasternal, and right parasternal to avoid this error, taking the greatest peak pressure drop.

Congenital aortic stenosis shows distortion of valve morphology (usually two instead of three cusps) with or without calcification (Fig. 8.17). Degenerative disease shows normal morphology invaded by annular to leaflet thickening and calcification (Fig. 8.18). Rheumatic disease manifests itself by leaflet tip thickening extending into valve leaflets with or without calcification.

Aortic Regurgitation

Aortic regurgitation may be congenital, degenerative, infectious, rheumatic, traumatic, or the result of distortion of the aortic root. Views used for aortic stenosis

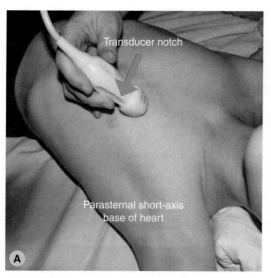

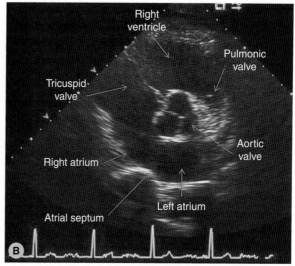

Obtaining the parasternal short-axis view (base of heart)

• From the parasternal long-axis view, rotate the transducer notch clockwise to approximately 2 o'clock.
• Tilt the transducer superiorly toward the patient's right shoulder while maintaining the notch position at 2 o'clock.

Figure 8.7. Correlation between transducer, notch position **(A)** and image **(B)** from parasternal short-axis view of the base of the heart. (*Courtesy of Jim Underwood.*)

serve well for aortic regurgitation. In addition, attention to suprasternal views may help identify important changes in the ascending aorta such as dissection, aneurysm, atherosclerotic change, and syphilitic "tree bark" thickening.

In acute cases, the left ventricular dimensions may be normal or nearly normal. Early closure of the mitral valve may be seen on two-dimensional (2D) image and quantified with M mode. Color Doppler will show brief, torrential flow confirmed by CW Doppler with

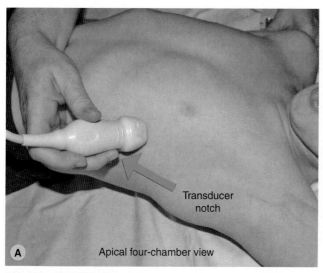

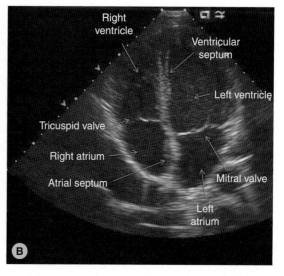

Obtaining the AP4 view

• Find the patient's point of maximal impulse (PMI).
• Place the transducer on the PMI, with the notch at approximately 3 o'clock.
• Slowly slide the transducer along rib space while maintaining the notch position; the transducer may have to be moved up or down a rib space.

Figure 8.8. **(A)** Correlation between the transducer (start at point of maximal impulse and slide transducer along rib space; the transducer may have to be moved up or down a rib space) and notch positions (approximately 3 o'clock) and **(B)** image obtained in the apical four-chamber (AP4) view. (*Courtesy of Jim Underwood.*)

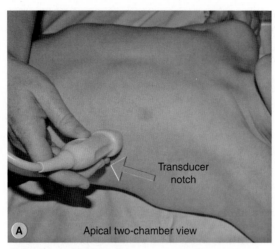
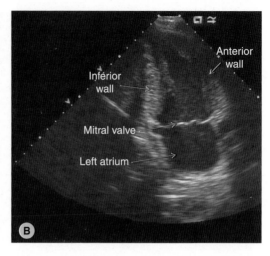

A — Transducer notch — Apical two-chamber view

B — Anterior wall — Inferior wall — Mitral valve — Left atrium

Obtaining the AP2 view
• From the AP4 view, rotate the transducer notch from the 3 o'clock to the 12 o'clock position.
• The AP3 view can be obtained by rotating the transducer notch slightly toward the 11 o'clock position.

Figure 8.9. **(A)** Correlation between the transducer (start at point of maximal impulse and slide the transducer along the rib space; the transducer may have to be moved up or down a rib space) and notch positions (approximately 12 o'clock) and **(B)** image obtained in the apical two-chamber view. AP, apical. (*Courtesy of Jim Underwood.*)

cessation of flow prior to the next systole. In this situation, dissection of the aorta, traumatic disruption of the aortic valve, or infectious vegetation may be anticipated.

In chronic cases, left ventricular dilatation will advance as the severity of the regurgitation increases. Color Doppler will provide an estimate of severity (Fig. 8.19). Larger jets are wider in the left ventricular outflow tract and fill the left ventricle to a larger extent. Estimates are best made as mild, moderate, or severe. Larger amounts of regurgitation are associated with greater degrees of left ventricular enlargement. CW Doppler images show more rapid decrease in diastolic flow with larger jets. Although M-mode and 2D volume measurements can prove helpful, these are best used for more painstaking, formal study.

Mitral Stenosis

Calcific mitral stenosis occurs when calcification extends from the mitral annulus into the valve leaflets. Usually this is seen in older, hypertensive patients. Often, dialysis accelerates the process. Moderate and severe calcific mitral stenosis is quite uncommon. Rheumatic mitral stenosis appears as leaflet thickening starting at the tips and extending into the valve leaflets with commissural fusion and progressive calcification. Chordae tendineae and papillary muscles are often involved. In the left parasternal long-axis

view, the anterior leaflet gives a "hockey stick" appearance in diastole (Fig. 8.20). In the left parasternal short-axis view at the base, the classic "fish mouth" appearance is seen (Fig. 8.21). Often, the diastolic valve area can be estimated with accuracy in this view, provided that distortion from calcification is limited. "Doming" appears in the apical and subxiphoid views. Pulsed interrogation at the level of the valve opening in these views will show a characteristic diastolic flow velocity curve with slower decay and tighter valve areas. Presystolic accentuation occurs in patients remaining in sinus rhythm and disappears with atrial fibrillation. In either case, an estimate of mitral valve area can be made by measuring the pressure half-time and using the equation: MVA = 220 / PHT, where MVA is the mitral valve area in square centimeters and PHT (pressure half-time) is the time in milliseconds for peak pressure to decay to 50% (or peak frequency shift to decay to 70%) (Fig. 8.22). This formula can be applied readily at the bedside in the absence of significant mitral and/or aortic regurgitation. Finally, an estimate of peak and mean gradient can be made by applying the equation used for aortic stenosis.

Mitral Regurgitation

Whereas mitral stenosis is now rare, mitral regurgitation is frequent. Murmur intensity and location often do not correlate well with regurgitant severity.

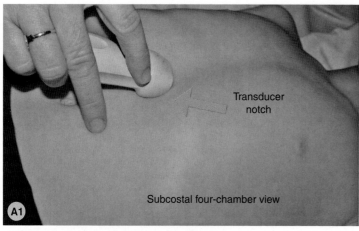

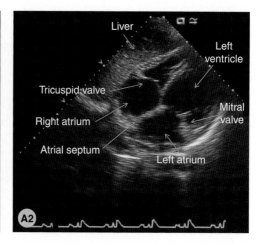

Obtaining the subcostal four-chamber view

- Place the transducer subxiphoid.
- The transducer notch should be at the 3 o'clock position.
- Try not to use too much pressure.

Obtaining the inferior vena cava view

- Rotate the transducer notch to the 12 o'clock position.

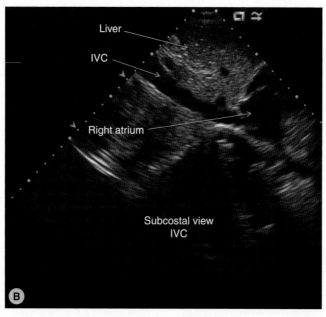

Figure 8.10. **(A)** Correlation between the transducer (subxiphoid) and notch positions (approximately 3 and 12 o'clock positions) **(A1)** and images obtained in the subcostal four-chamber view **(A2)**. **(B)** Inferior vena cava (IVC) view. (*Courtesy of Jim Underwood.*)

History, physical examination, electrocardiography, and chest radiography often do not adequately define the etiology and/or severity.

One should anticipate acute mitral regurgitation when heart failure or a new murmur accompanies ischemia or myocardial infarction. Papillary muscle dysfunction and rupture may be best appreciated from the apical and subxiphoid views. In the case of severe mitral regurgitation from rupture of a papillary

muscle head, emergent surgical repair improves survival. A point-of-care study can be lifesaving in these cases. Endocarditis and trauma may also lead to acute mitral regurgitation and require timely diagnosis and early intervention.

Mitral valve prolapse, coronary artery disease, dilated cardiomyopathy, mitral annular calcification, rheumatic heart disease, and endocarditis may all lead to chronic mitral regurgitation. With increasing volume

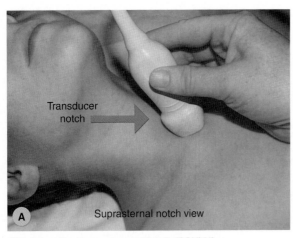

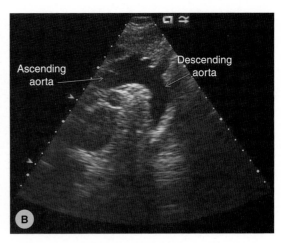

Obtaining the Suprasternal Notch (SSN) View

• Place the transducer in the suprasternal notch, with the transducer notch at the 12 o'clock position (notch to nose).
• Tilt the transducer laterally or medially to view the descending or ascending aorta.

Figure 8.11. (A) Correlation between the transducer (suprasternal) and notch positions at 12 o'clock (notch to nose) and **(B)** image obtained in the suprasternal notch view. Tilt the transducer laterally or medially to view the descending and ascending aorta. (*Courtesy of Jim Underwood.*)

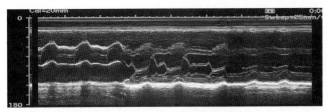

M-mode sweep in the parasternal long-axis view

Figure 8.12. M-mode sweep in the parasternal long-axis view position. (*Courtesy of Jim Underwood.*)

overload, the left ventricle dilates and then fails. With repair, the course of left ventricular failure can be arrested. This is not the case with mitral valve replacement, making serial studies essential for patients with mitral regurgitation. Repairable valves with severe regurgitation can be identified at the bedside and during an office visit. Progressive left ventricular dilatation and early deterioration in ejection fraction can be identified. Once again, color Doppler (Fig. 8.23) plays a large role in differentiating mild, moderate, and severe regurgitation. An eccentric jet should prompt

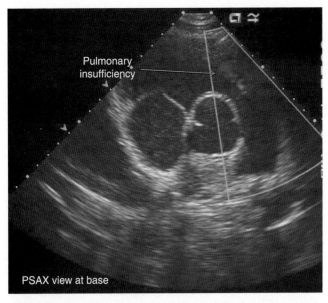

Figure 8.13. Pulmonary insufficiency (PI) diagnosed by color Doppler (mild PI is not an uncommon normal finding). PSAX, parasternal short axis. (*Courtesy of Jim Underwood.*)

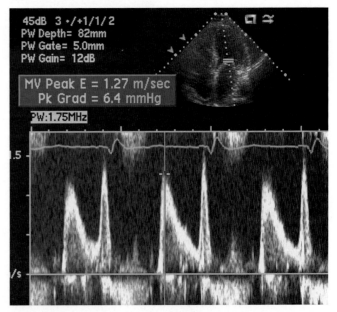

Figure 8.14. Pulsed wave Doppler image of the mitral valve flow. (*Courtesy of Jim Underwood.*)

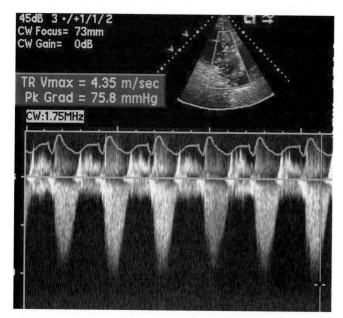

Figure 8.15. Continuous wave Doppler image of severe tricuspid insufficiency caused by chronic pulmonary hypertension due to repeated pulmonary emboli. Pulmonary artery pressure is greater than 75 mm Hg. (*Courtesy of Jim Underwood.*)

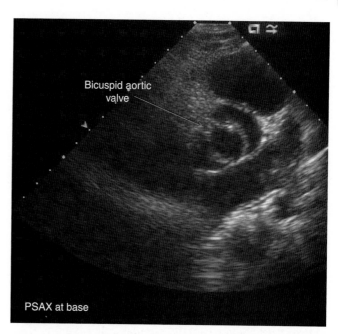

Figure 8.17. Parasternal short-axis (PSAX) view of the bicuspid aortic valve (note typical "football" appearance of the valve in systole). (*Courtesy of Jim Underwood.*)

extra caution because color Doppler study may underestimate the volume of the regurgitation. Efforts to quantify the regurgitant fraction are best left to a traditional full study. Comparison of pulsed Doppler left ventricular inflow and left ventricular outflow time velocity integrals multiplied by respective cross-sectional valve areas might be helpful for highly skilled operators. Similarly, interrogation of pulmonary vein

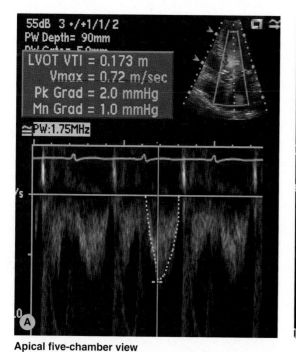

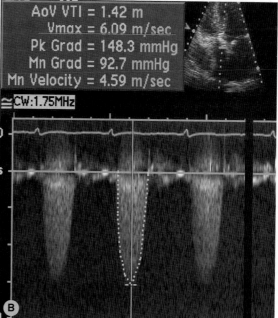

Apical five-chamber view

Image A: Doppler image of the left ventricular outflow tract.
Image B: Doppler image of the aortic valve.

Figure 8.16. Continuous wave Doppler image of the aortic valve flow. **(A)** Normal flow velocity. **(B)** Abnormally high flow velocity due to aortic stenosis. (*Courtesy of Jim Underwood.*)

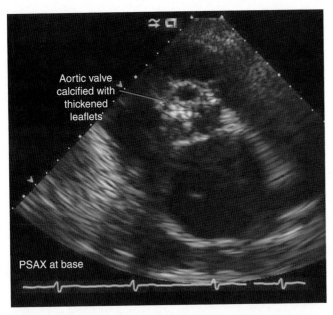

Figure 8.18. Severe aortic valvular calcification particularly involving the noncoronary cusp of the aortic valve. PSAX, parasternal short axis. (*Courtesy of Jim Underwood.*)

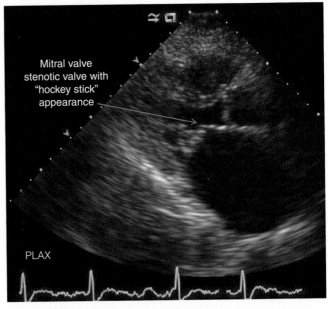

Figure 8.20. Rheumatic mitral stenosis, demonstrating the typical "hockey stick" appearance of the mitral valve in the parasternal long-axis view (PLAX). Note the grossly dilated left atrium. (*Courtesy of Jim Underwood.*)

patterns may be attempted. Serial 2D-directed M-mode measurement of mid–left ventricular dimensions at end diastole and end systole proves much easier to obtain and follow serially.

Pulmonic Stenosis

Pulmonic stenosis is best viewed in the left parasternal short-axis view at the base or the left parasternal right ventricular outflow tract view (Fig. 8.24). Pulmonic stenosis is most commonly congenital and may occur alone or in association with other etiologies. CW Doppler interrogation may give a good estimate of valve gradient, provided that care is taken to ensure the angle of interrogation does not exceed 30°. Unlike aortic stenosis, mild to moderate pulmonic stenosis usually does not progress. Severe pulmonic

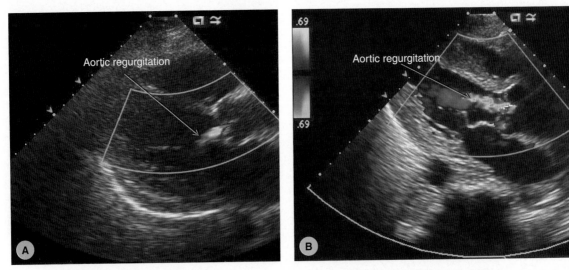

Figure 8.19. Parasternal long axis view Examples of aortic insufficiency (AI) (regurgitation) in the parasternal long-axis view. **(A)** Mild AI. **(B)** Moderate AI. (*Courtesy of Jim Underwood.*)

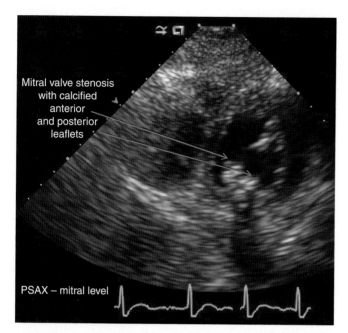

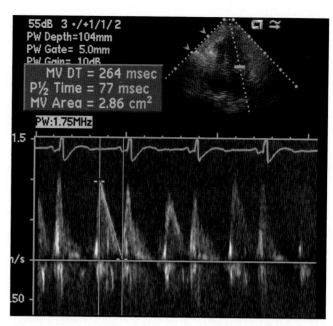

Figure 8.21. Calcific mitral valve stenosis in the parasternal short-axis (PSAX) view (mitral valve level). Severe mitral calcifications involve both the anterior and posterior leaflet. (*Courtesy of Jim Underwood.*)

Figure 8.22. A pressure half-time measurement in a patient with mitral stenosis is used to estimate mitral valve surface area. (*Courtesy of Jim Underwood.*)

stenosis with secondary right ventricular hypertrophy may require relief with balloon valvuloplasty, open valvotomy, or, in rare cases, prosthetic valve replacement.

Pulmonic Regurgitation

Small amounts of pulmonic regurgitation are commonly seen in normal hearts (Fig. 8.13). Larger amounts may be estimated by using Doppler techniques similar

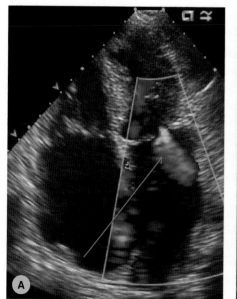
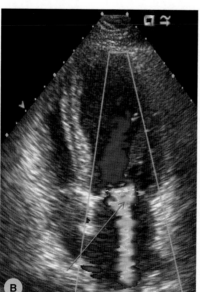
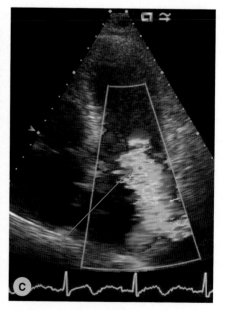

Figure 8.23. Apical four-chamber view. Mild **(A)**, moderate **(B)**, and severe **(C)** mitral regurgitation demonstrated by color Doppler in the apical four-chamber views during systole (*arrow*). Note the dilated left atrium in A and C. (*Courtesy of Jim Underwood.*)

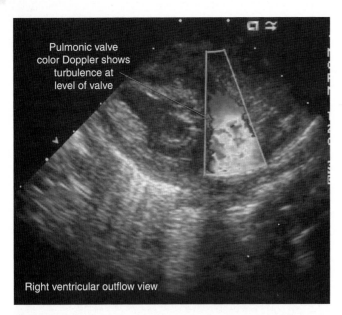

Pulmonic valve color Doppler shows turbulence at level of valve

Right ventricular outflow view

Figure 8.24. Pulmonic stenosis demonstrated by color Doppler in the right ventricular outflow view. (*Courtesy of Jim Underwood.*)

to those used in aortic insufficiency, taking into account secondary right ventricular enlargement. Color Doppler jet size, depth of penetration, and width of the vena contracta relative to the width of the right ventricular outflow tract are all helpful in judging the severity of regurgitation. Etiologies include congenital, infectious, idiopathic dilatation of the annulus, pulmonary hypertension, and trauma.

Tricuspid Valve Disease

With three leaflets of varying sizes, the tricuspid valve provides plenty of imaging challenge. The anterior leaflet is the largest and the septal leaflet the smallest, inserting in a more apical position than the anterior leaflet of the mitral valve. Anterior and posterior leaflets are seen in the right ventricular inflow tract view. Anterior and septal leaflets are seen in the left parasternal short-axis view at the base, the apical four-chamber view, and the subcostal four-chamber view.

Tricuspid Insufficiency

Small amounts of tricuspid insufficiency are common in normal hearts. Pathologic tricuspid regurgitation most often occurs from annular dilatation from pulmonary hypertension of any cause. Myxomatous change may lead to prolapse. Endocarditis may disrupt the valve or supporting structures. Trauma may lead to a chordal rupture.

Estimation of tricuspid regurgitation severity depends largely on study of the regurgitant jet with color Doppler imaging (Fig. 8.25). Jet width, depth of penetration, and jet area as compared to the right atrial area all help to estimate the severity of tricuspid incompetence. Examination of the inferior vena cava with increasing tricuspid regurgitation will reveal enlargement, systolic pulsation, blunting of respiratory variation, and retrograde systolic flow. Finally, in chronic states, right ventricular and atrial enlargement will occur commensurate with the degree of regurgitation.

CW interrogation of the tricuspid regurgitation jet can be used to estimate right ventricular peak systolic pressure using the equation: RV systolic pressure = $4 \times (V_{max} TR^2)$ + RAP, where RV systolic pressure is the right ventricular peak systolic pressure, $V_{max} TR^2$ is the peak CW velocity shift of the tricuspid regurgitant jet squared, and RAP is the estimated right atrial pressure (Fig. 8.15).

Tricuspid Stenosis

Congenital tricuspid stenosis is rare. Rheumatic involvement may be seen when rheumatic mitral stenosis is present. Carcinoid syndrome may lead to tricuspid stenosis without left-sided valvular involvement. Valve thickening is seen with restriction of valve opening. Pulsed and CW interrogation may be used to estimate valve gradient and valve area as with mitral stenosis.

CHAMBERS

Left Ventricle

Study of the left ventricle should be attempted in each standard view in the left parasternal, apical, and subxiphoid windows. Ultrasound unit settings must be optimized in each view to ensure adequate definition of the endocardium. If the endocardium is not visualized, measurements cannot be made in that segment, and wall motion abnormalities cannot be described. With good images, M-mode measurements can be made, and the ejection fraction can be estimated from visual inspection, M-mode–calculated estimation, and application of area-length formulas to apical four- and two-chamber views. Thickness of the mid–left ventricular intraventricular septum and posterior wall may be made using M mode (Fig. 8.26). M-mode assumptions and 2D volume calculations break down in the face of significant segmental wall motion abnormalities. For practical purposes, the point-of-care examiner might do well to describe subjective hypertrophy

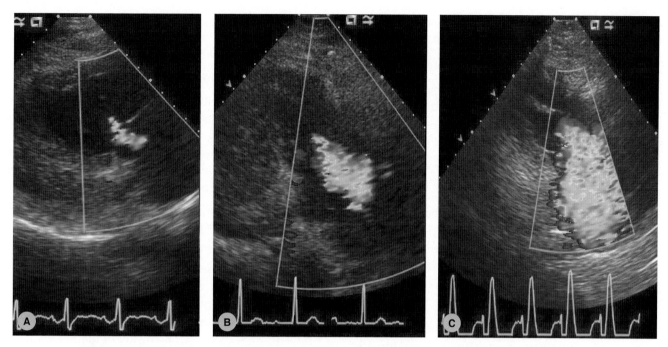

Figure 8.25. Parasternal long axis view (RV inflow view). Mild **(A),** moderate **(B),** and severe **(C)** tricuspid regurgitation demonstrated by color Doppler in the right ventricular inflow view. Note the dilated right atrium in B and C. (*Courtesy of Jim Underwood.*)

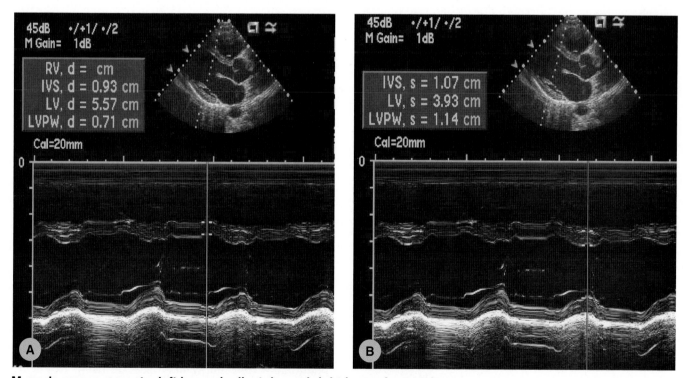

M-mode measurements; left image is diastole, and right image is systole.

Figure 8.26. Left ventricular diameter measurements by M mode in the parasternal long-axis view. **(A)** Diastole. **(B)** Systole. (*Courtesy of Jim Underwood.*)

(whether concentric or eccentric), enlargement, and decrements in systolic function as normal, mild, moderate, or severe, avoiding attempts at more precise quantification.

Cardiac output can be determined most easily by using Doppler interrogation. For example,

$$CO = \text{Stroke volume} \times HR = VTI\ lvot \times CSA\ lvot \times HR,$$

where

CO = cardiac output

VTI lvot = velocity time integral of the left ventricular outflow tract

CSA lvot = cross-sectional area of the left ventricular outflow tract = $(lvot\ radius)^2 \times 3.14$

HR = heart rate

Left Ventricle with Coronary Artery Disease

Using all available windows and with careful attention to endocardial definition, the examiner should identify each myocardial segment and describe motion as normal, hypokinetic (reduced motion), akinetic (no motion), or dyskinetic (reverse-direction motion). Filling defects (thrombus) should be sought, especially at the apex and in areas of akinesis and dyskinesis (Fig. 8.27). Although an estimate of left ventricular ejection fraction may be made, more formal measurement of ejection fraction using an area-length formula usually will not be pursued during a point-of-care

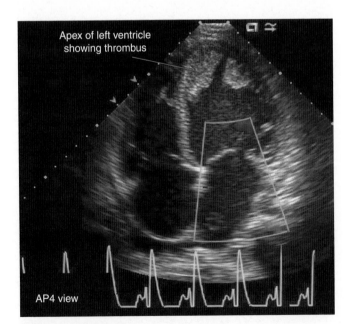

Figure 8.27. Apical thrombus in the left ventricle (*arrow*) is likely the result of apical akinesis due to the myocardial infarction. AP4, apical four-chamber. (*Courtesy of Jim Underwood.*)

examination. When endocardial definition proves inadequate, more formal study with intravenous contrast should be considered (Fig. 8.28).

Dilated Cardiomyopathy

Images of idiopathic dilated cardiomyopathy show as expected, left ventricular enlargement with myocardial thinning and generalized hypokinesis (Fig. 8.29). Left ventricular thrombi and enlargement of the left atrium, right ventricle, and right atrium are often seen as well. Because of annular dilatation and distortion of dynamic valve support structures, varying degrees of mitral insufficiency may be expected.

Hypertrophic Cardiomyopathy

Most cases of hypertrophic cardiomyopathy exhibit asymmetric septal hypertrophy, where the proximal intraventricular septum extending into the midseptum measures greater than 1.4 times the thickness of the opposite wall. Dynamic narrowing of the left ventricular outflow tract in systole often results, with accompanying systolic anterior motion of the anterior leaflet of the mitral valve with a gradient in systole (Fig. 8.30). Less common variants include apical and midventricular hypertrophic cardiomyopathy.

Restrictive Cardiomyopathy

Restrictive cardiomyopathies usually exhibit preserved systolic function, concentric left ventricular hypertrophy, and restrictive filling patterns seen with pulsed Doppler interrogation of the left ventricular inflow tract. With amyloidosis, a speckled myocardial pattern may be seen, although this pattern may be artifactually produced with excessive gain.

Noncompaction of the Left Ventricle

Noncompaction of the left ventricle is a cardiomyopathy characterized by systolic and diastolic dysfunction. This rare pathology can be readily diagnosed with 2D echocardiography (Fig. 8.31).

Left Ventricular Diastolic Function

Echocardiographic opportunities for the study of left ventricular diastolic function continue to emerge. For practical point-of-care applications, however, pulsed interrogation of the left ventricular inflow tract just distal to the tips of the mitral valve in diastole will produce four patterns (Fig. 8.32). A pseudonormal pattern may be unmasked by interrogating before, during, and after a Valsalva maneuver. Although interrogation of pulmonary vein inflow may also be used, this technique often proves difficult and unrewarding at the bedside with highly portable equipment, limited time, and less-than-expert transducer skills.

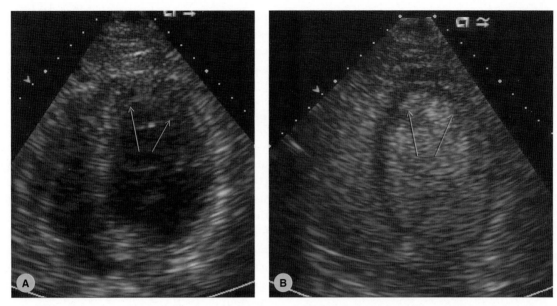

Figure 8.28. Apical 4 Chamber View **(A)** Left ventricle endocardium is difficult to visualize (*arrows*). **(B)** Use of the intravenous echo contrast to better visualize the left ventricular chamber and endocardium. (*Courtesy of Jim Underwood.*)

Left Atrium

The left atrium is best studied from the apical and sub-costal views and the volume estimated from these views (Fig. 8.33). The subcostal four-chamber view and the left parasternal short-axis view at the base provide good definition of the interatrial septum. An atrial myxoma may rarely be seen emanating from the septum. Left atrium thrombi are quite rare and are usually associated with tight mitral stenosis. Pulmonary veins prove more difficult to visualize. The left atrial appendage proves most difficult to image through a transthoracic approach unless three-dimensional echocardiography is employed.

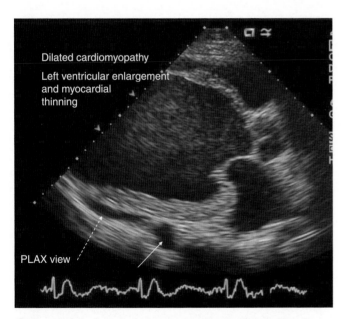

Figure 8.29. Severe dilative cardiomyopathy in the parasternal long-axis (PLAX) view. Note the left ventricular dilatation, myocardial thinning, pericardial effusion (*interrupted arrow*), and coronary sinus (*solid arrow*). (*Courtesy of Jim Underwood.*)

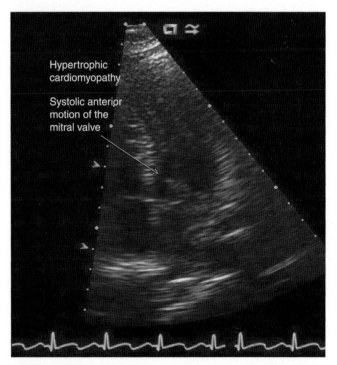

Figure 8.30. Hypertrophic cardiomyopathy with typical systolic anterior motion of the mitral valve in systole, demonstrated in the apical four-chamber view. (*Courtesy of Jim Underwood.*)

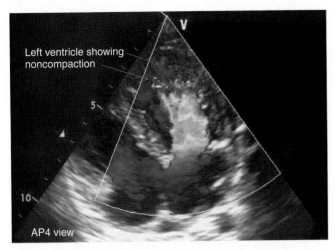

Figure 8.31. Noncompaction of the left ventricle. AP4, apical four-chamber. (*Courtesy of Jim Underwood.*)

Right Ventricle

The right ventricle (RV) can be well seen in apical and subcostal views plus the left parasternal right ventricular inflow tract view. RV free wall thickness can be measured using M mode with upper limits of normal at 5 mm. Chamber enlargement can be estimated. In general, the transverse diameter at the atrioventricular valve level of the RV should not exceed 40% of the total transverse diameter of the RV and left ventricle combined at that level (Fig. 8.34). A moderator band is commonly seen. Pacemaker leads and right heart catheters are easily identified. In right ventricular dysplasia, enlargement and thinning are seen.

Right Atrium

Views that show the RV well also show the right atrium (RA) well. The proximal inferior vena cava (IVC) can often be well defined with rotation of the transducer notch to 12 o'clock in the subxiphoid window (Fig. 8.10B). The interatrial septum can be studied with ease. A eustachian valve or Chiari network must be recognized as normal variants. Right heart catheters, pacemaker leads, thrombi, and rare tumors such as renal cell carcinomas and atrial myxomas may be seen in the RA.

PERICARDIUM

Normal pericardium, visceral and parietal, forms a thin, membranous, serosal sac extending from posterior attachments and encircling the majority of the heart. Only a very small amount of fluid is present in this sac in the normal state, just enough to "lubricate" as the myocardium constantly moves in the thorax. Pericardium and fluid are not usually seen unless fluid

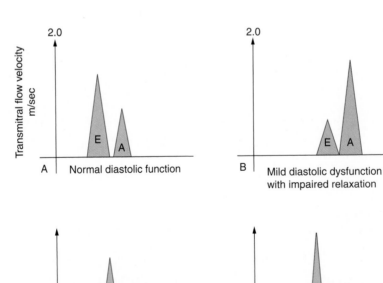

Figure 8.32. Diastolic flow patterns showing normal versus impaired dilatation. The E wave represents passive filling of the ventricle and the A wave represents active filling of the ventricle during atrial systole. (*Courtesy of Jim Underwood.*)

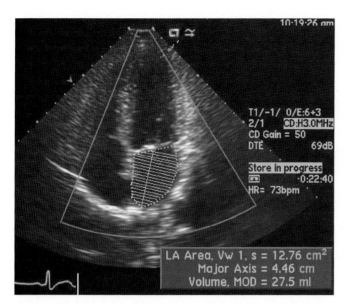

Figure 8.33. Left atrial surface calculation in the apical four-chamber view. (*Courtesy of Jim Underwood.*)

accumulates and/or thickening of the membranes occurs.

Pericardial Effusion

Pericardial effusions are easily seen in left parasternal, apical, and subxiphoid views. Effusions are described as small (<1 cm), moderate (1–2 cm), or large (>2 cm) as measured posteriorly (Fig. 8.35). Shaggy-appearing adherent tissue in some cases may represent involvement by chronic infection or inflammation. Masses imply neoplastic involvement. Pericardial effusion must be differentiated from chronic obstructive pulmonary disease, anterior mediastinal masses or adiposity, and pleural effusion. Although loculated pericardial effusions occur, most often after cardiac surgery, an anterior clear space without other evidence of pericardial fluid can usually be attributed to the other etiologies, with further study dictated by the clinical situation. When pleural and pericardial effusions coexist, identification of parietal pericardium allows differentiation (Fig. 8.36).

Effusion and Tamponade

When enough pericardial fluid accumulates, pressure within the pericardial sac increases, and restriction to normal cardiac filling occurs. This may occur with rapid accumulation of small to moderate amounts of fluid or with slow accumulation of large amounts of fluid. This state of cardiac tamponade leads to diastolic collapse of the right atrium and right ventricle (Fig. 8.37). This state increases with inspiration and leads to concomitant compromise of left ventricular filling. Apical and subxiphoid four-chamber views prove

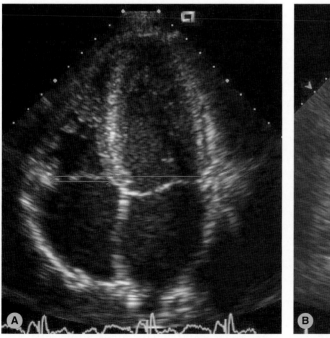
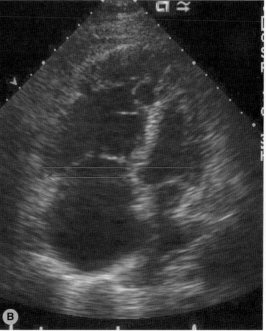

Figure 8.34. Normal **(A)** versus dilated **(B)** right ventricle. (*Courtesy of Jim Underwood.*)

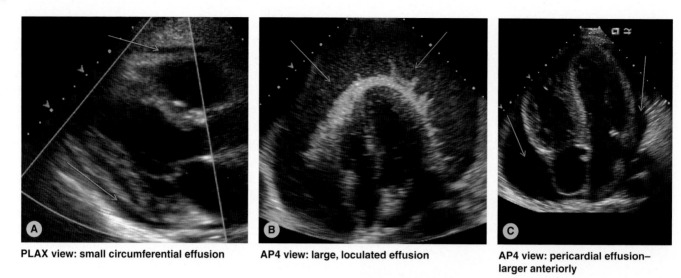

PLAX view: small circumferential effusion **AP4 view: large, loculated effusion** **AP4 view: pericardial effusion–larger anteriorly**

Figure 8.35. **(A)** Small pericardial effusion in parasternal long-axis view (PLAX) (*arrow*). **(B)** Large effusions in apical four-chamber (AP4) views. Large, loculated effusion. **(C)** Pericardial Effusion larger anteriorly. (*Courtesy of Jim Underwood.*)

particularly helpful in seeing the right heart diastolic compromise. The left parasternal short-axis view demonstrates systolic flattening of the intraventricular septum, which also shows respiratory variation. Finally, pulsed and CW interrogation of left ventricular inflow and outflow tracts show greater than 10% respiratory variation in diastolic and systolic frequency shifts, respectively, when a cardiac tamponade state occurs (Fig. 8.38).

Constriction

Pericardial constriction ensues when pericardial stiffening occurs secondary to fibrosis, thickening, and/or calcification. A chronic process, constriction may follow tuberculosis, other infection, collagen vascular disease, trauma, radiation, and cardiac surgery. If both pericardial and pleural effusions are present, pericardial

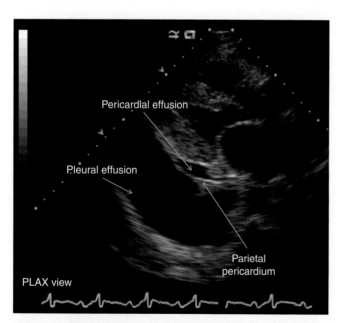

Figure 8.36. Large pleural and small pericardial effusions. PLAX, parasternal long-axis. (*Courtesy of Jim Underwood.*)

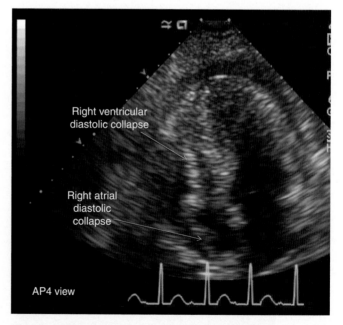

Figure 8.37. Pericardial tamponade is defined by restrictive diastolic filling. Note the right ventricular and right atrial collapse in diastole. AP4, apical four-chamber. (*Courtesy of Jim Underwood.*)

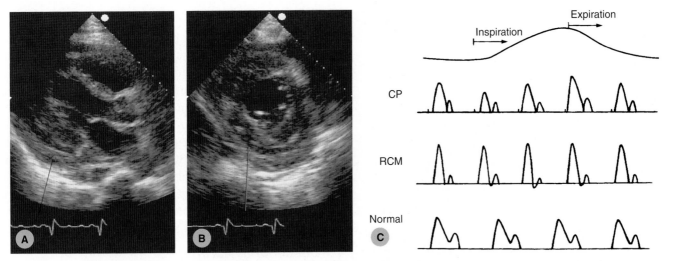

Figure 8.38. Combination of pericardial effusion and pericardial constriction in parasternal long-axis **(A)** and parasternal short-axis **(B)** views. **(C)** Restrictive versus constrictive versus normal Doppler flow pattern through the mitral valve. RCM, restrictive cardiomyopathy; CP, constrictive pericarditis. (*Image courtesy of David Adams, Duke University.*)

thickening can be diagnosed if parietal pericardium exceeds 2 mm. M-mode study may show abrupt movement of the posterior wall of the left ventricle in diastole with little movement thereafter. The septum may show an early diastolic notch. Study of inferior vena cava (IVC) may show dilatation and lack of respiratory variation in IVC diameter.

With Doppler interrogation of left ventricular inflow, an increase in the E/A waves ratio with rapid deceleration time and greater than 25% respiratory variation of E velocity can be seen. Significant respiratory distress may mimic these findings, and hypovolemia and hypervolemia may mask them. When available, tissue Doppler study shows rapid early diastolic relaxation.

Effusive-Constrictive Pericarditis

The point-of-care echocardiographer must remember that significant pericardial effusion with or without tamponade may coexist with constriction. From a practical standpoint, removal of pericardial fluid and relief of tamponade lead to partial or no relief of hemodynamic compromise, and the clinical, echocardiographic, and Doppler pictures afterward point to constriction (Fig. 8.38).

Constriction versus Restriction

With restrictive cardiomyopathy (i.e., amyloid), ventricular thickening and biatrial enlargement are seen. There is little respiratory variation in E velocity, and little variation is seen in hepatic vein flow. Tissue Doppler diastolic velocities are normal or reduced, not increased, as seen with constriction.

GREAT VESSELS

Aorta

Ascending Aorta

The best imaging of the ascending aorta may be attained from the left parasternal short- and long-axis plus suprasternal notch views. Apical and subxiphoid windows provide only limited images of the aortic root. Atherosclerotic change and increased reflectance from calcification are often seen. In cases of dissection involving the ascending aorta, a dissection flap with true and false lumens may be seen (Fig. 8.39). Use of color Doppler and several views reduces the likelihood of a false-positive diagnosis from reverberation artifact. Concomitant aortic insufficiency and pericardial effusion may also be defined. These findings prompt further emergency imaging confirmation, consultation, and potential lifesaving emergency surgical repair.

Similar views are employed in the identification and follow-up of aneurysms of the ascending aorta and sinuses of Valsalva. In general, ascending aortic aneurysms of greater than 5 cm in transverse diameter should be considered for surgical repair. Sinus of Valsalva aneurysms may be quite large. They often lead to associated aortic insufficiency and may rupture into the right atrium more often than into the left atrium.

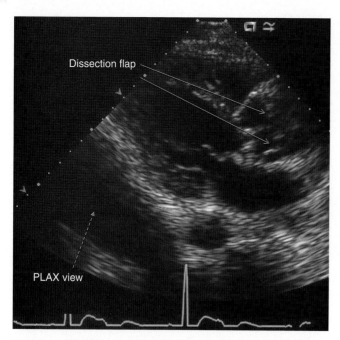

Figure 8.39. Dissection of the thoracic aorta at the knob in the parasternal long-axis view (PLAX) (*solid arrows*). Note the pleural effusion (*interrupted arrow*). (*Courtesy of Jim Underwood.*)

Transverse Aorta

In adult patients, only the suprasternal window provides reasonable access to transthoracic study of the aortic arch. Dissection, aneurysm, atherosclerotic change, and major branch compromise may be seen. On occasion, coarctation may be seen, particularly when aided by color Doppler. CW Doppler can be used to estimate the systolic gradient across the coarctation (Fig. 8.40). Similarly, patent ductus arteriosus can be seen. This anomaly also may be seen with color Doppler–aided interrogation of the pulmonary artery from the left parasternal short-axis view with the transducer angulated to focus on the pulmonary artery.

Descending Aorta

Left parasternal long- and short-axis views provide good visualization of the descending thoracic aorta. Atherosclerotic change, dissection, and aneurysm may all be seen. Fluid posterior to the aorta in this view is most likely pleural effusion; fluid anterior to the aorta is most likely pericardial effusion. An intra-aortic balloon counterpulsation device may be readily imaged when present.

Main Pulmonary Artery

The main pulmonary artery and proximal left and right pulmonary arteries are best seen from the left

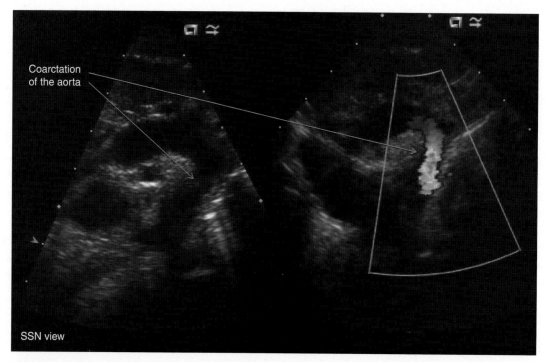

Figure 8.40. Aortic coarctation in the jugular notch view is confirmed by color Doppler demonstrating increased flow velocity through the coarctation (*arrows*). SSN, suprasternal notch. (*Courtesy of Jim Underwood.*)

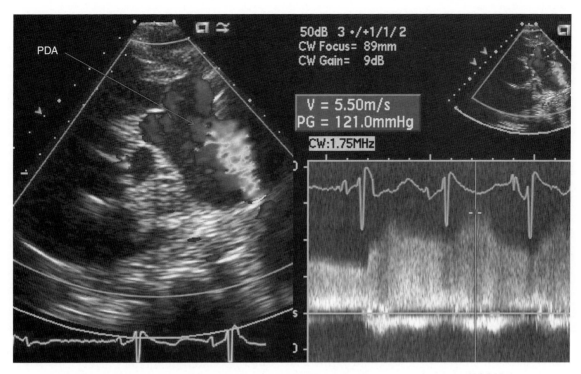

Figure 8.41. Patent ductus arteriosus in the parasternal short-axis view (PSAX) confirmed by color Doppler. (*Courtesy of Jim Underwood.*)

parasternal short-axis view with the transducer angulated superiorly. Aneurysms may be seen on rare occasions. A patent ductus arteriosus also may appear (Fig. 8.41). Very rarely, a large thrombus (saddle embolus) may be defined (Fig. 8.42). This finding may prove lifesaving in an acutely and severely ill patient, but such study should not be used to exclude pulmonary embolism, nor should it delay more definitive imaging or treatment.

Inferior Vena Cava and Hepatic Veins

The subxiphoid window with the transducer notch angulated to 12 o'clock usually gives a good look at the inferior vena cava extending from the inferior right atrium to the hepatic veins (Fig. 8.10B). In adults, the IVC measures less than 20 mm in greatest transverse diameter. Larger measurements imply pressure or volume overload. Blunting of respiratory variation in this measurement indicates further increase in right atrial filling pressure. A normal IVC implies an RAP equal to 5 mm Hg; a dilated IVC implies an RAP equal to 10 mm Hg; and a dilated IVC without respiratory variation implies an RAP equal to 15 mm Hg. Similarly, hepatic vein interrogation may show systolic flow dominance with mild tricuspid regurgitation, systolic blunting with moderate tricuspid regurgitation, and systolic reversal with severe tricuspid regurgitation.

SHUNTS

Two-dimensional echocardiography coupled with color Doppler provides a powerful tool for the detection, localization, and subjective quantification of shunts. Further, an estimate of unidirectional shunt severity for ventricular and atrial septal defects can be made by comparing right ventricular outflow tract to left ventricular outflow tract velocity time integrals:

$$Qp/Qs = VTI\ rvot \times CSA\ rvot\ /\ VTI\ lvot \times CSA\ lvot$$

where Qp is pulmonary flow, Qs is systemic flow, VTI rvot is the velocity time integral of the right ventricular outflow tract, CSA rvot is the cross-sectional area of the right ventricular outflow tract, VTI lvot is the velocity time integral of the left ventricular outflow tract, and CSA lvot is the cross-sectional area of the left ventricular outflow tract.

Most shunts are best detected using apical and subxiphoid windows (Figs. 8.43 and 8.44). In all cases, the transducer should be carefully angulated and rotated

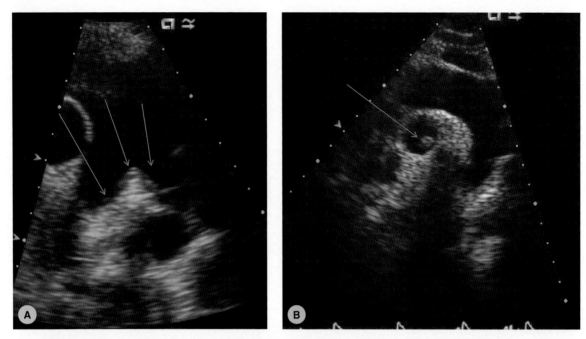

Figure 8.42. **(A)** Pulmonary saddle embolism in the parasternal short-axis view (PSAX) above the aortic valve level (*arrows*). Note the dilated pulmonary artery. **(B)** Additional thrombus in the right pulmonary artery in the same patient. (*Courtesy of Jim Underwood.*)

through standard views to cover the entire cardiac anatomy. Left parasternal short-axis views may prove crucial when studying shunts involving the base of the heart and those involving sinus of Valsalva aneurysms, endocarditis, and membranous ventricular septal defects. Finally, as noted previously, study of patent ductus arteriosus in the adult may require use of suprasternal notch imaging (Fig. 8.45).

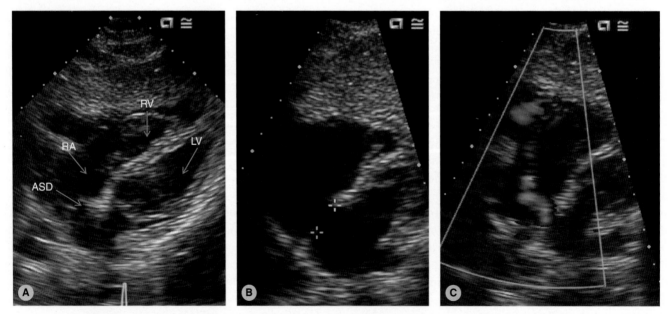

Figure 8.43. Atrial septal defect (ASD) in the subcostal (subxiphoid) views **(A, B)** is confirmed by Doppler flow **(C)** across the atrial septum. LV, left ventricle; RA, right atrium; RV, right ventricle. (*Courtesy of Jim Underwood.*)

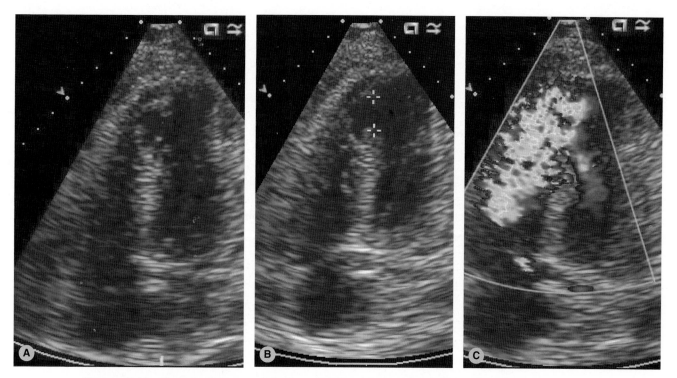

Figure 8.44. Ventricular septal defect (VSD). **(A, B)** confirmed by Doppler flow **(C)** across the ventricular septum. (*Courtesy of Jim Underwood.*)

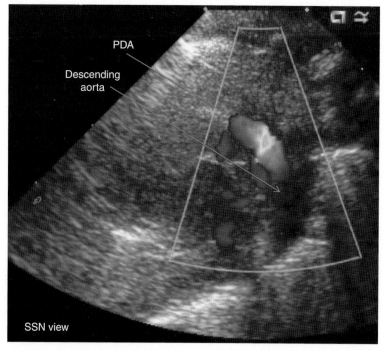

Figure 8.45. A patent ductus arteriosus (PDA) in an adult patent is demonstrated in a suprasternal notch (SSN) view. (*Courtesy of Jim Underwood.*)

Suggested Readings

Beaulieu Y, Marik P. Bedside ultrasonography in the ICU, part 1. *Chest.* 2005;128:881.

Beaulieu Y, Marik P. Bedside ultrasonography in the ICU, part 2. *Chest.* 2005;128:1766.

Fiegenbaum H, Armstrong W, Ryan T. *Feigenbaum's Echocardiography.* 6th ed. Philadelphia, PA: Lippincott Williams & Wilkins; 2005.

Lang R, Bierig M, Devereux R, et al. Recommendations for chamber quantification: a report from the American Society of Echocardiography's Guidelines and Standards Committee and the Chamber Quantification Writing Group, developed in conjunction with the European Association of Echocardiography, a branch of the European Society of Cardiology. *J Am Soc Echocardiogr.* 2005;18:1440.

Levitov A, Mayo P, Slonim A. *Critical Care Ultrasonography.* New York, NY: McGraw-Hill; 2009.

Nagueh S, Appleton C, Gillebert T, et al. Recommendations for the evaluation of left ventricular diastolic function by echocardiography. *J Am Soc Echocardiogr.* 2009;22:107.

Otto C. *Textbook of Clinical Echocardiography.* 3rd ed. Philadelphia, PA: WB Saunders; 2004.

CHAPTER 9

Stress Echocardiography

Michael Wiid, MD, FACP; Marguerite Underwood, RN, RDCS;
Sharan Ramaswamy, PhD; and Krish Ramachandran, MD

INTRODUCTION

Stress echocardiography is a well-established, extensively used technique in cardiology. Its application, specifically for the detection of coronary artery disease (CAD), and the implications that can be inferred for prognosis in a variety of clinical settings are reviewed here to familiarize the primary care provider with this technique.

Oxygen consumption of the heart muscle is determined by heart rate, systolic blood pressure, left ventricular end-diastolic volume, wall thickness, and contractility.[1] The heart is predominantly dependant on aerobic metabolism, with minimal capacity to generate energy through anaerobic metabolism. Coronary circulation exhibits maximal oxygen extraction at rest. Increasing perfusion is the only mechanism available to the heart to increase oxygen consumption. Myocardial oxygen consumption and coronary blood flow in normal individuals are linearly related. Decreasing the resistance at the coronary arteriolar level is the main mechanism to increase coronary blood flow during exercise. In patients with CAD, a threshold exists for ischemia and exercise. Beyond this threshold, additional limitations to blood flow can produce abnormalities in systolic and diastolic ventricular function, electrocardiographic changes, and chest pain. Because of the additional demand imposed by increased wall tension, the subendocardium is more susceptible to myocardial ischemia than the subepicardium. Increases in myocardial oxygen demand during exercise and inadequate coronary flow resulting from obstructive CAD or the inability of vessels to sufficiently vasodilate because of abnormal endothelial function result in regional myocardial ischemia.

Myocardial ischemia causes electrical gradients resulting in ST-segment depression or elevation, depending on the surface electrocardiographic leads being monitored, but usually results in ST-segment depression; ST-segment elevation is an uncommon occurrence indicative of more severe coronary flow reduction. Exercise-induced wall motion abnormality (WMA) precedes angina or ST-segment changes.

Stress echocardiography was introduced in 1979 and has developed into a robust technique for identifying patients with CAD and determining prognosis[2-7] (Fig. 9.1). The rationale for its use is that cardiovascular stress will result in ischemia, which in turn is manifested as a regional WMA distal to an obstructive coronary lesion. In addition to its role in CAD, stress echocardiography can be used to assess the severity of valvular heart disease and to detect occult pulmonary hypertension and the development of dynamic left ventricular outflow tract obstruction with exercise. In 1990, the American College of Cardiology endorsed stress echocardiography as a "valuable adjunct to the workup of patients with known or suspected CAD as a valid, clinically useful and accepted procedure."[2,7] Figure 9.2 demonstrates an algorithm for the evaluation and management of patients suspected of having an acute coronary syndrome. The versatility, rapid availability of results, relatively low cost, and excellent diagnostic yield of stress echocardiography have brought this procedure to the forefront of noninvasive evaluation of CAD.

METHODOLOGY

Either exercise or pharmacologic stress with dobutamine or atropine can be used.[3,4,6-12] Although supine and upright bicycles have been used, treadmills are the most widely used exercise modality in the United States.[13] The most frequently used pharmacologic agent for stress echocardiography in the United States is dobutamine, possibly with the addition of atropine if an adequate heart rate response during peak dobutamine infusion cannot be achieved. If postexercise imaging is used, it is imperative that the imaging be completed within 60 seconds to avoid the resolution of stress-induced WMA.[14] For those unable to exercise, dobutamine can be infused in 3-minute stages from 5 µg/kg/min up to 40 µg/kg/min; atropine 0.25 to 1 mg intravenous push can be administered during peak dobutamine infusion for an

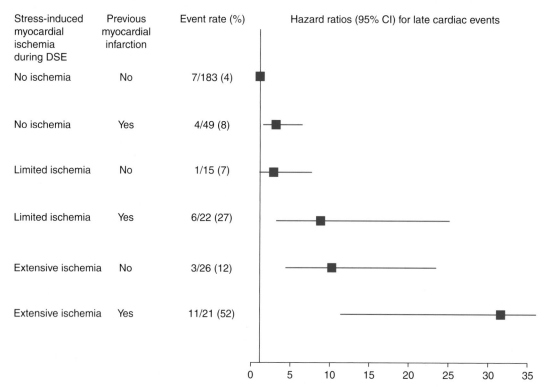

Stress-induced myocardial ischemia during DSE	Previous myocardial infarction	Event rate (%)	Hazard ratios (95% CI) for late cardiac events
No ischemia	No	7/183 (4)	
No ischemia	Yes	4/49 (8)	
Limited ischemia	No	1/15 (7)	
Limited ischemia	Yes	6/22 (27)	
Extensive ischemia	No	3/26 (12)	
Extensive ischemia	Yes	11/21 (52)	

Figure 9.1. Long-term prognostic value of dobutamine stress echocardiography (DSE) results in addition to a history of myocardial infarction in patients undergoing major vascular surgery. (*Reproduced with permission from Kertai MD, Poldermans D. The utility of dobutamine stress echocardiography for perioperative and long-term cardiac risk assessment.* J Cardiothorac Vasc Anesth. *2005;19:520–528.*)

inadequate heart rate response. Age-predicted maximum predicted heart rate (AMPHR) of at least 85% is desirable to detect CAD with optimal sensitivity.

Stress echocardiography requires a comparison of echocardiographic data obtained at the time of or after stress with baseline resting data.[15,16] It is essential to review resting and stress images side by side using digital acquisition and display. By allowing several successive cardiac cycles to be captured and stored in memory, digitized echocardiography enhances the capability of acquiring satisfactory comparative postexercise images. The most satisfactory poststress images are selected and compared with baseline images using side-by-side quadruple-screen displays.[4,6–12,17–20] If contrast is used for endocardial enhancement, the contrast harmonics preset has to be switched.[20–22] Harmonic imaging by itself offers clinically significant improvement in endocardial visualization. Tissue harmonic imaging allows the clinician to detect higher frequencies than the one transmitted, resulting in a dramatic reduction in image artifacts, haze, and clutter and a significant enhancement in endocardial visualization.[21–24]

EQUIPMENT AND PERSONNEL NEEDS

1. The examination room should be equipped with resuscitation equipment.

2. Two-dimensional (2D) Doppler echocardiographic instrumentation with fundamental, harmonic, contrast harmonics package with digital acquisition and storage capability that can display images side by side in a quadruple-screen format.[3,6–9,20]

3. Motorized treadmill.

4. Twelve-channel electrocardiographic (ECG) monitoring device.

5. Specially designed echocardiographic beds with cutout windows to facilitate imaging from the apex. Spatial organization of the room's equipment is essential for minimizing the time for the patient to get off the treadmill to the bed and assume a left lateral decubitus position.

6. Intravenous infusion pump and syringes to administer contrast and atropine and other necessary medications as needed.

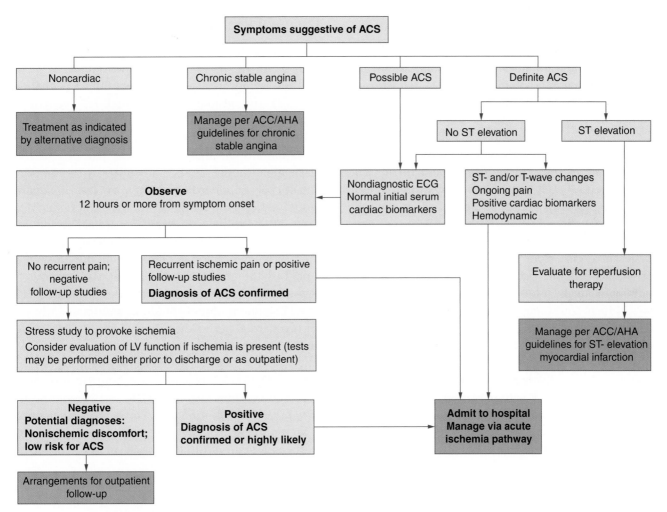

Figure 9.2. American College of Cardiology (ACC)/American Heart Association (AHA) algorithm for evaluation and management of patients suspected of having acute coronary syndrome (ACS). ECG, electrocardiogram; LV, left ventricular. (*Reproduced with permission from Anderson JL, Adams CD, Antman EM, et al. 2007 guidelines for the management of patients with unstable angina/non–ST-elevation myocardial infarction: executive summary: a report of the American College of Cardiology/American Heart Association Task Force on Practice Guidelines. Circulation. 2007;116:803–877. [© 2007 American Heart Association, Inc.]*)

The 12-lead ECG is monitored by an ECG technician while the sonographer obtains images before and after exercise. The study can be supervised by a registered nurse who is trained in exercise physiology.[4]

A physician who is well trained in stress testing, both performing and interpreting stress echocardiograms, should be present in the building where stress testing is performed and must be immediately available for any assistance and in making appropriate clinical and management decisions.

PATIENT PREPARATION

The patient should abstain from oral intake for 2 hours before the procedure. Unless requested by the clinician, the patient's medications are not interrupted before exercise testing; however, it is imperative to hold beta blockers for 24 hours prior to a dobutamine stress test. A brief history that is focused on the documentation of risk factors for CAD, past events related to CAD, chest pain pattern, and medications should be obtained before the exercise test. Results of relevant laboratory tests including hemoglobin, electrolyte panel, and cardiac enzyme markers should be reviewed as appropriate.[3,6,7] The patient is then oriented to the room and instructed to return to the examination table as quickly as possible after exercising. The 12 ECG leads are positioned; lead V2 is moved one space higher than normal, and leads V5 and V6 are placed one interspace lower to avoid interference with the usual echocardiographic windows.

IMAGING

Resting echocardiographic images are obtained from the parasternal and apical windows. Four standard views are acquired: (1) parasternal long axis, (2) parasternal short axis, (3) apical four chamber, and (4) apical two chamber[2–4,6,7,9–12,19] (Fig. 9.3). In some laboratories, additional apical long-axis and apical short-axis views are acquired, especially if the visualization of the apex is suboptimal on apical four-chamber and apical two-chamber views.[3,6,7] The study is recorded on a videotape, a simultaneous representative cardiac cycle is acquired and digitized, and each of the views is stored digitally. These same four views are acquired immediately postexercise. Four sets of images are acquired with a dobutamine protocol (i.e., rest, low-dose dobutamine, peak dobutamine, and recovery). Each view will have four images in a quadruple-screen format demonstrating the same view in four different stages of the dobutamine stress protocol. The acquisition of poststress images is challenging because of lung and motion artifacts and the limited time window after exercise; however, with current instrumentation, several consecutive cardiac cycles can be captured and the images from the best cycle selected and compared with resting images.

DIAGNOSTIC CRITERIA

The interpretation of the test has two parts: (1) the results of the exercise test (workload achieved, AMPHR, symptoms, arrhythmias, and ECG changes) and (2) the global and regional left ventricular response to stress.[2–4,6–9,12,19] Interpretation of the echocardiographic study necessitates a detailed semiquantitative analysis with the use of either the 16-segment model, as recommended by the American Society of Echocardiography,[25] or the 17-segment model, as recommended by the American Heart Association Writing Group on Myocardial Segmentation and Registration for Cardiac Imaging in 2002.[26] The 17-segment model differs from the 16-segment model by the addition of the apical cap, which is the segment beyond the end of the left ventricular cavity. The 17-segment model should be predominantly used for myocardial perfusion studies,[25] and the 16-segment model is appropriate for studies assessing WMAs, since the tip of the normal apex (segment 17) does not move.[25] Figure 9.4 provides a schematic representation of the various segments. The corresponding coronary artery distribution of the myocardial segments is depicted in Fig. 9.5. Each segment is analyzed individually and scored on the basis of its motion and

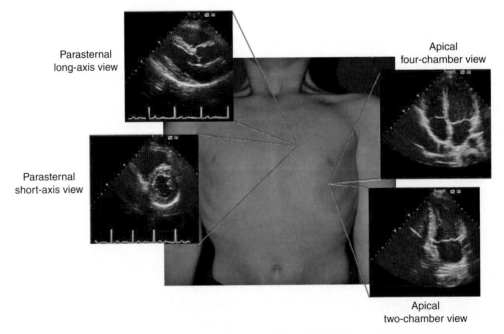

Parasternal long-axis view

Apical four-chamber view

Parasternal short-axis view

Apical two-chamber view

Figure 9.3. Approximate probe positioning and representative still images of standard parasternal long-axis, parasternal short-axis, apical four-chamber, and apical two-chamber views.

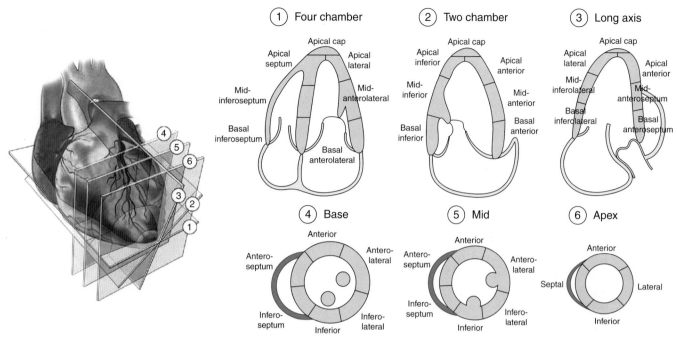

Figure 9.4. Segmental analysis of left ventricular walls based on schematic views, in a parasternal short- and long-axis orientation, at three different levels. The "apex segments" are usually visualized from apical four-chamber, apical two-chamber, and apical three-chamber views. The apical cap can be appreciated only on some contrast studies. (*Reproduced with permission from Lang RM, Bierig M, Devereux RB et al. Recommendations for chamber quantification: a report from the American Society of Echocardiography's Guidelines and Standards Committee and the Chamber Quantification Writing Group, developed in conjunction with the European Association of Echocardiography, a branch of the European Society of Cardiology.* J Am Soc Echocardiogr. *2005;1:1440–1463.*)

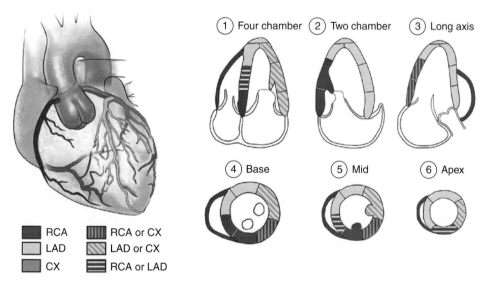

Figure 9.5. Typical distributions of the right coronary artery (RCA), the left anterior descending (LAD) artery, and the circumflex (CX) coronary artery. The arterial distribution varies between patients. Some segments have variable coronary perfusion. (*Reproduced with permission from Lang RM, Bierig M, Devereux RB, et al. Recommendations for chamber quantification: a report from the American Society of Echocardiography's Guidelines and Standards Committee and the Chamber Quantification Writing Group, developed in conjunction with the European Association of Echocardiography, a branch of the European Society of Cardiology.* J Am Soc Echocardiogr. *2005;1:1440–1463.*)

systolic thickening: 1 = normal; 2 = hypokinetic; 3 = akinetic; 4 = dyskinetic; and 5 = aneurysmal. Worsening of WMAs or development of new ones is the hallmark of stress-induced myocardial ischemia. The lack of hyperdynamic motion may indicate ischemia but is less specific.[1] However, an akinetic segment that becomes dyskinetic during stress has not been found to have any diagnostic or prognostic implication.[1] By dividing the sum of the scores by the total number of segments analyzed, a global left ventricular wall motion score index, both at rest and after exercise, can be generated.[3,6–9,16,18,27] A WMA that remains fixed after exercise is often related to a previous myocardial infarction.[1,9] Other adjunctive diagnostic criteria for a positive stress echocardiography result include left ventricular (LV) cavity dilatation and a decrease in global systolic function.[1,3] Biplane and three-dimensional (3D) imaging may shorten the acquisition period of postexercise or peak exercise images, and this will further improve the sensitivity of stress echocardiography.[28–30] The physician who is responsible for reporting the results of the test must analyze the images in a systematic fashion. The workload achieved and the time between completion of exercise and image acquisition must be considered.[7,28,29]

DIAGNOSTIC ACCURACY

The sensitivity and specificity of stress echocardiography, with the use of wall motion criteria, are comparable to those of stress thallium or technetium-99 sestamibi single photon emission computed tomography (SPECT).[31–35] In a large comparison study, the overall sensitivity and specificity of exercise echocardiography were 85% and 88%, respectively, compared with 85% and 81% for exercise thallium imaging.[5–7,16,31–42] The sensitivities of exercise echocardiography and exercise thallium imaging for CAD in patients with single-, double-, and triple-vessel involvement were also similar: 58%, 86%, and 94% versus 61%, 84%, and 94%, respectively.[1] The diagnostic accuracy of a test depends on the patient population (pretest probability of disease), image quality, and expertise of the interpreter. When a threshold of 70% for stenosis significance was used, the sensitivity of both techniques was 85%. The specificities were 88% and 81% for exercise echocardiography and SPECT, respectively.[7] SPECT appears to have marginally higher sensitivity to detect single-vessel disease.[9] The diagnostic accuracy of dobutamine stress echocardiography (DSE) appears comparable to that of exercise echocardiography and SPECT.[3,4,6,9,17,42–44] Both stress echocardiography and stress-gated SPECT nuclear imaging appear

to perform similarly for the detection of CAD in women,[17,37,44–49] (Fig. 9.6), and both were given similar recommendations for stress testing in women in the American Heart Association position statement.[37] The negative predictive value of exercise echocardiography is excellent and clearly in excess of 95% (96% in men and 98% in women), with annualized event rates of 0.75% in women and 1.24% in men.[33,40,42,45,47,50–60] The annualized event rates for normal DSE are at least twice that of normal exercise echocardiography.[49]

ADVANTAGES

Stress echocardiography is a versatile, portable, and cost-effective technique that offers immediate availability of results.[2–4,9,16,31–34,36–39,43–45,47,50,53–55,57–59,61–62] The accuracy of CAD detection appears comparable to that of stress SPECT.[31–35,37,44,59] The specificity of stress echocardiography appears marginally superior to that of stress SPECT, especially in women.[37] Extensive data are also available for using this technique for preoperative risk stratification.[33,35,43]

LIMITATIONS

Inadequate endocardial visualization due to poor acoustic windows can be a significant problem in patients with chronic obstructive pulmonary disease, chest deformities, and morbid obesity.[3,6,7,12,19] Distinguishing scar from peri-infarct ischemia can be challenging compared to stress SPECT. Stress echocardiography is a highly operator-dependent technique. Hence, expertise and experience in image acquisition and interpretation is necessary for the sonographer and physician to achieve accurate results.

CONCLUSIONS

Stress echocardiography is an excellent technique for accurately detecting CAD and has the attractive features of versatility, portability, and relatively low cost.[3,4,6,7,16,17,21,31–36,39,43–45,47–50,53,59,61,62] In an era where there is considerable radiation exposure from medical imaging, stress echocardiography has the added benefit of not involving any exposure to radiation. Most of the literature on the sensitivity of stress echocardiography is from an era prior to the development and availability of harmonic imaging, contrast for endocardial enhancement, and contrast harmonics. Many studies also lacked information regarding digital acquisition, display, and storage.

Developments in biplane 2D imaging and 3D volumetric imaging are likely to shorten the poststress

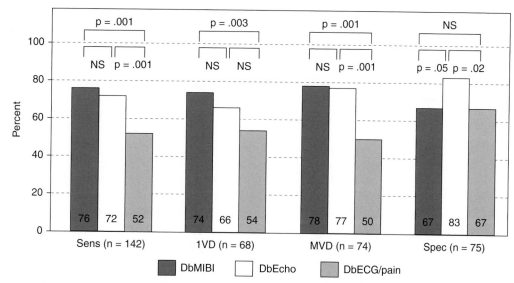

Figure 9.6. Comparison of dobutamine single photon emission computed tomography (SPECT; DbMIBI), dobutamine echocardiography (DbEcho), and dobutamine electrocardiographic (DbECG) changes or angina (DbECG/pain) for the diagnosis of coronary artery disease (CAD). Dobutamine technetium sestamibi SPECT and dobutamine echocardiography have similar overall sensitivities for the detection of CAD, but dobutamine echocardiography has a significantly higher overall specificity. Both tests are diagnostically superior to dobutamine ECG. Dobutamine technetium sestamibi SPECT has a higher sensitivity than dobutamine echocardiography or dobutamine ECG in patients with single-vessel disease. 1VD, single-vessel disease; MVD, multivessel disease; Sens, sensitivity; Spec, specificity. (*Reproduced with permission from DeCara JM. Noninvasive cardiac testing in women.* J Am Med Womens Assoc. *2003;58:254–263.*)

image acquisition and further improve the sensitivity and accuracy of stress echocardiography to detect CAD.[14,20,23,24,29,30] Future advances in myocardial contrast echocardiography may permit the simultaneous evaluation of myocardial regional function and perfusion, which is the ideal goal of noninvasive physiologic evaluation of CAD at the bedside.[2,3] It is hoped that this will also be significantly more cost efficient than contemporary technology.

References

1. Libby P, Bonow RW, Mann DL, Zipes DP. *Braunwald's Heart Disease: A Textbook of Cardiovascular Medicine.* 8th ed. Philadelphia, PA: Saunders Elsevier; 2008.

2. Armstrong WF, Ryan T. Stress echocardiography from 1979 to present. *J Am Soc Echocardiogr.* 2008;21: 22–28.

3. Armstrong WF, Zoghbi WA. Stress echocardiography: current methodology and clinical applications. *J Am Coll Cardiol.* 2005;45:1739–1747.

4. Gottdiener JS. Overview of stress echocardiography: uses, advantages, and limitations. *Curr Probl Cardiol.* 2003;28:485–516.

5. Marwick TH. Current status of stress echocardiography for diagnosis and prognostic assessment of coronary artery disease. *Coron Artery Dis.* 1998;9:411–426.

6. Pellikka PA, Roger VL, Oh JK, Miller FA, Seward JB, Tajik AJ. Stress echocardiography. Part II. Dobutamine stress echocardiography: techniques, implementation, clinical applications, and correlations. *Mayo Clin Proc.* 1995;70: 16–27.

7. Roger VL, Pellikka PA, Oh JK, Miller FA, Seward JB, Tajik AJ. Stress echocardiography. Part I. Exercise echocardiography: techniques, implementation, clinical applications, and correlations. *Mayo Clin Proc.* 1995;70:5–15.

8. Becher H, Chambers J, Fox K, et al. BSE procedure guidelines for the clinical application of stress echocardiography, recommendations for performance and interpretation of stress echocardiography: a report of the British Society of Echocardiography Policy Committee. *Heart.* 2004;90 (suppl 6):vi23–vi30.

9. Geleijnse ML, Fioretti PM, Roelandt JR. Methodology, feasibility, safety and diagnostic accuracy of dobutamine stress echocardiography. *J Am Coll Cardiol.* 1997;30: 595–606.

10. Hachamovitch R, Di Carli MF. Methods and limitations of assessing new noninvasive tests: part I: anatomy-based validation of noninvasive testing. *Circulation.* 2008;117: 2684–2690.

11. Hachamovitch R, Di Carli MF. Methods and limitations of assessing new noninvasive tests: part II: outcomes-based validation and reliability assessment of noninvasive testing. *Circulation.* 2008;117:2793–2801.

12. Sicari R, Nihoyannopoulos P, Evangelista A, et al. Stress echocardiography expert consensus statement: European Association of Echocardiography (EAE) (a registered branch of the ESC). *Eur J Echocardiogr.* 2008;9:415–437.

13. Presti CF, Armstrong WF, Feigenbaum H. Comparison of echocardiography at peak exercise and after bicycle exercise in evaluation of patients with known or suspected coronary artery disease. *J Am Soc Echocardiogr.* 1988;1:119–126.

14. Peteiro J, Garrido I, Monserrat L, Aldama G, Calvino R, Castro-Beiras A. Comparison of peak and postexercise treadmill echocardiography with the use of continuous harmonic imaging acquisition. *J Am Soc Echocardiogr.* 2004;17:1044–1049.

15. Mairesse GH, Vanoverschelde JL, Robert A, Climov D, Detry JM, Marwick TH. Pathophysiologic mechanisms underlying dobutamine- and exercise-induced wall motion abnormalities. *Am Heart J.* 1998;136:63–70.

16. Roger VL, Pellikka PA, Oh JK, Bailey KR, Tajik AJ. Identification of multivessel coronary artery disease by exercise echocardiography. *J Am Coll Cardiol.* 1994;24: 109–114.

17. Geleijnse ML, Krenning BJ, Soliman OI, Nemes A, Galema TW, ten Cate FJ. Dobutamine stress echocardiography for the detection of coronary artery disease in women. *Am J Cardiol.* 2007;99:714–717.

18. Hoffmann R, Lethen H, Marwick T, et al. Standardized guidelines for the interpretation of dobutamine echocardiography reduce interinstitutional variance in interpretation. *Am J Cardiol.* 1998;82:1520–1524.

19. Pellikka PA, Nagueh SF, Elhendy AA, Kuehl CA, Sawada SG. American Society of Echocardiography recommendations for performance, interpretation, and application of stress echocardiography. *J Am Soc Echocardiogr.* 2007;20:1021–1041.

20. Thomas JD, Adams DB, Devries S, et al. Guidelines and recommendations for digital echocardiography. *J Am Soc Echocardiogr.* 2005;18:287–297.

21. Flachskampf FA, Rost C. Stress echocardiography in known or suspected coronary artery disease: an exercise in good clinical practice. *J Am Coll Cardiol.* 2009;53: 1991–1992.

22. Mulvagh SL, Rakowski H, Vannan MA, et al. American Society of Echocardiography consensus statement on the clinical applications of ultrasonic contrast agents in echocardiography. *J Am Soc Echocardiogr.* 2008;21: 1179–1201; quiz 1281.

23. Skolnick DG, Sawada SG, Feigenbaum H, Segar DS. Enhanced endocardial visualization with noncontrast harmonic imaging during stress echocardiography. *J Am Soc Echocardiogr.* 1999;12:559–563.

24. Zaglavara T, Norton M, Cumberledge B, et al. Dobutamine stress echocardiography: improved endocardial border definition and wall motion analysis with tissue harmonic imaging. *J Am Soc Echocardiogr.* 1999;12:706–713.

25. Lang RM, Bierig M, Devereux RB, et al. Recommendations for chamber quantification: a report from the American Society of Echocardiography's Guidelines and Standards Committee and the Chamber Quantification Writing Group, developed in conjunction with the European Association of Echocardiography, a branch of the European Society of Cardiology. *J Am Soc Echocardiogr.* 2005;1:1440–1463.

26. Cerqueira MD, Weissman NJ, Dilsizian V, Jacobs AK, Kaul S, Laskey WK, et al. Standardized myocardial segmentation and nomenclature for tomographic imaging of the heart: a statement for healthcare professionals from the cardiac imaging committee of the council on clinical cardiology of the American Heart Association. *Circulation.* 2002;105:539–542.

27. Elhendy A, van Domburg RT, Bax JJ, et al. Optimal criteria for the diagnosis of coronary artery disease by dobutamine stress echocardiography. *Am J Cardiol.* 1998;82:1339–1344.

28. Ahmad M, Xie T, McCulloch M, Abreo G, Runge M. Real-time three-dimensional dobutamine stress echocardiography in assessment stress echocardiography in assessment of ischemia: comparison with two-dimensional dobutamine stress echocardiography. *J Am Coll Cardiol.* 2001;37:1303–1309.

29. Corsi C, Lang RM, Veronesi F, et al. Volumetric quantification of global and regional left ventricular function from real-time three-dimensional echocardiographic images. *Circulation.* 2005;112:1161–1170.

30. Takeuchi M, Otani S, Weinert L, Spencer KT, Lang RM. Comparison of contrast-enhanced real-time live 3-dimensional dobutamine stress echocardiography with contrast 2-dimensional echocardiography for detecting stress-induced wall-motion abnormalities. *J Am Soc Echocardiogr.* 2006;19:294–299.

31. Elhendy A, Geleijnse ML, Roelandt JR, et al. Comparison of dobutamine stress echocardiography and 99m-technetium sestamibi SPECT myocardial perfusion scintigraphy for predicting extent of coronary artery disease in patients with healed myocardial infarction. *Am J Cardiol.* 1997;79:7–12.

32. Elhendy A, Geleijnse ML, van Domburg RT, et al. Comparison of dobutamine stress echocardiography and technetium-99m sestamibi single-photon emission tomography for the diagnosis of coronary artery disease in hypertensive patients with and without left ventricular hypertrophy. *Eur J Nucl Med.* 1998;25:69–78.

33. Shaw LJ, Eagle KA, Gersh BJ, Miller DD. Meta-analysis of intravenous dipyridamole-thallium-201 imaging (1985 to 1994) and dobutamine echocardiography (1991 to 1994) for risk stratification before vascular surgery. *J Am Coll Cardiol.* 1996;27:787–798.

34. Shaw LJ, Marwick TH, Berman DS, et al. Incremental cost-effectiveness of exercise echocardiography vs. SPECT imaging for the evaluation of stable chest pain. *Eur Heart J.* 2006;27:2448–2458.

35. Smart SC, Bhatia A, Hellman R, et al. Dobutamine-atropine stress echocardiography and dipyridamole sestamibi scintigraphy for the detection of coronary artery disease: limitations and concordance. *J Am Coll Cardiol.* 2000;36:1265–1273.

36. Marwick TH, Anderson T, Williams MJ, et al. Exercise echocardiography is an accurate and cost-efficient technique for detection of coronary artery disease in women. *J Am Coll Cardiol.* 1995;26:335–341.

37. Mieres JH, Shaw LJ, Arai A, et al. Role of noninvasive testing in the clinical evaluation of women with suspected coronary artery disease: consensus statement from the Cardiac Imaging Committee, Council on Clinical Cardiology, and the Cardiovascular Imaging and Intervention Committee, Council on Cardiovascular Radiology and Intervention, American Heart Association. *Circulation.* 2005;111:682–696.

38. Peteiro J, Monserrrat L, Pineiro M, et al. Comparison of exercise echocardiography and the Duke treadmill score for risk stratification in patients with known or suspected coronary artery disease and normal resting electrocardiogram. *Am Heart J.* 2006;151:1324e1–1324e10.

39. Quinones MA, Verani MS, Haichin RM, Mahmarian JJ, Suarez J, Zoghbi WA. Exercise echocardiography versus 201Tl single-photon emission computed tomography in evaluation of coronary artery disease. Analysis of 292 patients. *Circulation.* 1992;85:1026–1031.

40. Smart SC, Knickelbine T, Malik F, Sagar KB. Dobutamine-atropine stress echocardiography for the detection of coronary artery disease in patients with left ventricular hypertrophy. Importance of chamber size and systolic wall stress. *Circulation.* 2000;101:258–263.

41. Southard J, Baker L, Schaefer S. In search of the false-negative exercise treadmill testing evidence-based use of exercise echocardiography. *Clin Cardiol.* 2008;31:35–40.

42. Sozzi FB, Elhendy A, Roelandt JR, et al. Prognostic value of dobutamine stress echocardiography in patients with diabetes. *Diabetes Care.* 2003;26:1074–1078.

43. Kertai MD, Poldermans D. The utility of dobutamine stress echocardiography for perioperative and long-term cardiac risk assessment. *J Cardiothorac Vasc Anesth.* 2005;19:520–528.

44. Kwok Y, Kim C, Grady D, Segal M, Redberg R. Meta-analysis of exercise testing to detect coronary artery disease in women. *Am J Cardiol.* 1999;83:660–666.

45. Arruda-Olson AM, Juracan EM, Mahoney DW, McCully RB, Roger VL, Pellikka PA. Prognostic value of exercise echocardiography in 5,798 patients: is there a gender difference? *J Am Coll Cardiol.* 2002;39:625–631.

46. DeCara JM. Noninvasive cardiac testing in women. *J Am Med Womens Assoc.* 2003;58:254–263.

47. Elhendy A, Shub C, McCully RB, Mahoney DW, Burger KN, Pellikka PA. Exercise echocardiography for the prognostic stratification of patients with low pretest probability of coronary artery disease. *Am J Med.* 2001;111:18–23.

48. Shaw LJ, Mieres JH. The role of noninvasive testing in the diagnosis and prognosis of women with suspected CAD. *J Fam Pract.* 2005;suppl:4–5, 7.

49. Wenger NK, Shaw LJ, Vaccarino V. Coronary heart disease in women: update 2008. *Clin Pharmacol Ther.* 2008;83:37–51.

50. Arruda AM, Das MK, Roger VL, Klarich KW, Mahoney DW, Pellikka PA. Prognostic value of exercise echocardiography in 2,632 patients > or = 65 years of age. *J Am Coll Cardiol.* 2001;37:1036–1041.

51. Biagini E, Elhendy A, Bax JJ, et al. Seven-year follow-up after dobutamine stress echocardiography: impact of gender on prognosis. *J Am Coll Cardiol.* 2005;45:93–97.

52. Bouzas-Mosquera A, Peteiro J, Alvarez-Garcia N, et al. Prediction of mortality and major cardiac events by exercise echocardiography in patients with normal exercise electrocardiographic testing. *J Am Coll Cardiol.* 2009;53:1981–1990.

53. Colon PJ 3rd, Guarisco JS, Murgo J, Cheirif J. Utility of stress echocardiography in the triage of patients with atypical chest pain from the emergency department. *Am J Cardiol.* 1998;82:1282–1284, A10.

54. Das MK, Pellikka PA, Mahoney DW, et al. Assessment of cardiac risk before nonvascular surgery: dobutamine stress echocardiography in 530 patients. *J Am Coll Cardiol.* 2000;35:1647–1653.

55. Elhendy A, Arruda AM, Mahoney DW, Pellikka PA. Prognostic stratification of diabetic patients by exercise echocardiography. *J Am Coll Cardiol.* 2001;37:1551–1557.

56. Geleijnse ML, Elhendy A, van Domburg RT, et al. Cardiac imaging for risk stratification with dobutamine-atropine stress testing in patients with chest pain. Echocardiography, perfusion scintigraphy, or both? *Circulation.* 1997;96:137–147.

57. Geleijnse ML, Elhendy A, van Domburg RT, Cornel JH, Roelandt JR, Fioretti PM. Prognostic implications of a normal dobutamine-atropine stress echocardiogram in patients with chest pain. *J Am Soc Echocardiogr.* 1998;11:606–611.

58. Marwick TH, Shaw L, Case C, Vasey C, Thomas JD. Clinical and economic impact of exercise electrocardiography and exercise echocardiography in clinical practice. *Eur Heart J.* 2003;24:1153–1163.

59. Metz LD, Beattie M, Hom R, Redberg RF, Grady D, Fleischmann KE. The prognostic value of normal exercise myocardial perfusion imaging and exercise echocardiography: a meta-analysis. *J Am Coll Cardiol.* 2007;49:227–237.

60. Smart SC, Sagar KB. Diagnostic and prognostic use of stress echocardiography in stable patients. *Echocardiography.* 2000;17:465–477.

61. Cortigiani L, Sicari R, Bigi R, et al. Usefulness of stress echocardiography for risk stratification of patients after percutaneous coronary intervention. *Am J Cardiol.* 2008;102:1170–1174.

62. Elhendy A, van Domburg RT, Bax JJ, et al. Noninvasive diagnosis of coronary artery stenosis in women with limited exercise capacity: comparison of dobutamine stress echocardiography and 99mTc sestamibi single-photon emission CT. *Chest.* 1998;114:1097–1104.

ULTRASOUND USE FOR EVALUATION OF ORGANS OF THE ABDOMEN AND PELVIS

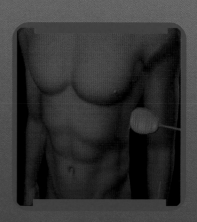

CHAPTER 10

Abdominal Ultrasound

Jonathan M. Dort, MD, FACS; Gary C. Clagett, RT, RVT, RDMS;
William R. Fry, MD, FACS, RVT, RDMS; and Alexander B. Levitov, MD, FCCM, RDCS

INTRODUCTION

Abdominal complaints can be challenging for physicians. Although bedside ultrasound is being used extensively by trauma surgeons for the Focused Assessment with Sonography for Trauma (FAST) examinations, other practitioners are less likely to use ultrasound in their day-to-day assessment of abdominal complaints and verification of physical findings related to the abdomen. In its guidelines, the American Institute of Ultrasound in Medicine lists multiple indications for the performance of abdominal ultrasonography that the reader may use for reference (Table 10.1). Ultrasonography can identify potential causes of abdominal pain, pinpoint abdominal sources of infection, and provide information on bowel function. The presence of physical findings such as shifting dullness or palpable hepatomegaly also can be instantly verified. Anatomy and blood flow through major abdominal vessels (aorta, inferior vena cava) can be visualized and ultrasound guidance for invasive procedures can be used to reduce the risk of complications.

The FAST examination has become the most common form of abdominal examination used by nonradiologists. The following sections will describe the FAST examination and address the application of ultrasound in each of the intra-abdominal organs. For most abdominal examinations, a 5-MHz curvilinear probe will provide satisfactory images and is implied, unless otherwise noted.

FOCUSED ASSESSMENT OF SURGICAL TRAUMA EXAMINATION

FAST examination is used when assessing trauma patients with or without hemodynamic instability. It is aimed at identifying the presence of intra-abdominal fluid (i.e., blood) and is 90% to 95% sensitive, but the specificity is low because of the high prevalence of ascites in trauma patients. Generally speaking however, in an appropriate clinical scenario the presence of fluid will be an indication for laparotomy. The examination is performed in four views and is sometimes combined with ultrasound of the lung and subcostal views of the

heart to rule out pericardial tamponade (Fig. 10.1). Hepatorenal and splenorenal recesses are interrogated with longitudinal (long-axis) views of the right and left upper quadrant, respectively (Fig. 10.2A, B). Respiratory motions are used when possible. The pelvis and bladder are visualized in the transverse view to identify fluid in the dependent pelvis (Fig. 10.2C, D). It is worth noting that common causes of intra-abdominal catastrophe, such as duodenal bleeding, cannot be identified by an ultrasound examination.

ASCITES

Transudative ascitic fluid appears as an anechoic area between the abdominal wall and the bowel; however, hemoperitoneum and peritonitis (secondary or spontaneous) will be more echogenic in appearance and reminiscent of falling snow (Fig. 10.3). The presence or absence of cirrhosis might help to differentiate between the two.

LIVER

Hepatic pathology that is often suspected on the history and physical examination (i.e., palpation and percussion for hepatomegaly) can be confirmed or ruled out with ultrasound imaging. Right upper quadrant pain, jaundice, gastrointestinal bleeding, and concern for hepatic tumors are several reasons to consider ultrasound evaluation of the liver. Nonmalignant states such as cirrhosis, hepatic steatosis, and cysts and solid masses such as arteriovenous malformations, hepatomas, and metastases can all be visualized.

While in some thin patients a linear probe can be used, in general a curved linear or sector probe in the 2- to 5-MHz frequency range is best. Any systematic approach works, as long as the entire liver is evaluated. In general, the patient may remain in a supine position for the entire examination, although sometimes a left lateral decubitus or upright position may also be beneficial. One approach is to start at the costal margin at the right midclavicular line. The midclavicular line roughly marks the middle of the gallbladder fossa and the anatomic division of the right

TABLE 10.1. American Institute of Ultrasound in Medicine Indications for Abdominal Ultrasonography

Abdominal, flank, and/or back pain

Signs/symptoms referred from abdominal organs, such as jaundice

Palpable abnormalities, such as a mass

Abnormal laboratory test result values suggestive of abdominal pathology

Follow-up of known or suspected abdominal pathology

Search for metastatic disease or occult primary neoplasm

Evaluation of suspected congenital abnormalities

Abdominal trauma

Pre- and posttransplantation evaluation

Planning and guidance for an invasive procedure

Search for the presence of free or loculated peritoneal and/or retroperitoneal fluid

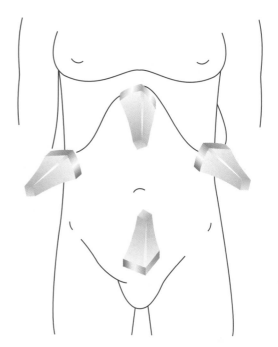

Figure 10.1. Ultrasound probe positioning for Focused Assessment with Sonography for Trauma examination of the abdomen.

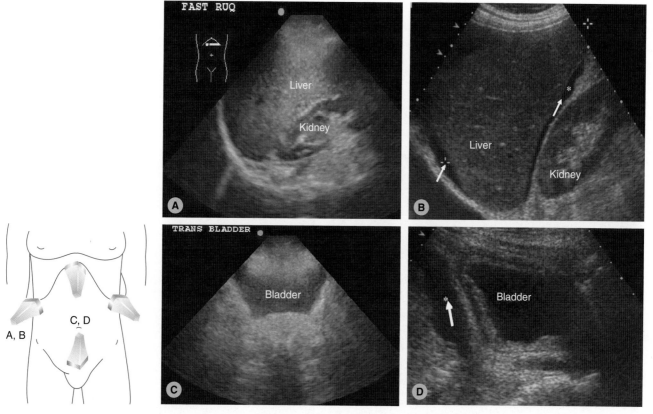

Figure 10.2. Focused Assessment with Sonography for Trauma (FAST) examination of right upper quadrant (RUQ) and pelvis. **(A)** Normal. **(B)** Fluid in hepatorenal recess and around the liver (*solid white arrows*). **(C)** Normal suprapubic image of the full bladder. **(D)** Pelvic fluid located behind the bladder (*asterisk*).

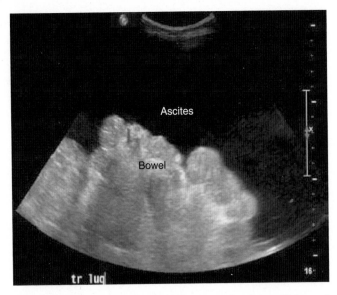

Figure 10.3. Large amount of ascitic fluid (small bowel is well visualized and marked).

Normal Anatomy

The surface of the liver should be smooth. The parenchyma of the liver should be uniform in echogenicity, which is lower than that of the adjacent kidney. Hypoechoic portal and hepatic veins can be differentiated by the portal venous structures, which have a hyperechoic stripe in their walls, whereas the hepatic veins do not (Fig. 10.4A). Bile ducts may not be visualized in the normal liver. Bile ducts run parallel to the portal veins, so a dilated intrahepatic biliary tree will differ from the portal venous system because it does not have hyperechoic walls. Using Doppler imaging, color or power preferably, one can identify the vein and the bile duct. In normal anatomy, the echogenicity of the liver parenchyma and the right renal cortex should be similar. Differentiations in echogenicity between the liver and the kidney can suggest disease states.

Diseases of the liver can be generally divided into diffuse (cirrhosis, hepatic steatosis) and focal (cysts, masses, etc.).

Cirrhosis

Cirrhosis is a scarring of the liver that increases the amount of collagen in the liver (Fig. 10.4B). This generally increases the echogenicity of the liver relative to the kidney. In more advanced states of cirrhosis, the liver can become nodular and lose its smooth surface. A heterogeneous echogenic appearance of the liver

and left lobes of the liver. Angling laterally and medially, having the patient take a medium to deep breath, and moving the probe superiorly and often to the midaxillary line or more posteriorly are required to fully evaluate the right lobe then the left lobe. Both sagittal and transverse images should be taken. Because of its location, both subcostal and intercostal views are necessary to fully evaluate the liver.

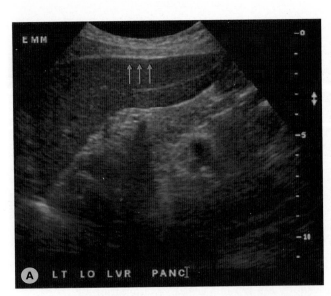
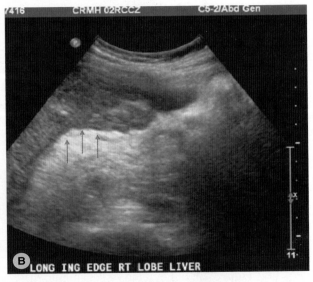

Figure 10.4. Right upper quadrant ultrasound of the normal left lobe of the liver. **(A)** Note the smooth liver edge (*blue arrows*) and cirrhotic right lobe. **(B)** Note the irregular edge (*blue arrows*) and hyperechoic appearance of the liver parenchyma.

can also be seen with cirrhosis but is nonspecific because it is also seen in acute hepatitis and fatty metamorphosis of the liver.

Hepatic Steatosis

As the incidence of obesity in the U.S. population increases, so does the incidence of nonalcoholic steatorrheic hepatitis and liver steatosis. This can be seen as either a diffuse hyperechoic or a mixed pattern of relative hyperechoic and hypoechoic patches (Fig. 10.5A). It is assumed that the hyperechoic areas have fatty infiltration and the hypoechoic areas are spared fatty infiltration. Comparing echogenicity to the right renal cortex can again be helpful. When focal sparing is present, there is generally not a discrete mass but more diffuse margins between fatty infiltration and spared areas. Focal disease states can be further subdivided by their ultrasound appearance into hypoechoic, hyperechoic, and isoechoic.

Cysts

Cysts of the liver are seen as hypoechoic, spherical structures (Fig. 10.6A). They are usually uniform with and without septations. Posterior enhancement is usually present. Cysts may be singular or multiple. They are often congenital, and in the case of multiple cysts, polycystic hepatic disease should be considered. If there are septations within the cyst, traumatic cysts or a liver abscess should be considered (Fig. 10.6B). Isoechoic masses can occasionally be

identified because of the distortion of the liver's contour or a substance that distorts the local anatomy. Isoechoic masses include hepatic adenomas, regenerating nodules, hepatocellular carcinoma, and metastatic disease. Hyperechoic hepatic masses usually fall within the following categories.

Hemangioma

Liver hemangiomas are the most common hyperechoic masses seen in the liver (Fig. 10.6C). Because they are primarily venous in nature, they often do not demonstrate flow on Doppler examination. If the diagnosis is uncertain, computed tomography (CT) or magnetic resonance imaging (MRI) can confirm the diagnosis.

Hepatocellular Carcinoma (Hepatoma)

Hepatomas can appear on ultrasound as hyperechoic, hypoechoic, or of a mixed pattern, particularly if they are large, where some tumor necrosis may have occurred (Fig. 10.5B). CT and MRI can be done to further define the mass, but if possible, biopsy is the best way to make the diagnosis.

Metastatic Disease

Liver metastases of various tumors are not uncommon, and ultrasound can alert the practitioner of their presence. Ultrasound can also help to stage the primary tumor and assist with the choice of therapy (i.e., surgical or medical). Metastatic lesions can also appear on ultrasound as hyperechoic, hypoechoic, or of a mixed pattern, particularly if they are large, where

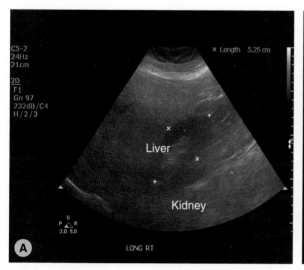
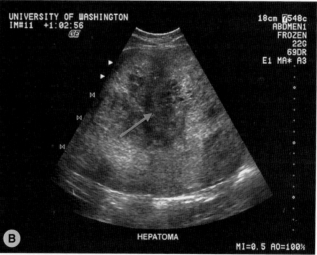

Figure 10.5. Right upper quadrant ultrasound of liver steatosis. **(A)** Increased liver echogenicity compared with that of the adjacent normal kidney. **(B)** Hepatocellular carcinoma with hyperechoic and hypoechoic areas (*blue arrow*). Background liver echogenicity is increased due to cirrhosis.

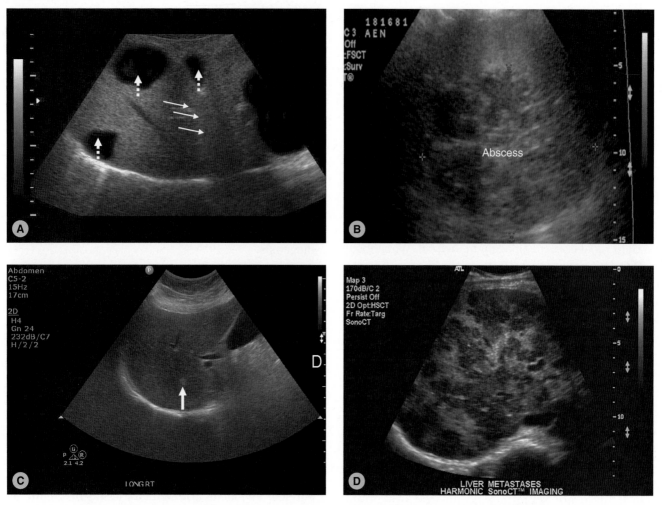

Figure 10.6. Right upper quadrant ultrasound. **(A)** Liver cysts (*interrupted white arrows*). Note the characteristic acoustic enhancement artifact (*solid white arrows*). **(B)** Liver abscess. Note the presence of septations and inhomogeneous echogenicity of the lesion. **(C)** Hemangioma (*solid white arrow*). **(D)** Liver parenchyma is virtually replaced by multiple metastases.

some tumor necrosis may have occurred (Fig. 10.6D). Metastases are commonly multiple lesions, and CT and MRI can be performed to further define the masses; however, biopsy is the preferred method for establishing the diagnosis.

ABDOMINAL AORTA

While history and the presence of a pulsatile mass on physical examination may suggest abdominal aortic pathology, an abdominal aortic aneurysm (AAA) may have no symptoms prior to rupture. Occasionally, a patient with a leaking AAA or dissection may have initial symptoms thought to be renal in nature. AAA and occlusive disease of the aorta can lead to emboli in the legs and feet. A dissection usually begins in the thoracic aorta but can go progress to the femoral

arteries. Because the descending thoracic aorta is not well visualized by transthoracic scanning, evaluation of the abdominal aorta may provide insight, if positive, into the patient's diagnosis.

Using a curved, liner, or phased array transducer in the 2- to 5-MHz range, one can image the aorta just to the left of the midline. It can be obscured by bowel gas in the nonfasting patient over most of its length. Starting near the xiphoid, the aorta can be visualized using the liver as an acoustic window. Both longitudinal and transverse images should be taken (Fig. 10.7A, B). The aorta bifurcates into the iliac arteries usually at the level of the umbilicus.

Normal Anatomy

The aorta extends from the diaphragmatic hiatus to the level of the umbilicus, where it bifurcates into the

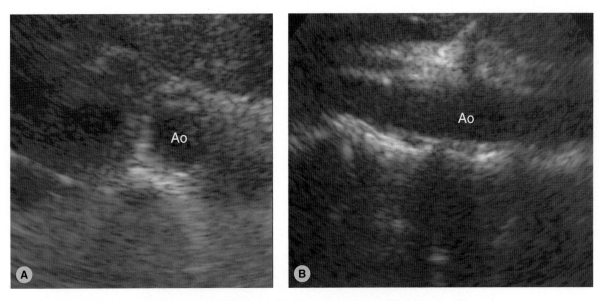

Figure 10.7. Normal abdominal aorta (Ao) in transverse (short-axis, **A**) and longitudinal (long-axis, **B**) views.

iliac arteries (Fig. 10.7A, B). The aorta divides into five main branches in the abdomen: the celiac artery, the superior mesenteric artery, the two renal arteries (10% of patients have multiple renal arteries), and the inferior mesenteric artery. The normal diameter of the abdominal aorta is less than 2 cm.

Abdominal Aortic Aneurysm

An AAA is defined as 1.5 times the normal aortic diameter or greater than 3 cm (Fig. 10.8A, B [see also color insert]). Most AAAs originate below the level of the renal arteries, although some may encompass some or all of the visceral arteries. Thrombus may be contained in a portion of or the entire circumference of the aneurysm. This thrombus can embolize to the lower extremities and lead to arterial insufficiency or occlusion. Size is measured transversely from the outer walls. A rupture or leaking AAA may have a better acoustic window because of surrounding fluid, but large retroperitoneal bleeds may make actual dimensions difficult to determine. Free blood in the abdomen (see section on FAST examination) and the presence of an AAA mandate immediate surgical consultation.

Aortic Occlusive Disease

Occlusive disease of the abdominal aorta may manifest itself with a normal to slightly enlarged aortic diameter. There is often a significant amount of hyperechoic calcium deposition in the aortic wall, with ultrasound shadowing making luminal visualization difficult. Significant irregularities in the aortic lumen

are often seen. These irregularities can be a source for emboli. Doppler examination can determine whether flow is still maintained through the aorta.

Abdominal Aortic Dissections

Abdominal aortic dissections as an isolated finding are rare. Most dissections of the aorta originate in the thoracic aorta and continue down to the abdominal aorta (Fig. 10.8C). The caliber of the abdominal aorta with a dissection can initially be normal, but can dilate to a significant aneurysmal size. Color Doppler may be helpful in distinguishing between a true and false lumen, with the flow pattern being somewhat better organized in a true lumen. Imaging of the thoracic aorta and even the aortic valve needs to be performed to rule out proximal involvement and to better plan strategy. Doppler modalities can also be used to determine whether perfusion of intra-abdominal organs and the spine is being jeopardized.

INFERIOR VENA CAVA

Evaluation of the inferior vena cava (IVC) may be performed if there is a concern for deep vein thrombosis and pulmonary emboli or to evaluate a patient's intravascular volume. Normal respiratory variations are usually associated with euvolemia (Fig. 10.9A), while inspiratory collapse is a sign of hypovolemia. Lack of respiratory variation is a sign of congestion, particularly when pulsatile flow is present. Advanced renal cell carcinoma appears particularly thrombogenic and may result in renal vein thrombosis and

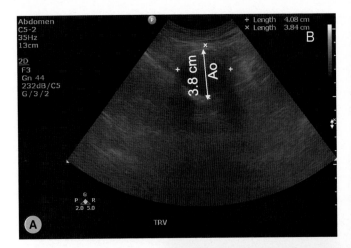

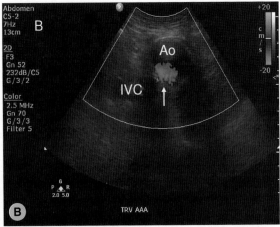

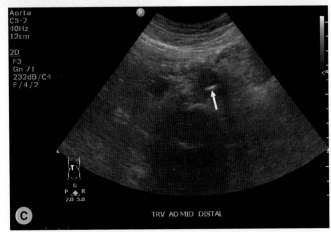

Figure 10.8. **(A)** Abdominal aortic spelling for consistency aneurysm (AAA). **(B)** AAA with thrombus (*solid white arrow*). **(C)** Short-axis view of abdominal aortic dissection (the arrow indicates an intimal flap within the aortic lumen). Ao, aorta; IVC, inferior vena cava.

subsequent extension proximal into the IVC or even as far as the right atrium (Fig. 10.9C). Extension of the clot into the IVC may significantly alter the therapeutic plan and require IVC interruption. With the advent of temporary inferior vena cava filters, patients may not know they have one, forget they have one, or forget they had it removed. To that end, one should be familiar with the appearance of an IVC filter on ultrasound.

A curvilinear or phased array transducer in the 2- to 5-MHz frequency range is used, although higher-frequency 7- to 10-MHz linear sequential array probes can be used in the thin or pediatric patient. The inferior vena cava is imaged just to the right of the midline. It can be obscured by bowel gas in the nonfasting patient over most of its length. Starting near the xiphoid, one can visualize the aorta using the liver as an acoustic window. A right lateral view at the midaxillary line allows visualization of the intrahepatic portion of the vena cava (Fig. 10.9B). Both longitudinal and transverse images should be taken. The vena cava

is formed by the confluence of the iliac veins at the level of the umbilicus.

Normal Anatomy

The inferior vena cava extends from the right atrium to the level of the umbilicus (Fig. 9A, B). Branches include the hepatic veins, renal veins, and right gonadal vein. The diameter of the vena cava depends on intravascular volume status and can be difficult to see in severe hypovolemia.

Thrombus

Thrombus in the inferior vena cava is less common than deep vein thrombosis, and its true incidence is not known but may be between 5% and 15% of the patients with deep vein thrombosis. A thrombus can arise from either blood clots or tumors. Blood clots can be found in any location within the inferior vena cava or its branches (Fig. 10.10A). Tumor thrombi

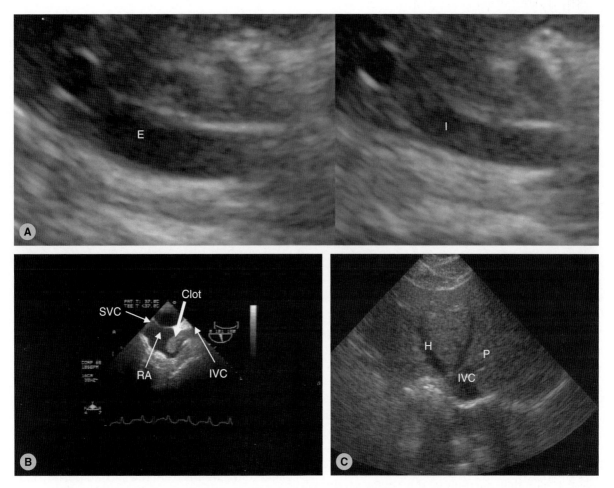

Figure 10.9. (A) Longitudinal (long-axis) view of the inferior vena cava (IVC). Note the change in IVC diameter with inspiration (I) and expiration (E). **(B)** Transesophageal echocardiogram in bicaval view. The IVC is filled with a clot extending into the right atrium. **(C)** IVC on the level of the liver. Note the "playboy bunny" appearance of IVC and portal (P) and hepatic (H) veins. This patient's thrombophilia is due to renal cell carcinoma. RA, right atrium; SVC, superior vena cava.

occur most commonly from renal tumors. They are usually seen in conjunction with renal vein thrombosis. It should be kept in mind that extrinsic compression from tumors could also cause occlusion and/or a thrombus to form within the vena cava. Leg swelling is associated with a significant thrombus in the vena cava.

Inferior Vena Cava Filters

Many types of IVC filters are available. An IVC filter is most often placed below the renal veins (Fig. 10.10B). Echogenicity of the filter is variable, and they may be difficult to image.

PANCREAS

Because of its posterior position, the pancreas can be difficult to palpate on physical examination. Epigastric or right upper quadrant pain, painless jaundice, suspicion

of an endocrine neoplasm, and staging of a known lesion are all reasons to consider ultrasound evaluation of the pancreas. The use of endoscopic ultrasound allows for improved resolution because of the ability to use a high-frequency transducer. This is also true for intraoperative ultrasound, which offers superior spatial resolution of the pancreas when compared to CT, transabdominal ultrasound, and MRI.

Transabdominal imaging of the pancreas can be challenging because of the presence of bowel gas or obesity. With the patient in the supine position, the pancreas can be recognized by surrounding anatomic landmarks, anterior to the splenic vein, superior mesenteric artery, superior mesenteric vein, and aorta. The right lateral decubitus position can be employed to view the tail. With transabdominal imaging, a curved linear 2.5- to 4-MHz probe is used. For endoscopic or intra-abdominal imaging and in small

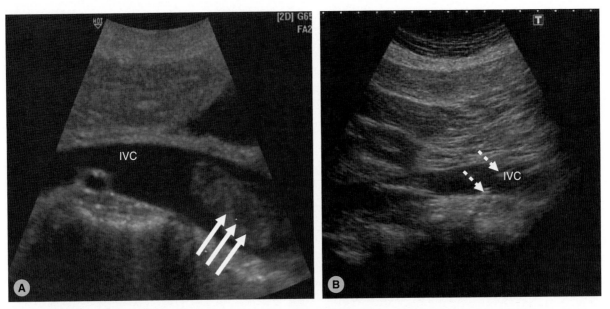

Figure 10.10. (A) Large mobile thrombus in the inferior vena cava (IVC; long-axis view, *solid white arrows*). **(B)** IVC filter (*interrupted white arrows*). (*Image courtesy of James Foster, MD, RPVI, RVT.*)

children, a higher-frequency probe in the 7.5- to 10-MHz range may be used. One should use the liver and spleen as acoustic windows. One approach is to start at the xiphoid process and sweep toward the head and neck of the pancreas, which wrap around an echogenic fat pad that surrounds the origin of the superior mesenteric artery, and then sweeps towards the tail, which runs superiorly and backward toward the left maxilla. Do not forget to look at the uncinate process. Transverse and longitudinal scanning of the entire pancreas should be performed.

Normal Anatomy

The pancreas lies directly behind the gastric antrum and transverse colon. It lies anterior and inferior to the splenic vein. It is a nonencapsulated, multilobar gland that extends from the second portion of the duodenum to the splenic hilum. It typically appears hyperechoic compared to the liver in adults and hypoechoic in children. The normal pancreas is a homogenous structure, 15 to 20 cm in length (Fig. 10.11A). The pancreatic duct is usually seen as a

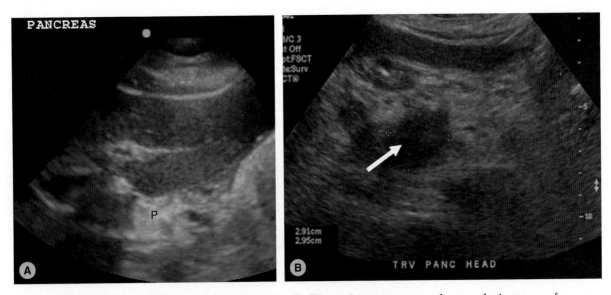

Figure 10.11. (A) Normal pancreas (P). **(B)** This inhomogeneous, hypoechoic mass of the head of the pancreas is pancreatic cancer (*solid white arrow*).

sinusoidal, parallel-lined, echogenic structure in the middle of the gland. On transverse section, the duct can appear anechoic. Disease states of the pancreas can be divided into diffuse and localized.

Fatty Infiltration

When the pancreas becomes more infiltrated with fat, as it does in obese and elderly patients, the gland can become more hyperechoic. This can make it isoechoic with the surrounding retroperitoneal fat, and therefore more difficult to size.

Acute Pancreatitis

Pancreatitis is an inflammatory process, mainly diffuse, with multiple etiologies. The most common causes are gallstone disease, which blocks the common channel of entry from the common bile duct into the duodenum are alcoholism, congenital anomalies, medications, and lipid disorders. The typical ultrasound appearance is one of glandular enlargement and decreased echogenicity (Fig. 10.12A). In early stages of the disease, the appearance may be normal. Dilation of the duct may be seen. A collection of fluid may also be seen within the gland or in the peripancreatic spaces, such as the lesser sac. It is important to look for gallstones, as they remain the most common cause of acute pancreatitis. These would appear hyperechoic with posterior shadowing.

Chronic Pancreatitis

The appearance of the gland in chronic pancreatitis is more heterogeneous (Fig. 10.12B). It can have irregular borders, with areas of hyperechoic fibrosis and ductal dilatation. A ductal stricture or multiple strictures can be seen, as can patchy inflammatory areas with reduced echogenicity.

Cysts

Pancreatic pseudocysts, the most common pancreatic cysts, most likely occur as a result of acute pancreatitis. They also can occur as a result of trauma or may be idiopathic. They appear as anechoic structures within or adjacent to the pancreas (Fig. 10.12B). As they mature, their well-defined borders thicken. Posterior enhancement is also seen, as well as occasional internal echoes from a clot or debris. A mucinous cystic neoplasm is typically seen as a large, multilocular cyst containing mucinous or hemorrhagic material. Serous cystadenoma, is typically visualized in the pancreatic head and most often appears as numerous small cysts separated by fibrous septae radiating from the center.

Masses

Pancreatic carcinoma generally appears as a hypoechoic lesion, although a small percentage can be isoechoic or hyperechoic. The majority of tumors are

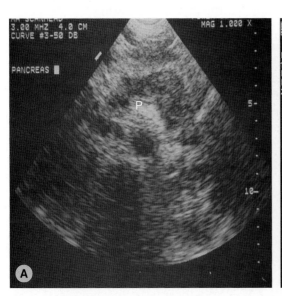
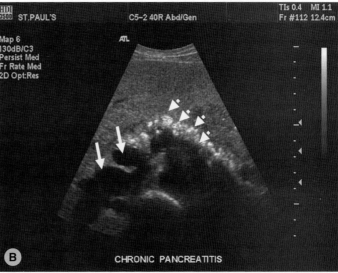

Figure 10.12. **(A)** Acute pancreatitis. Note the glandular enlargement, areas of fluid collection within the pancreas (P), and areas of decreased echogenicity. **(B)** Chronic pancreatitis. Note the pancreatic calcifications (*interrupted white arrows*) and multiple cyst (pseudocyst) formation (*solid white arrows*). (*Image courtesy of Corky Hecht, RDMS, RDCS, RVT.*)

found in the head of the pancreas. Heterogeneity increases as the tumor, and central necrosis develops. Endoscopic ultrasound has excellent sensitivity for finding lesions, even those less than 2 cm. Endoscopic ultrasound is also the most sensitive modality for evaluating portal vein involvement and thus helps in the choice of therapy. In tumors in which it is difficult to evaluate the borders, compression of the vein or other vascular structures may provide the diagnosis. The finding of dilation of the biliary and pancreatic ducts, as well as the gallbladder, may aid in the diagnosis but is not always present. Rarely, primary pancreatic neoplasias can appear hyperechoic.

Although rare, pancreatic metastases from other primary tumors are most often isoechoic or slightly hypoechoic. They can be homogenous and well circumscribed. Occasionally, primary pancreatic carcinoma can be isoechoic. In this instance, the ability to detect irregularity, ductal dilatation, or compression of surrounding structures becomes increasingly important.

THE BILIARY TREE

Ultrasonography is useful in the evaluation of right upper quadrant pain, screening for biliary tract abnormalities, and differentiating extrahepatic from intrahepatic causes of jaundice. It is also the procedure of choice for the evaluation of gallbladder pathology. Transabdominal, endoscopic, laparoscopic, and intraoperative evaluations can all provide useful diagnostic information.

It is important to have the patient fast to reduce bowel distention and increase gallbladder distention.

Evaluation in the supine and left lateral decubitus positions is important. Longitudinal and transverse imaging should be routinely performed. A 2.5- to 4-MHz probe is generally used transabdominally. For endoscopic or intra-abdominal evaluations, higher-frequency probes, 7.5- to 10-MHz, may be utilized to improve resolution.

Normal Anatomy

The gallbladder fossa is typically found at the midclavicular line. The normal gallbladder is seen as a pear-shaped structure containing anechoic bile (Fig. 10.13A, B). It is typically up to 10 cm in length and 5 cm in width. The cystic duct entrance to the common bile duct is difficult to evaluate and not often seen. The common bile duct can be traced anterior to the portal vein and lateral to the hepatic artery to the insertion in the duodenum. The distal end of the common bile duct can be obscured by duodenal gas and is often difficult to see transabdominally.

Biliary Colic

Biliary colic is thought to be caused by intermittent obstruction of the cystic duct by a gallstone (Fig. 10.14A). Ultrasound has high sensitivity for gallstones, which are seen as hyperechoic intraluminal structures with anechoic posterior shadowing. Unless impacted, they are mobile and will move with a change in patient position. Gallbladder polyps can be distinguished by their fixed position on the gallbladder wall and the lack of shadowing.

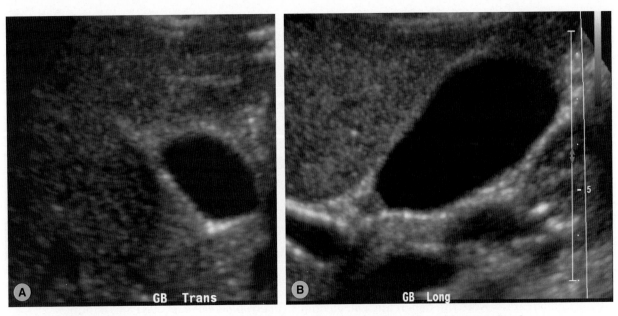

Figure 10.13. Normal gallbladder in transverse (short-axis, **A**) and longitudinal (long-axis, **B**) views.

Cholecystitis

If gallbladder outlet obstruction persists, biliary colic may progress to acute cholecystitis (Fig. 10.14B, C). While this remains a clinical diagnosis, there are several sonographic findings that support the diagnosis. These include the presence of gallstones, gallbladder wall thickening (>3 mm), maximum tenderness over the gallbladder when scanning (Murphy's sign), pericholecystic fluid, and a distended gallbladder. Complications of acute cholecystitis can also be evaluated. Gangrenous cholecystitis can be determined by the presence of fibrinous material within the wall of the gallbladder as well as mucosal sloughing, pericholecystic fluid, and a lack of an ultrasonographic Murphy's sign. In emphysematous cholecystitis, air can be seen in the wall as a hyperreflective area with acoustic shadowing. It is highly suggestive of gangrenous cholecystitis.

Choledocholithiasis

It is difficult to see distal common bile duct stones by transabdominal imaging because of overlying bowel gas in the duodenum. When stones are seen, they appear as hyperechoic filling defects with acoustic shadowing (Fig. 10.14D). Laparoscopic evaluation carries a much higher sensitivity for common bile duct stones. More commonly seen is dilation of the ductal system proximal to the obstruction. Normal duct diameter is less than 6 mm but increases with age and can reach 10 mm postcholecystectomy. Any dilation beyond that is strongly suggestive of distal obstruction.

Choledochal Cysts

Choledochal cysts are seen as large cystic masses in continuity with the bile duct, both intrahepatic and

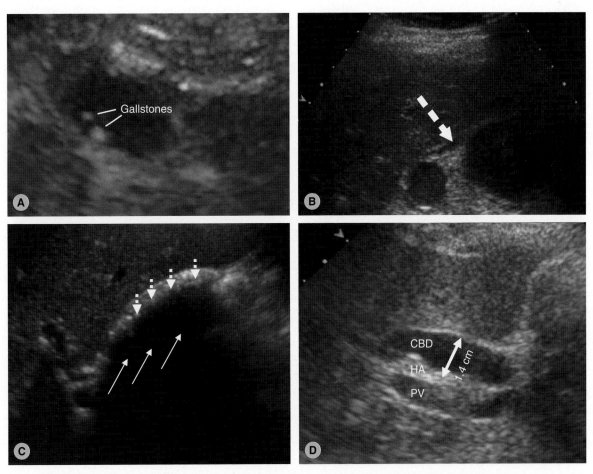

Figure 10.14. **(A)** Gallstones within the gallbladder lumen. **(B)** Pericholecystic fluid indicating cholecystitis (*interrupted white arrow*). **(C)** Gallbladder wall thickening (cholecystitis, *interrupted white arrows*) and multiple stones in the gallbladder as evidenced by extensive acoustic shadowing obscuring all deeper structures (*solid white arrows*). **(D)** Dilated common bile duct (CBD). Any dilation beyond 1 cm (10 mm) is strongly suggestive of distal obstruction. HA, hepatic artery; PV, portal vein. (*Image courtesy of Thomas Stoecker, MD.*)

extrahepatic, based on the classification. Dilation of the ductal system can also be seen entering the mass, or the mass may be secondary to that dilation.

Primary Sclerosing Cholangitis

Primary sclerosing cholangitis leads to progressive jaundice and has a strong association with inflammatory bowel disease. It appears as mural thickening of the common bile duct without acoustic shadowing. Fibrous strictures are seen, as a hyperechoic finding, with segmental dilation.

Neoplasms

Klatskin tumors are slow-growing malignant tumors of the common bile duct, seen most often at the confluence of the hepatic ducts. It is most often echogenic, with proximal hepatic dilation and a nondilated distal common bile duct. Dilation of the entire biliary system is seen with tumors of the ampulla, distal duct, duodenum, and pancreatic head.

SPLEEN

Ultrasonography has been proven beneficial in the evaluation of splenomegaly, focal splenic lesions, anemia, hematologic disorders, and trauma. In addition, ultrasound is widely utilized for guided biopsy or abscess drainage. The spleen can be difficult to access because it lies behind the lower left ribs. With the patient turned to the right, a 2.5- to 4-MHz probe is utilized along the intercostal spaces and along the costal margin. Having the patient take a deep breath can help push the spleen into view but may also hinder evaluation by inflating lung tissue between the body wall and spleen. Sagittal and transverse views should be obtained.

Normal Anatomy

The spleen lies between the 9th and 12th left ribs. It is a homogenous, finely textured organ, approximately 11 cm in longest diameter (Fig. 10.15A). However, the size can be variable but should be less than 14 cm. From the splenic vessels at the hilum, it can be traced

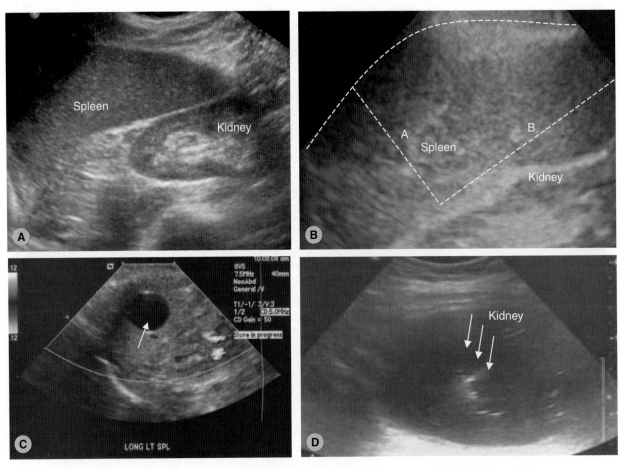

Figure 10.15. Spleen. **(A)** Normal spleen. **(B)** Splenomegaly noted in both transverse (A) and longitudinal (B) dimensions. **(C)** Splenic cyst. Note the anechoic appearance. **(D)** Splenic abscess. Note the internal acoustic signals within the abscess cavity and increased echogenicity, when compared to the cyst.

to the diaphragm, kidney, and pancreatic tail. The capsule of the spleen is smooth and highly echogenic.

Splenomegaly

Splenomegaly may be defined as a length greater than 14 cm (Fig. 10.15A). Other findings may include overlap of the splenic tip and the lower pole of the left kidney. There are many etiologies for splenomegaly, including neoplasia, congestion, lymphoproliferative disorders, infections, and inflammatory disorders. Noninvasive scanning may not be able to distinguish between these disorders because the echogenicity can be variable.

Fluid-filled lesions such as hematomas, cysts, and abscesses are most likely to appear without internal echoes (Fig. 10.15C, D [see also color insert]). Acute infarcts will start as well-defined hypoechoic lesions but will increase in echogenicity after 24 hours. Ultimately, these infarcts may return to normal echogenicity. A subcapsular hematoma will appear as a hypoechoic lesion under an intact echogenic capsule. Intraparenchymal hematomas can have varying echogenicity. Abscesses and neoplasms can appear hypoechoic. However, this is unreliable because they can have variable echogenicity. Lymphoma that presents as a focal lesion will most often appear hypoechoic. Neoplasms and chronic infarcts may appear hyperechoic. Splenic calcifications will appear as echogenic densities with acoustic shadowing and without an associated mass.

SMALL BOWEL

Because ultrasound waves are disrupted by bowel air, ultrasonography has had limited application in the evaluation of small-bowel diseases. However, it has recently seen increased utilization in the evaluation of the acute abdomen, inflammatory bowel disorders, infections, and neoplasms. Ultrasonography of the small bowel offers the standard advantages of ultrasound, including safety, portability, and cost.

The patient is best evaluated in the supine position. Fasting can help to reduce intestinal air and motility. A standard 3.5- to 5-MHz transducer will allow evaluation of large lesions of the intestine. A higher frequency probe, 7- to 10-MHz, can help delineate the layers of the bowel with better resolution. Endoscopic evaluation is also a useful and common method of evaluating the foregut and rectal walls.

Normal Anatomy

The bowel is a long and mobile organ with variable wall anatomy (Fig. 10.3). High-frequency linear array transducers will show layers of the bowel wall by contrasting echogenicity that generally correspond to the anatomic layers of the wall. The muscularis propria, submucosa, and mucosa all give echogenic signals that are separated by echo-poor interfaces.

Acute Appendicitis

The normal appendix is tubular, compressible, and nonperistaltic. The diameter should be less than 6 mm. The appendix may be difficult to find, but a normal finding can help rule out appendicitis. Findings in acute appendicitis can include a widened diameter, a lack of compressibility, and evidence of complications such as fluid around the appendix or the presence of an abscess (Fig. 10.16A).

Crohn's Disease

No single sonographic finding is pathognomonic of Crohn's disease, but there are several associated findings. The most sensitive and specific of these is wall thickening of the small bowel (Fig. 10.16B). Thickening of greater than 3 to 4 mm is indicative of active disease. A loss of wall layer stratification, hypervascularity by duplex scanning, ulceration, and surrounding enlarged lymph nodes all can be suggestive findings.

Intussusception

Intussusception appears as concentric circles when visualized in the transverse plane. When evaluated longitudinally, two multilayered structures are seen with an echogenic layer of mesentery in between. Adults will often have separate pathology at the site of intussusception.

Neoplasia

Small-intestine tumors are rare but can have some identifiable characteristics. Lymphoma often has wall thickening with loss of normal layer stratification. Carcinoid is more likely seen as an intraluminal mass, typically homogeneous, hypoechoic, and smooth bordered with disruption of the submucosa and thickening of the muscularis propria. Mesenchymal tumors are hypoechoic with little involvement of the bowel wall.

Celiac Disease

The typical findings of celiac disease are continuous peristalsis of fluid-filled loops after the patient has fasted. Other findings can include increased gallbladder size, reduced jejunal mucosal folds, thickened small-bowel wall, enlarged mesenteric lymph nodes, and free abdominal fluid. These findings must be correlated with the clinical scenario.

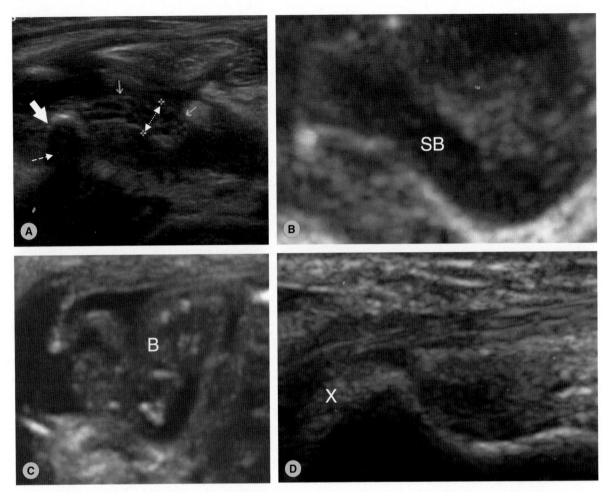

Figure 10.16. **(A)** Acute appendicitis and appendicolith (*large solid arrow*). Note the acoustic shadow of the appendicolith (*interrupted white arrow*) and dilated, inflamed, noncompressible appendix (*small white arrows*). **(B)** Dilated loop of small bowel (SB) with thickened bowel wall (compare to normal-caliber small bowel in Fig. 10.3). This finding is consistent with bowel inflammation but is nonspecific. **(C)** Bowel (B) within the hernia sack. **(D)** Fascial dehiscence with *X* marking the edges of fascia.

Hernia

Ultrasonography has been increasingly used for the evaluation of hernias, both internal and through the abdominal wall. The findings with internal hernia are those of bowel obstruction, with an area of dilated bowel seen transitioning to an area of collapsed bowel. Visualizing peristalsing bowel, fatty tissue, or other abdominal organs protruding through normal layers of the abdominal wall can confirm abdominal wall hernias. Fascia is seen as an echogenic line adjacent to the muscle layer (Fig. 10.16D). The contents can be seen pushing through this layer, either at rest or with a Valsalva maneuver.

Suggested Readings

American College of Surgeons. FAST examination. Available at: http://www.facs.org. Accessed November 2, 2009.

American Institute of Ultrasound in Medicine. AIUM practice guidelines for the performance of an ultrasound examination of the abdomen and/or retroperitoneum. Laurel, MD: American Institute of Ultrasound in Medicine; 1994, revised 2008. Available at: http://www.aium.org. Accessed November 2, 2009.

Gill KA. *Abdominal Ultrasound*: A Practitioner's Guide. Philadelphia, PA: WB Saunders; 2000.

John Ma O, Mateer JA. Emergency Ultrasound. New York, NY: McGraw-Hill Professional; 2007.

Levitov A, Mayo P, Slonim A. *Critical Care Ultrasonography*. New York, NY: McGraw-Hill; 2009.

CHAPTER 11

Pelvic Ultrasound

Creagh T. Boulger, MD, RDMS and David P. Bahner, MD, RDMS

INTRODUCTION

Pelvic ultrasound is a useful tool for any physician who treats women, especially those of reproductive age. It can be used to identify a wide range of conditions including adnexal masses, free fluid in the pelvis, extrauterine pregnancy, fibroids, ovarian torsion, and, most commonly, intrauterine pregnancies.

The use of ultrasound in medicine has existed for more than 60 years and has encompassed many clinical uses. Pelvic ultrasound's inception and expansion increased when Dr. Ian Donald, of Glasgow, Scotland, used it to help both pregnant and nonpregnant patients in the 1960s. Donald used early ultrasound equipment and published his work on imaging the uterus and adnexa.[1] Its practical utility spread, and it has become a standard tool within obstetrics and gynecology and those specialties that treat patients with pelvic complaints. As the scope of practice with diagnostic ultrasound becomes codified within the primary care community, operators will have to demonstrate technical and interpretive skills in understanding pelvic ultrasound images, just as Donald did so many years ago. Now, with the luxury of high-end equipment with superior resolution, wireless connectivity, and portability, modestly priced equipment can allow clinicians to utilize bedside ultrasound within their practices to improve patient care and satisfaction.

Pelvic imaging has evolved into a highly advanced, technological examination that can be delivered portably and wirelessly to a network of care providers. Usually, the primary care clinician is not routinely trained on how to comprehensively image the pelvis, and thus will often refer the patient for pelvic imaging. Under the traditional imaging model, the examination is performed by a sonographer and then interpreted by a specialist. The clinician as the sonologist is an alternative that allows the use of transabdominal and transvaginal imaging to aid the real-time management of the patient. Since the sonographic pelvic examination has not fully been realized outside of some obstetric, radiologic, and emergency medicine practices, more education is clearly needed. Developing into a sonologist or even a sonographer requires significant training that depends on the individual operator and his or her specialty or institutional privileging.

This chapter presents information on this highly advanced, relatively easy-to-use, diagnostic and therapeutic tool for assessing patients with pelvic complaints. Anatomy, transducers and technique, normal images and common pathology, coding and reimbursement, and the future of pelvic ultrasound will be covered. Other considerations include understanding how to achieve full utility, operator-dependent issues, and concerns regarding a general lack of educational infrastructure for how to integrate this tool into clinical practice.

ANATOMY

Before beginning, one must understand the relevant anatomy and essential landmarks of the pelvis including the vessels, ovaries, uterus, and bladder (Fig. 11.1A). Three components of understanding an ultrasound image are recognizing the relative anatomy of the patient, choosing the appropriate probe, and knowing how to read the picture on the ultrasound screen. Probe choice for transabdominal and transvaginal ultrasound, technique, probe and patient positioning, and probe manipulation will be covered to highlight how to visualize pelvic landmarks. The suggested protocol outlines how to standardize the collection of images and hopefully the diagnostic process.

The primary pelvic anatomy one must interrogate when performing a pelvic ultrasound includes the bladder, vaginal vault, cervix, posterior cul-de-sac, uterus, adnexa, and ovaries. In the pelvis, the bladder lies most anteriorly and is a landmark for the cervix, which lies posteriorly. The anterior cul-de-sac, or the vesicouterine pouch, resides between the bladder and the uterus. The posterior cul-de-sac, also known as the pouch of Douglas, resides posterior to the uterus. Since it is the most dependent area in the supine patient, it is the first location where free fluid collects.

The normal uterus consists of the fundus, corpus, cornua, and cervix. Laterally, the fallopian tubes, ovaries, and iliac vessels are usually surrounded by bowel within the true pelvis. The uterus is suspended from the pelvic wall by the broad ligament. The superior portion of this broad ligament is the fallopian tube, while the mesovarium encompasses the ovary. The ovarian ligament connects the ovary to the uterus. These ligaments are not commonly visualized on ultrasound unless there is a significant amount of free fluid in the pelvis. The vasculature of the uterus arises from the iliac arteries, while the vascular supply for the ovary arises from the abdominal aorta and receives arterial blood from just below the renal arteries. The left ovary drains into the left renal vein, while the right ovary drains into the inferior vena cava.

Uterine version is determined by the incline of the cervix, while uterine flexion is based on the relationship of the body to the cervix; thus, an anteflexed anteverted uterus has the fundus pointing most anterior and the cervix pointing posterior, as it lies in a straight plane from the fundus to the tip of the cervix. The anteverted and retroverted uterus will appear on transabdominal and transvaginal ultrasound examinations in relation to the surrounding structures. Transvaginally, the anteverted fundus is normally displayed on the left of the screen, the leading edge, while the fundus of the retroverted uterus will be on the right of the screen, the receding edge (Fig. 11.1B, C). The most common orientation of the uterus is anteverted and anteflexed however, it can also be retroverted or retroflexed or a combination of positions. The positioning of the ovaries is dependent on the position of the uterus. Thus, if the uterus is tilted to one side, the ipsilateral ovary will more often be located posterior to the uterus. The ovaries are walnut-sized structures located posterior and lateral to the uterus and anteromedial to the iliac vasculature. They consist of a central medulla and an outer cortex where follicles mature during the ovarian cycle. The position of the ovary is variable because the mobility of the mesovarium, the filling of the bladder, and the overlying bowel can alter its position within the same patient.

ANATOMIC VARIANTS

The female gynecologic system is subject to complete and partial duplication and has several potential developmental variants. These variants include the bicornuate uterus, where the uterus is Y-shaped, with two fundi and one cervix. Didelphia, another variant, can best be described as two uterine bodies, a double cervix, and two vaginas. Duplication may be best visualized transabdominally because a wider field of view can be helpful in visualizing the entire pelvis.

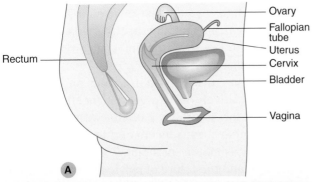

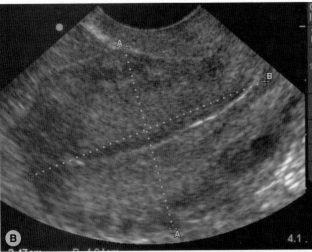

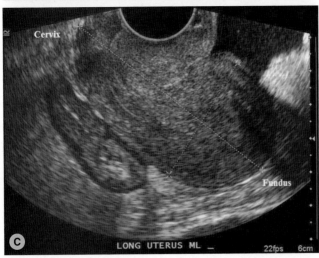

Figure 11.1. **(A)** Sagittal section of gross pelvis. **(B)** Sagittal view of the uterus at the cervix. **(C)** Sagittal view of an anteverted uterus. Note that the fundus is toward the leading edge.

TRANSDUCER CHOICE AND MANEUVERS

In addition to understanding the anatomy, it is as important to understand the ultrasound equipment, technique, and protocol to obtain and interpret adequate images. Early pelvic ultrasound utilized transabdominal imaging, while the transvaginal approach, although invented years before, came into common use only in the 1980s when better equipment and resolution were developed. Both techniques share some of the same concepts of probe movements to obtain images and improve quality by manipulating the knobs. It is important to select the probe that will produce the best picture of the anatomy one is trying to interrogate. For transabdominal sonography, a low-frequency curvilinear probe is preferred, whereas the higher-frequency endoluminal probe is best suited for transvaginal scanning. The key to acquiring good images is to understand the cardinal movements of the ultrasound probe. The probe has two main axes. The first is the axis parallel to the indicator, the long axis. The other axis is perpendicular to the indicator, the short axis. These Cartesian demarcations help one orient the probe position to the image on the screen and understand how best to move the probe in response to the corresponding anatomic landmarks. When imaging a structure, it is possible to obtain sagittal, coronal, and oblique sonographic cuts of the target. This is accomplished with fine motor movements, which can be mastered after more fully understanding the axes of the transducer probe. For example, when imaging a blood vessel, these cardinal motions allow one to transform a circular vessel into an elliptical cigar or eventually a long tube. One accomplishes this by rotating the probe, rocking and sliding, or sweeping the probe through the target area. The first motion we will discuss is the sweep. The sweep is a broad motion in the short axis of the probe. One does this to interrogate a large region and to subsequently identify an area of interest. The next motion is a rock and slide. The rock and slide is a sliding or tilting motion in the long axis of the probe. One performs the rock and slide to center an area of interest. The last cardinal motion is rotation. One rotates the probe on an axis to transition between the orthogonal planes (sagittal, oblique, and coronal), remove shadows, obtain a better acoustic window, or obtain a clearer or more complete view of the area of interest. Rotating the probe with the indicator toward the patient's right or the patient's head is usually the standard maneuver. A key point to note is that the operator should perform only one cardinal motion at a time when first scanning and that often these become very fine, subtle motions.

Transabdominal Sonography

For transabdominal pelvic ultrasound examinations, the probe of choice is a 2- to 5-MHz curvilinear probe with a large footprint (Fig. 11.2). For this examination, the patient is placed in a supine position. The probe is placed on the abdomen below the umbilicus and just above the pubic bone. Longitudinal or sagittal images are obtained by identifying the anechoic bladder, which should point to the cervix of the uterus (Fig. 11.3A). Once this is visualized, the operator rocks and slides the probe to center the bladder and uterus. Transverse or coronal images are obtained by rotating the probe 90° with the indicator (leading edge) pointing to the patient's right. With the probe perpendicular to the midline, the operator performs a transverse sweep and identifies the caudal bladder and the cephalad uterus (Fig. 11.3B). Again, the operator performs a sweep to

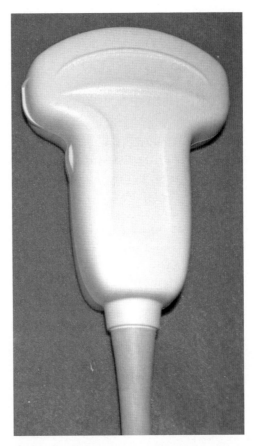

Figure 11.2. A 2- to 5-MHz curvilinear probe with a large footprint is best for transabdominal pelvic ultrasound.

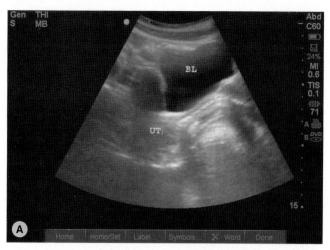

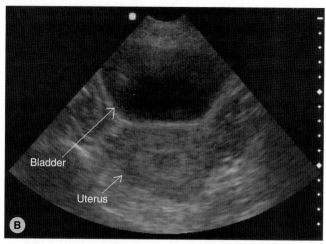

Figure 11.3. Image taken of Blue Phantom Normal IUP Endovaginal Simulator in the first trimester. **(A)** Transabdominal view of bladder "pointing to" cervix and vaginal vault. **(B)** The operator performs a transverse sweep and identifies the caudal bladder and the cephalad uterus.

identify the entire bladder and uterus, remembering to rock and slide to center the image. Saving video clips of the uterus is performed with the sweeping motion in either orientation. Transabdominal pelvic ultrasound is more commonly utilized in children, trauma, and the second and third trimester of pregnancy. If possible, this examination should ideally be performed with the patient having a full bladder.

Transvaginal Ultrasound

Transvaginal ultrasound is the preferred method of imaging for first-trimester pregnancy and for more detailed images of the pelvic organs, especially the adnexa. The probe of choice for endovaginal ultrasound is a high-frequency endocavitary probe (Fig. 11.4). Ultrasound gel should be placed directly on the probe to reduce the air interface, and the probe itself should be covered with a condom. On top of the condom on the probe tip, one should place sterile ultrasound gel or sterile lubricating gel. Some standard

ultrasound gels have been reported to cause vaginitis and possibly infection.[2]

For optimal scanning, the patient should be supine with her legs in the lithotomy position. The probe is then inserted into the patient's vagina with the indicator of the probe facing anterior (Fig. 11.5). This approach allows the operator to obtain sagittal, longitudinal images of the uterus. The first step is to identify the bladder, which should point to the cervix (Fig. 11.6A). If this is not visualized, one can try gently inserting the probe further or slightly removing the probe, as it may be in the posterior fornix. The next step is to rock and slide to visualize the whole uterus from cervix to fundus. This is essential to visualize the entire posterior cul-de-sac and interrogate this area

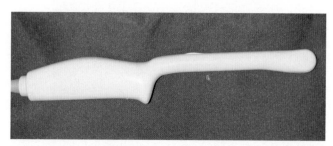

Figure 11.4. A high-frequency endoluminal probe for transvaginal ultrasound.

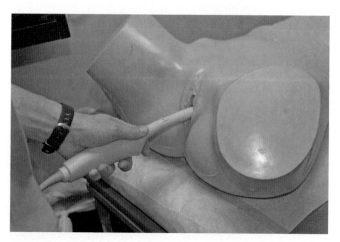

Figure 11.5. The probe is inserted into the patient's vagina with the indicator of the probe facing anteriorly.

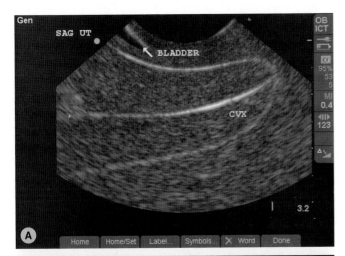

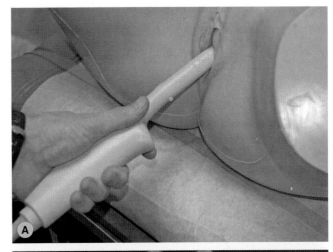

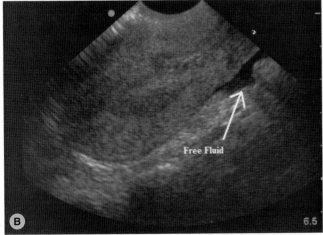

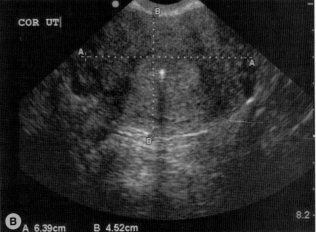

Figure 11.6. (A) Identify the bladder, which should point to the cervix. **(B)** An image of the posterior cul-de-sac demonstrating the collection of free fluid.

Figure 11.7. (A) Rotate the probe counterclockwise 90°, with the indicator to the patient's right, to obtain coronal images. **(B)** Transvaginal, coronal view of nongravid uterus, with measurements.

for free fluid (Fig. 11.6B). Following this is a sweep to visualize the uterus laterally in its entirety. It is good practice to save both stills and clips of the images obtained with both of these maneuvers. A video of these maneuvers can be viewed on the accompanying DVD. Next, one will rotate the probe counterclockwise 90°, with the indicator to the patient's right, to obtain coronal images (Fig. 11.7A). From this orientation, the operator repeats the rock-and-slide maneuver to center the uterus on the screen and then performs a sweep from anterior to posterior to view the coronal cuts of the uterus in its entirety. Again, one should save both stills and clips of the uterus in the coronal plane (Fig. 11.7B). If a gestational sac or target area is identified, these images should be centered, amplified with the zoom feature, and saved. Additional clips of the coronal sweep can be saved, as video allows the operator to visualize the real-time relationship of the structures within the pelvis.

After obtaining sagittal and coronal images of the uterus, one should proceed to interrogate each adnexa. This can be done with the indicator to the right. The probe should be in this position once imaging of the coronal view is complete. As one sweeps anteriorly, the uterine cornua can be identified as a takeoff point toward each adnexa. To view the adnexa, one will rock and slide the probe from the cornua, in coronal orientation, to the right. In doing this, the operator's hand will be near the patient's left thigh and the probe tip will be toward the patient's right adnexa. The ovary should be located anteromedial to the iliac vessels and lateral to the uterus. After the rock and slide to the side is complete, one then should perform a sweep through the entire adnexa, anterior to posterior, to identify the ovary. Once the ovary is visualized, the operator should save images with measurements; this can be done by using the dual-screen feature as shown in Fig. 11.8A. The probe is then rotated clockwise 90° so that the indicator is once again anterior to obtain the sagittal view of the ovary. One may need to perform a sweep again to relocate the ovary as it may come out of plane when the probe is moved. Once the ovary is identified, sagittal images and measurements should be saved. To image the left ovary, one slides the probe and identifies the coronal uterus and sweeps anteriorly to find the cornua. Note, the probe is still rotated with the indicator toward the patient's right. With the cornua as the take-off point, the operator slides the probe over to the patient's left. As mentioned previously, this means that the operator's hand will be near the patient's

right thigh and the probe tip angled toward the patient's left adnexa. A sweeping motion from anterior to posterior will identify the ovary. A rock and slide is performed to visualize the left adnexa and center the ovary between the uterus medially and the iliac vessels laterally, as shown in Fig. 11.8B and C. Once the ovary is visualized, one should save images and measurements, preferably in two planes. If the ovaries cannot be visualized, one should save a clip of a sweep or rock and slide through the adnexa. It should also be mentioned that imaging of the ovaries and ovarian pathology are beyond the scope of a traditional focused pelvic ultrasound examination, and if there is concern for ovarian pathology, a formal

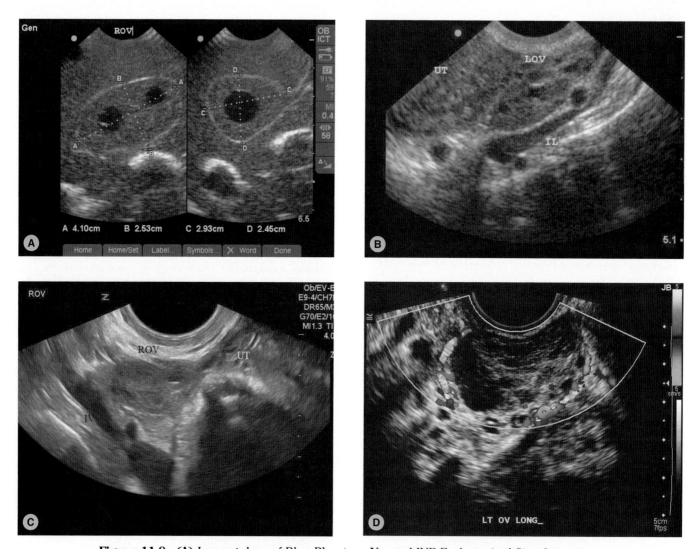

Figure 11.8. (A) Image taken of Blue Phantom Normal IUP Endovaginal Simulator in the first trimester. **(B)** Left ovary with iliac vessel lateral (receding edge) and uterus medial to it (leading edge). **(C)** Right ovary with iliac vessel lateral (leading edge) and uterus medial to it (receding edge). **(D)** Color flow of the ovary lights up the vasculature in the periphery of the ovary, which is sometimes referred to as the "ring of fire." The hues seen are indicative of the direction of vasculature flow relative to the probe (See color insert). This can be remembered with the mnemonic "BART": blue away, red toward.

comprehensive ultrasound examination should be obtained by a sonographer.

An additional image that can be obtained in a patient with a positive pregnancy test and hypotension is a right upper quadrant ultrasound, looking for fluid in the Morrison pouch. Traditionally, if fluid is present in this region in an unstable pregnant patient, a ruptured ectopic pregnancy should be suspected and early operative intervention should be initiated.

NORMAL ANATOMY

Sagittal Uterus

Figures 11.3A and 11.6A display the sagittal view of the bladder, cervix, and uterus in transabdominal and transvaginal views. Note the bladder, the anechoic structure in the near field, "pointing" to the cervix. Posterior to the cervix is the posterior cul-de-sac. This is the most dependent portion of the pelvis and is the region where free fluid in the pelvis will collect first (Fig. 11.6B). From the view of the bladder and cervix, the operator rocks and slides the probe to identify the fundus of the uterus while keeping the hyperechoic endometrial stripe in long axis to view the entirety of the posterior cul-de-sac. The operator measures the uterus in the sagittal plane from the fundus to the cervical os and across the widest portion of the fundus.

Coronal Uterus

The operator rotates the probe 90° to obtain the coronal image of the uterus and takes measurements at the widest margin (Fig. 11.7B).

Adnexa

Next, the operator interrogates the adnexa by following the cornua of the uterus laterally and finding the iliac vessels. The uterus and iliac vessels are the medial and lateral borders of the ovaries, respectively. Scanning from the levator ani muscle up to the bladder marks the area where most normal ovaries are found. Figure 11.8A is an example of a dual-screen image of the ovary from a pelvic phantom with accompanying measurements. Figure 11.8B and C demonstrates the relative anatomy of the ovary to the uterus and iliac vessels. Color flow Doppler can be used to determine whether the flow pattern is consistent with ovarian tissue (Fig. 11.8D [see also color insert]).

COMMON PATHOLOGY

In this section we discuss some of the common physiologic and pathologic processes one might encounter when performing pelvic ultrasound.

Intrauterine Pregnancy

First we will discuss the normal intrauterine pregnancy (IUP). An IUP should be visible when the quantitative β-human chorionic gonadotropin (β-HCG) level is between 1,000 and 2,000 mIU/mL, which occurs at approximately 5 weeks of gestational age. Table 11.1 describes the correlation between the ultrasound images, gestational age, and β-HCG level.

An IUP can be seen transvaginally when the β-HCG level is between 1,000 and 2,000 mIU/mL and transabdominally when it is 6,500 mIU/mL or higher. The β-HCG level should double every 48 hours for the first 8 weeks. After 8 weeks its rise becomes unpredictable as it begins to plateau. The double decidual sign can be seen in early pregnancy. This is demonstrated by the inner and outer layer of the decidual reaction surrounding the gestational sac (Figs. 11.9 and 11.10A, B). The outermost layer is known as the decidua vera; the innermost, along the gestational sac, is the decidua capsularis. The region

TABLE 11.1. The Correlation between Ultrasound Images, Gestational Age, and β-HCG Level

Gestational Age (weeks)	β-HCG (mIU/mL)	Transvaginal Ultrasound Findings
4–5	1,000–2,000	Intradecidual sac/gestational sac (Fig. 11.9)
5–6	>2,000	Gestational sac and yolk sac (Fig. 11.10A, B)
6	10,000–20,000	Fetal pole with yolk sac ± FHT (Fig. 11.11 and 11.12A, B)
6–7	>20,000	FHT (90–110 bpm), fetus will begin to develop recognizable anatomy

β-HCG, β-human chorionic gonadotropin; FHT, fetal heart tones.

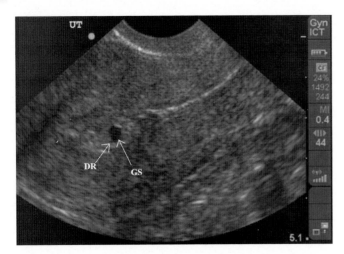

Figure 11.9. Note the anechoic, regular gestational sac (GS) and the hypoechoic ring around the gestational sac, the decidual reaction (DR).

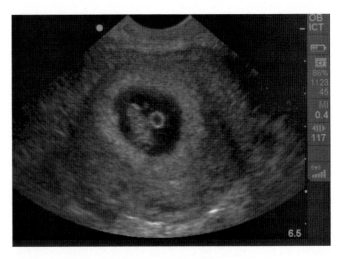

Figure 11.11. Fetal pole with yolk sac.

where the two converge is the decidua basalis, which is the site of future placental formation.

A double decidual sign is usually indicative of an IUP. However, it is present only in about 50% of all IUPs and thus is not 100% accurate.[3] If one visualizes only the gestational sac, this sign is not diagnostic for an IUP, and miscarriage or ectopic pregnancy must remain in the differential diagnosis.

Figures 11.11 and 11.12A and B demonstrate the presence of a fetal pole. This should be present by the time the gestational sac measures 16 mm (6 weeks' gestation).[3] Once a fetal pole is visualized, it is important

to perform a sweep and capture this on video to ensure that the gestational sac is completely surrounded by uterine tissue. The operator should zoom in to get clearer detail and to take measurements of both the gestational sac and the crown-rump length (Fig. 11.12B). The gestational sac measurement (inner to inner) and the crown-rump length are the common estimates for first-trimester fetal age. At 6 weeks' gestation, fetal cardiac activity should be detected. When this is present, M mode should be used to document the fetal heart rate by placing the M-mode trace over the area of cardiac activity and identifying the M-mode

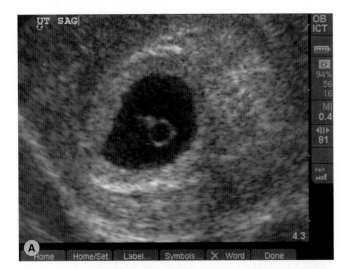

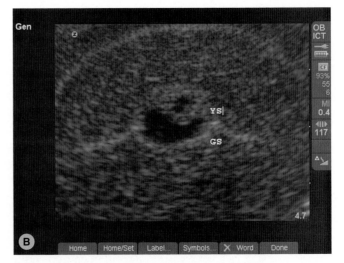

Figure 11.10. **(A)** Zoomed image of yolk sac, gestational sac, and decidual sign. **(B)** Coronal section of a gravid uterus. The double ring sign is demonstrated, which consists of a smaller inner ring, which is the yolk sac (YS), and a larger outer ring, which is the gestational sac (GS). When this is seen one must sweep through the uterus and save a clip to ensure that the entire gestational sac is surrounded by myometrium. One should also measure the gestational sac.

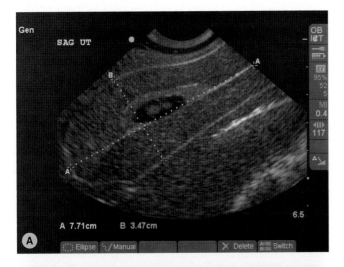

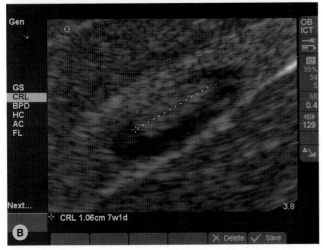

Figure 11.12. **(A)** Blue Phantom Normal IUP Endovaginal Simulator image in the first trimester. **(B)** Zoomed image of measured crown-rump length.

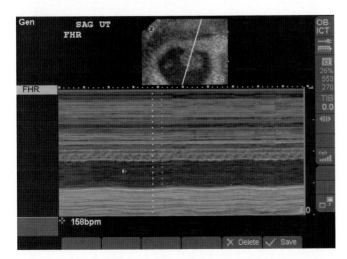

Figure 11.13. A zoomed-in image of the fetus with the fetal heart rate (FHR) measured by placing the M mode over the flicker of the heart beat. The calipers are then placed from one valley to the next, and the ultrasound machine calculates the FHR.

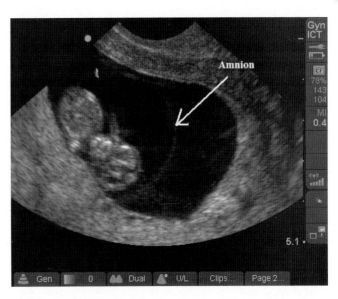

Figure 11.14. Intrauterine pregnancy with amnion and chorion visible.

waveform of the beating heart (Figure 11.13). Since pulsed wave Doppler focuses the ultrasound beam and can create more energy (and possible bioeffects) at the sample gate, this mode should not be used to measure the first-trimester heart rate. Later in the first trimester, both the amnion and chorion can be visualized (Fig. 11.14).

Multiple Gestations

Another variation of a normal IUP is multiple pregnancies (Fig. 11.15). When this is encountered, the operator should identify and label each fetus or gestational sac, take measurements of estimated gestational age, and document fetal heart tones for each fetus.

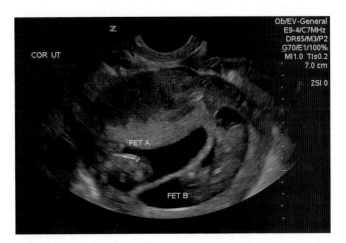

Figure 11.15. Dichorionic twins—two separate chorionic (gestational) sacs. FET, fetus.

Ectopic Pregnancy

An extrauterine pregnancy is an ectopic pregnancy and can be found in the fallopian tubes, cornua, and ovary and within the abdomen. Ectopic pregnancy is one of the pathologies that pelvic ultrasound may be most helpful in diagnosing. The single most important view is a sagittal view of the uterus that demonstrates an empty uterus without signs of a gestational sac or intrauterine pregnancy. Pelvic interrogation of the relevant structures can systematically assess the main areas where ectopic pregnancies implant and possibly identify a live ectopic pregnancy. Transvaginal ultrasound can detect extrauterine cardiac activity in 15% to 20% of ectopic pregnancies.[4,5] In many cases, secondary signs are often identified including a pseudo-gestational sac, a gestational sac incompletely surrounded by myometrium, thickened endometrium, and free fluid in the pelvis.

The presence of a tubal ring, a gestational sac in the adnex or other extrauterine location, is indicative of an ectopic pregnancy. The tubal ring is demonstrated in Fig. 11.16A. Ectopic pregnancies should be suspected in patients who have a positive pregnancy test, pelvic complaints, and no documented intrauterine pregnancy. The finding of an empty uterus (Fig. 16B) or a thickened endometrial stripe (Fig. 16C) in the context of a positive pregnancy test should heighten the suspicion for an ectopic pregnancy. Those patients with severe abdominal pain or unexplained hypotension should be evaluated quickly to determine if operative intervention is warranted. Peritoneal signs on physical examination, hemodynamic instability, or the presence of free fluid in the abdomen are commonly used to delineate those who need emergent surgical intervention. Patients at increased risk for ectopic pregnancy include those who have an intrauterine device, those with a history of tubal ligation or pelvic inflammatory disease, and those having fertility treatments. This last group of multiple implanted pregnancies can give rise to heterotopic pregnancies, a dangerous subset of ectopic pregnancies, where there may be an IUP as well as an ectopic pregnancy. Patients with a β-HCG level greater than 2,000 mIU/mL and without a confirmed IUP on transvaginal ultrasound and those at risk for heterotopic pregnancy should be investigated further for an ectopic pregnancy.

Miscarriages

Abortions or miscarriages are other diagnoses that are facilitated by pelvic ultrasound. In any female with a positive pregnancy test and vaginal bleeding, this should be on the differential diagnosis list. Some sonographic

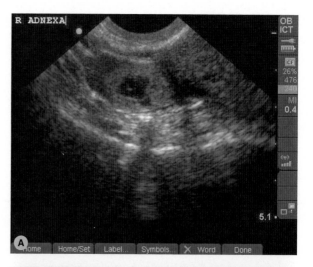

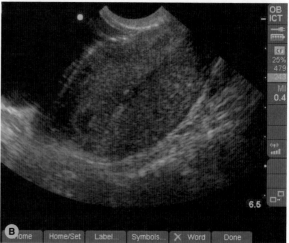

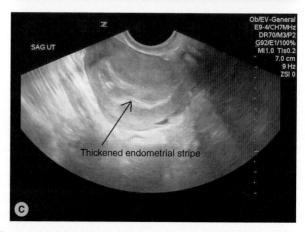

Figure 11.16. **(A)** Tubal ring, gestational sac, and yolk sac in the right adnexa. **(B)** An empty uterus in a patient with a positive urine pregnancy test, abdominal pain, and a β-human chorionic gonadotropin level greater than 2,000 mIU/mL. Figure 11.16A is from the same patient, which displays a tubal pregnancy. **(C)** Thickened endometrial stripe. This patient presented with abdominal pain and a positive pregnancy test and had a transvaginal ultrasound. She was found to have an ectopic pregnancy at exploratory laparotomy.

findings of embryonic demise are best defined on transvaginal high-resolution scans. Transabdominal ultrasound is less reliable in early pregnancy but should always be done first, as many times women are uncertain of their dates. One of the first sonographic indicators of a normal pregnancy is the presence of a gestational sac without a yolk sac. This can be a very early pregnancy, a pseudogestational sac, or a miscarriage, so one must be careful about how this is explained to the patient. The earliest accurate sign of pregnancy is the yolk sac. The first sign of a miscarriage is not so clearly defined. A sonographic sign of demise is an asymmetric gestational sac (Fig. 11.17). This often represents an incomplete abortion in the context of pelvic complaints. The distinction between an early gestational sac and an asymmetric incomplete abortion can be user dependent, so adhering to good technique can help illustrate distinguishing features.[4] Dating the pregnancy is done with measurements of the gestational sac, from the inner edge to inner edge, in either three planes or one plane, depending on vendor and measurement software packages. The crown-rump length (CRL) is usually 90° from the visualized yolk sac.

When the quantitative β-HCG level or last menstrual period suggests an estimated gestational age of greater than 6 weeks or if the CRL is greater than 5 mm, and no cardiac activity can be seen on ultrasound, especially when it has previously been detected, this often indicates embryonic demise (Fig. 11.18).[5–7] If embryonic demise is present, one may visualize this in several stages. An inevitable abortion can be seen as the uterus is expelling the pregnancy (Fig. 11.19) and the os is open. If the abortion is complete, the uterus should be empty with only small amounts of blood present. Blood can appear

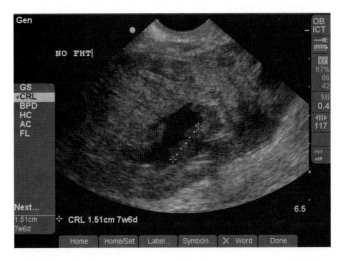

Figure 11.18. Crown-rump length greater than 5 mm without fetal heart tones. FHT, fetal heart tone.

hyperechoic with clots or even heterogenous, yet is usually anechoic when fresh.

When the size of the gestational sac is large, and there is no evidence of a fetal pole or yolk sac, this is referred to as an anembryonic pregnancy or historically as a "blighted ovum." This condition occurs when the pregnancy does not progress, yet the trophoblast does. It should be suspected when the mean gestational sac diameter (MGD) is greater than 13 mm, and there is no yolk sac or when the MGD is greater than 18 mm, and there is no fetal pole. Usually one should visualize a yolk sac by 15 mm MGD, a fetal pole by 20 mm MGD, and a fetal heart rate by 25 mm MGD. An anembryonic pregnancy is seen in Figure 11.20.

Ovarian Cysts

Ovarian cysts can be classified as physiologic (usually smaller and simple) or pathologic (usually larger and

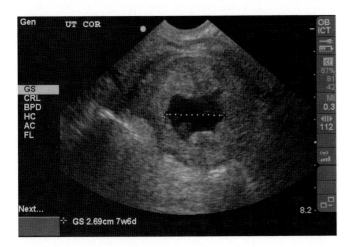

Figure 11.17. Asymmetric gestational sac.

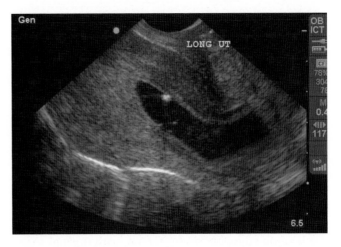

Figure 11.19. Open os, active miscarriage.

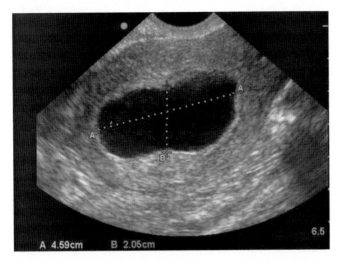

Figure 11.20. Anembryonic gestation. Gestational sac measured greater than 25 mm without a yolk sac.

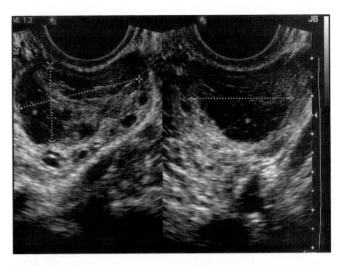

Figure 11.22. Hemorrhagic ovarian cyst.

complex). Ovarian cysts are an important type of pelvic pathology. Figure 11.21 demonstrates a corpus luteum cyst, and Figure 11.22 demonstrates a hemorrhagic ovarian cyst. There are subtle internal echoes within the hemorrhagic cyst, which are not seen in a normal corpus luteum cyst.

Fibroids (Leiomyomas)

Fibroids or leiomyomas are nonmalignant tumors within the uterine wall that can be visualized in both the nongravid and gravid uterus (Figs. 11.23 and 11.24).

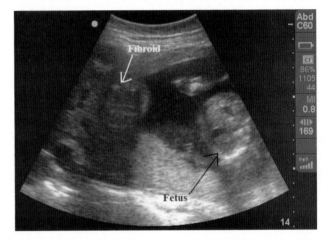

Figure 11.23. Gravid uterus with fibroid.

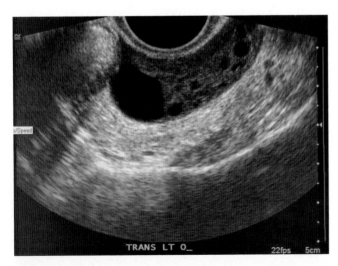

Figure 11.21. Corpus luteum cyst. Note the well-circumscribed, anechoic, black structure toward the leading edge, left of the screen, with normal ovarian tissue to its right.

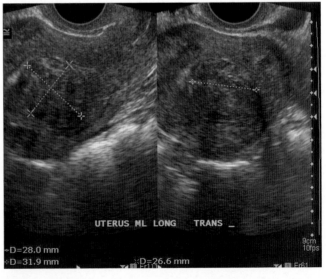

Figure 11.24. Nongravid uterus with fibroid.

Subchorionic Hemorrhage

A subchorionic hemorrhage is one of the most common abnormalities found in pregnancy. It is caused by separation of the chorion from the endometrium and subsequent bleeding. This is demonstrated in Figure 11.25. Patients with a subchorionic hemorrhage may present with vaginal bleeding but are often asymptomatic.

Gestational Trophoblastic Disease

One of the less common but interesting pathologies one might also see is a molar pregnancy. Partial moles versus complete moles depend on chromosomal aneuploidy. The appearance of a molar pregnancy within a uterus has been described as a cluster of grapes (Fig. 11.26).

Uterine Perforation

Another less common but important finding one may identify is uterine perforation, especially in the patient with abdominal pain with or without hypotension following an invasive procedure such as a dilation and curettage. Figure 11.27 demonstrates a patient with a miscarriage who underwent a dilation and curettage and suffered a perforation, with free fluid visualized near the uterine fundus.

Ovarian Torsion

The ovaries have a vascular pedicle that carries the ovarian artery and vein and reside within the broad ligament and mesovarium. Women of all ages are susceptible to torsion or twisting of this pedicle when the ovary rotates due to mass, vascular edema, or laxity in the ligament support to create a heterogenous clinical presentation.

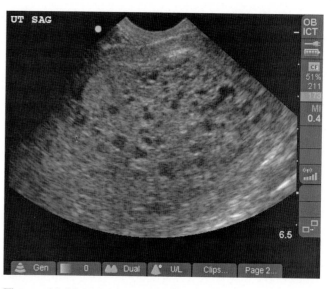

Figure 11.26. Molar pregnancy.

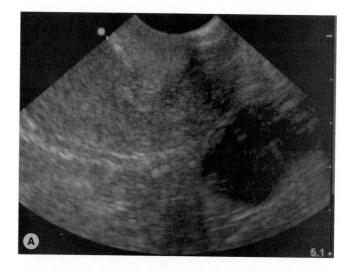

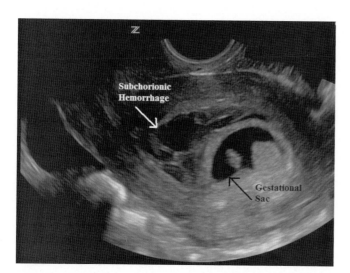

Figure 11.25. Subchorionic hemorrhage.

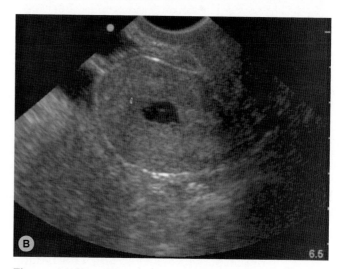

Figure 11.27. (A) Uterine perforation. **(B)**

Pelvic ultrasound should be utilized readily for suspected torsion. Those patients with intense sudden pain and ipsilateral symptoms should be considered high risk. However, multiple presentations have been described. Definitive diagnosis depends on Doppler interrogation of the ovary and its vascular network. Color Doppler can detect the presence of blood flow and direction, which can be remembered with the mnemonic "BART," blue away (from the transducer), red toward. Spectral Doppler can be used to place a gate in line with a vessel to measure blood flow. These spectral waveforms can display spectral patterns of low-resistance and high-resistance systolic and diastolic flow. The classic triphasic waveform is illustrative of a highly resistant vessel. Normal Doppler characteristics of the ovary are a ring of fire on color Doppler and a high-resistance artery on spectral Doppler.

If the operator is doing a scan and identifies an ovary measuring greater than 5 cm in any plane, the suspicion for torsion should be higher, and a comprehensive scan should be considered.[8] Conversely, patients with ovaries measuring less than 5 cm are less likely to be experiencing torsion. Ovarian torsion is beyond the scope of a focused transvaginal ultrasound and requires a comprehensive scan with Doppler flow and pulsed wave Doppler of the surrounding vessels to confirm the diagnosis.

PROTOCOLS AND BEST PRACTICES

Now that we have reviewed how to obtain pelvic ultrasound images and what one might encounter, the next step is how to apply this knowledge and consistently collect standard images from multiple operators. There are some common components of a standard pelvic ultrasound that include specific planes and demonstration of tissue in two orthogonal planes. The collection of video macro sweeps allows interpreting personnel a more complete assessment of the patient's anatomy. Micro sweeps are those small, finer movements that allow the sound beam to slightly move through a tiny gestational sac or a fetal thorax looking for a fetal heart rate. The necessary images one should save will vary across specialties and payers. The minimum number of scans in a protocol should be a long and short image of the structure, video sweeps, and measurements of relevant structures. In this manner, the same target is imaged from various planes and identified in still and video representation.

For a pelvic examination, images of the uterus in long (sagittal) and short (coronal) axis views are the starting point. From there, images of the adnexa bilaterally and the cul-de-sac for free fluid are needed for the minimal assessment. Zoomed images, measurements, labels, and other relevant annotations help to provide a richer context to any protocol designed to facilitate decision making. Pelvic ultrasound has a wide array of applicability depending on institution regulations, credentialing, and user comfort level. Having an organized approach to obtaining these images and interpreting them is essential to successful pelvic ultrasound. Figure 11.28 describes the essential components of a pelvic ultrasound examination, and Figure 11.29 illustrates an

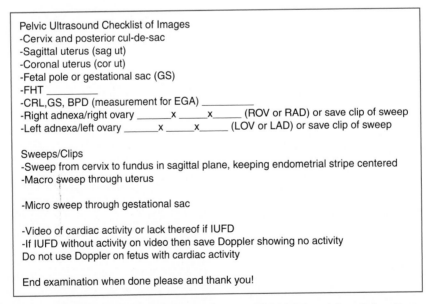

Pelvic Ultrasound Checklist of Images
-Cervix and posterior cul-de-sac
-Sagittal uterus (sag ut)
-Coronal uterus (cor ut)
-Fetal pole or gestational sac (GS)
-FHT _____
-CRL,GS, BPD (measurement for EGA) _____
-Right adnexa/right ovary _____x_____x_____ (ROV or RAD) or save clip of sweep
-Left adnexa/left ovary _____x_____x_____ (LOV or LAD) or save clip of sweep

Sweeps/Clips
-Sweep from cervix to fundus in sagittal plane, keeping endometrial stripe centered
-Macro sweep through uterus

-Micro sweep through gestational sac

-Video of cardiac activity or lack thereof if IUFD
-If IUFD without activity on video then save Doppler showing no activity
Do not use Doppler on fetus with cardiac activity

End examination when done please and thank you!

Figure 11.28. Sample protocol of images one should obtain with pelvic ultrasound. BPD, biparietal diameter; CRL, crown-rump length; EGA, estimated gestational age; FHT, fetal heart tones; IUFD, intrauterine fetal demise.

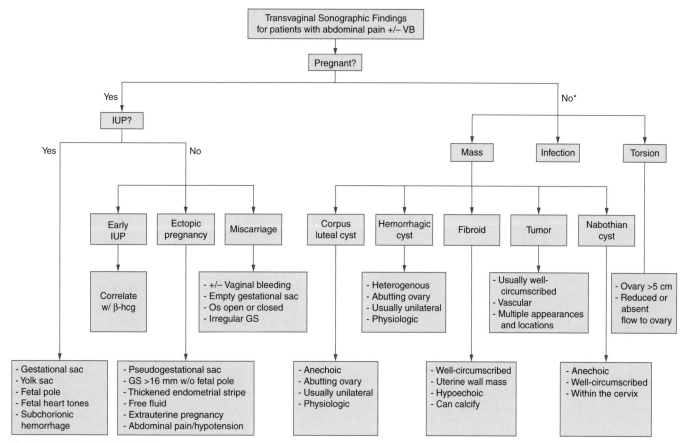

Figure 11.29. An algorithmic approach to interpreting the images one will obtain. β-HCG, β-human chorionic gonadotropin; GS, gestational sac; IUP, intrauterine pregnancy; VB, vaginal bleeding.

algorithm that can be used for medical decision making. If the transabdominal scan is clearly positive for a pregnancy, the transvaginal examination may not be warranted. Clinical context will dictate the use of transvaginal in addition to transabdominal ultrasound; transvaginal ultrasound is most commonly utilized in early first-trimester pregnancy because higher resolution is obtained from this approach.

COMMON TERMINOLOGY AND ABBREVIATIONS

- **SAG UT (sagittal uterus):** This view is demarcated by the endometrial stripe that appears hyperechoic and can be lengthened when manipulating the probe and aligning the long axis of the uterus.

- **COR UT (coronal uterus):** This view is obtained 90° from the sagittal uterus view, and the endometrial stripe once again marks the center of the uterus. In this view, the hyperechoic area is surrounded by myometrium and appears centrally tracked from the cervix toward the fundus.

- **Adnexa:** The lateral iliac vessels, ovarian tissue, and lateral half of the uterus make up the pelvic structures of the adnexa.

- **Cul-de-sac:** The potential pelvic space is oftentimes full of fluid, which can be described as a physiologic, small, medium, or large amount of free fluid.

- **RUQ (right upper quadrant): hepatorenal view:** In severe cases of hypotension, this ultrasound view can quickly demonstrate large amounts of intraperitoneal fluid, which can represent a ruptured ectopic pregnancy.

Once these images are obtained, one must utilize this information in medical decision making. At some academic institutions, backup coverage for pelvic consultation is available by obstetrics and gynecology. At other health care centers, there may not be backup for pelvic consultation, and the primary care physician must decide between operative and nonoperative interventions. Medical practice should defer to the national guidelines for practicing ultrasound and the local practice of delivering this care. One such plan is

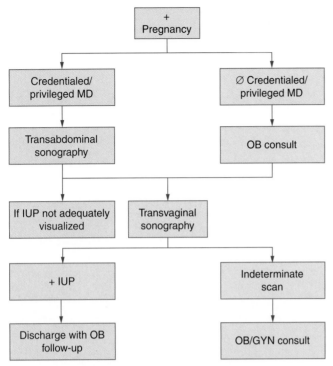

Figure 11.30. How to approach pelvic ultrasound in a facility where OB is available, a credentialing process is in place for ultrasound users, and there is a cohort of physicians with a mixed skill level in regard to ultrasound. Table 11.2 describes the images to obtain and how to proceed from the last level of the algorithm with these images. GYN, gynecology; IUP, intrauterine pregnancy; OB, obstetrics.

described here to utilize a framework of providers with mixed ultrasound privileges. Figure 11.30 describes an approach to pelvic ultrasound in a facility where obstetric care is available, an ultrasound credentialing process is in place, and there are physicians with varying skill levels. Table 11.2 describes the

images to obtain and how to proceed from the last level of the algorithm with these images.

FEASIBILITY

Pelvic ultrasound performed by emergency physicians can both minimize additional testing and expedite the disposition.[9,10] The service model of outpatient and emergency medicine means more point-of-care testing and bedside diagnostics and therapeutics. The performance of a sonography-enhanced pelvic examination can provide the clinician with important and timely clinical information. The practitioner's performance of this examination can be facilitated by introductory and basic pelvic techniques on how to obtain clinically relevant images and video. In this manner, even if the practitioner is unable to interpret the images, the images can be relayed to consultants and the information delivered back for appropriate patient care. This model is technically possible because the equipment and connectivity are available. However, two limitations to this model are standardized training and credentialing.

CODING AND REIMBURSEMENT

Diagnostic imaging has been viewed as an overpriced portion of health care, with magnetic resonance imaging and computed tomography scans the most expensive commonly used scans. Ultrasound is not nearly as expensive yet has a unique relationship in the commonly reimbursed components of a diagnostic study, the technical and the professional fee. Traditional imagers utilize sonography to acquire the images and thus this encompasses the technical fee. The images

TABLE 11.2. Medical Decision Making in Pelvic Ultrasound		
Follow-up with OB Outpatient	**Comprehensive Scan from ED**	**OB Consult in ED**
IUP + FHT	+β-HCG quantitative with inconsistent TVUS	Irregular gestational sac/ pseudogestational sac
IUP EGA consistent with β-HCG	Possible torsion	Possible miscarriage
Second-trimester pregnancy with FHT	Possible ectopic pregnancy	Possible subchorionic hemorrhage
Ovarian mass		
Vaginal bleeding with + IUP		
β-HCG, β-human chorionic gonadotropin; ED, emergency department; EGA, estimated gestational age; FHT, fetal heart tones; IUP, intrauterine pregnancy; OB, obstetric; TVUS, transvaginal ultrasound.		

are usually read by a medical physician and a report is generated to constitute the professional component. This process is a mainstay for those who perform comprehensive scans. A focused ultrasound is different from a comprehensive scan in that it is related to a direct complaint, is performed by the treating clinician, and is interpreted in real time to answer a focused question.

Focused ultrasound examination has been the crux of this chapter. A focused examination is performed with consent to answer a specific question in simple dichotomous yes-or-no terms. The clinician both acquires the images and interprets them contemporaneously. A focused examination involves a patient with a complaint that can be investigated with ultrasound to provide elements to aid in medical decision making. Focused examinations are performed at the bedside and for pelvic ultrasound involve both transabdominal and transvaginal approaches. Contrasting this is the comprehensive examination, which is performed by a sonographer and interpreted by a radiologist. The performance of any medical imaging procedure consists of technical and professional components. The technical component of ultrasound involves the acquisition of an image. The professional component is the interpretation of the examination by someone trained in sonology. Training, certification, credentialing, privileging, and accreditation are not uniformly connected with billing and collection of revenue from this procedure. The American College of Emergency Physicians has composed a document describing coding, reimbursement, and scope of practice for emergency physicians and the use of ultrasound. The *Current Procedural Terminology* (CPT) code for transvaginal echography is 76830; however, this describes a complete procedure, which would include interrogation of all of the following: the uterus, endometrium, adnexa, and ovaries. If transvaginal ultrasound is performed in the manner discussed earlier, as a more focused examination, the coding would need to have a modifier (–52), which would indicate that the examination was limited.[11] To bill for pelvic ultrasound, one must have a way to save images in hard copy or upload them to the electronic medical record. In addition, there must be documentation in the chart stating the indications for the examination, technical acquisition of the images, and findings and impressions.

FUTURE

Now that pelvic ultrasound is readily available, the question becomes, how can one integrate this into his or her practice? As with most aspects of ultrasound, there is an expansive future for pelvic ultrasound and its applicability to the general practitioner. One potential application is the concept of a virtual consult. A picture archiving computer system (PACS) with secure connectivity between groups of physicians is currently possible. In this system, images and video uploaded to the network can be viewed by anyone with access. Therefore, images at the patient site are transmitted to professionals able to interpret them, which allows asynchronous professional expertise to be given to the patient. Most times these relationships have not been fully realized since PACS is not universally available or affordable to primary care practices. Nonetheless, the technical challenges have been overcome; now the administrative protocol on how to manage these patients between different specialties must be locally developed. It is feasible that the emergency physician or general practitioner who becomes skilled in ultrasound could become the sonographer for the obstetrics/gynecology specialist physician. Depending on the credentials and privileging of the operator, straightforward cases could be managed without consultation, while more complicated findings could be referred to specialty consultants. In this model one could obtain images at the point of care, and if there was a question about the image and/or disposition, a phone call could be placed to the obstetrics/gynecology physician and he or she would be able to remotely view the images and aid in the plan for the patient. There are still limitations to this concept, such as appropriate documentation, report generation, and legal liability, but with ever-expanding technology, the concept of a virtual consult seems to be on the near horizon. Clearly, the improvements in ultrasound technology and resolution have made portable ultrasound a clinical reality. In fact, the education of operators has been outpaced by this evolving technology. The future should be focused on training those individuals who treat the pregnant patient. The sonographic pelvic examination is a robust method to interrogate the pelvic structures and provide the clinician with anatomic and pathologic relationships that can contribute to medical decision making. Consistent image acquisition and interpretation and developing these cross-disciplinary relationships can help provide this service for the patient. The future always has an unknown component, but as far as the possibilities, pelvic ultrasound will continue as a valuable adjunct in the assessment and management of patients with pelvic symptoms.

References

1. Donald I. Use of ultrasonics in the diagnosis of abdominal swelling. *Br Med J.* 1963;2:1154–1155.

2. Canadian Health and Food Branch. Risk of serious infection from ultrasound and medical gels. Available at: http://www.csdms.com/docs/ultrasoundgel_e.pdf. Accessed September 30, 2009.

3. Ma OJ, Mateer JR, Blaivas M. *Emergency Ultrasound.* 2nd ed. New York, NY: McGraw-Hill; 2008.

4. Parvey HR, Dubinsky TJ, Johnston DA, Maklad NF. The chorionic rim and low impedance intrauterine flow in the diagnosis of early intrauterine pregnancy: evaluation of efficacy. *Am J Roentgenol.* 1996;167:1479–1485.

5. Brown DL, Doubilet PM. Transvaginal sonography for diagnosing ectopic pregnancy: positivity criteria and performance characteristics. *J Ultrasound Med.* 1994;13(4):259–266.

6. Nyberg DA, Laing FC, Filly RA. Threatened abortion: sonographic distinction of normal and abnormal gestational sacs. *Radiology.* 1986;158:397–400.

7. Wilcox AJ. Incidence of early loss of pregnancy. *N Engl J Med.* 1998;319(4):189–194.

8. Houry D, Abbott JD. Ovarian torsion: a fifteen-year review. *Ann Emerg Med.* 2001;38:156–159.

9. Shea D, Aghababian R. The efficacy of abdominal and pelvic ultrasound in the emergency department. *Ann Emerg Med.* 1984;13(5):311–316.

10. Shih C. Effect of emergency physician-performed pelvic sonography on length of stay in the emergency department. *Ann Emerg Med.* 1997;29(3): 348–352.

11. Resnick J, Hoffenberg S, Tayal V, Dickman E. Ultrasound Coding and Reimbursement Document 2009. Available at: http://www.acep.org/WorkArea/DownloadAsset.aspx?id=33280 Accessed on February 28, 2010.

12. Cosby KS, Kendal JL. *Practical Guide to Emergency Ultrasound.* Philadelphia: Lippincott Williams & Wilkins; 2006.

13. Rumack CM, Wilson SR, Charboneau JW, Johnson JM. *Diagnostic Ultrasound.* Vol. 2, 3rd ed. St. Louis, MO: Elsevier Mosby; 2005.

14. Gilbert SG. *Pictoral Human Embryology.* Seattle, WA: University of Washington Press; 1989.

15. Levitov A, Mayo PH, Slonim AD. *Critical Care Ultrasonography.* New York, NY: McGraw-Hill; 2009.

16. American College of Obstetrics and Gynecology Statistics and Educational Pamphlets. Available at: www.acog.org. Accessed September 15, 2009.

CHAPTER 12

Ultrasound in Pregnancy for the Nonobstetrician

Patrice M. Weiss, MD, FACOG; Amanda B. Murchison, MD, FACOG;
Ross Hanchett, MD; and Eduardo Lara-Torre, MD, FACOG

INTRODUCTION

Ultrasound imaging has had an important impact on the practice of obstetrics and can be a powerful tool in the assessment of pregnancy.[1] In 2002, approximately 67% of all pregnant women had an ultrasound examination during pregnancy, making it a very common procedure. Ultrasound is currently recommended by the American College of Obstetricians and Gynecologists and the American Institute of Ultrasound in Medicine when there is a medical indication[1] but is not recommended for casual use in pregnancy (e.g., keepsakes and photograph albums).[2] The indications for ultrasound use in pregnancy are summarized in Table 12.1. In this chapter, ultrasound use by nonobstetricians and nonradiologists treating pregnant patients in the acute setting will be addressed.

SAFETY

Sonography is generally considered to be a safe imaging modality in pregnancy; however, the thermal effects of ultrasound can cause some concern. The high-frequency sound waves used in diagnostic ultrasound increase tissue temperatures by approximately 1°C.[3] These thermal effects have the greatest potential for harm. It is reassuring that no damaging effects to fetal tissue have been confirmed with over 30 years of ultrasound use. Nonetheless, the adherence to the following guidelines is important[4]:

- Ultrasound examinations should be performed only when clinically indicated.[4]
- The scanning process should be performed with the least amount of power and for the shortest duration possible.[4]
- Doppler ultrasound should be limited in the febrile patient because of the potential dangers of further increasing fetal tissue temperature.[3]

- Contrast agents should be avoided in pregnancy unless the risks outweigh the benefits.
- Ultrasound is a useful diagnostic tool but should not be used for entertainment or nonmedical uses.
- Three-dimensional (3D) ultrasound provides exquisitely detailed images but provides limited advantages over traditional ultrasound.

ULTRASOUND EQUIPMENT FOR PREGNANCY

The curvilinear and the vaginal ultrasound probes will be most commonly utilized in the basic assessment of pregnancy. Frequencies of 2 to 10 MHz are typically required for imaging pregnancy and the human pelvis.[4,5] The sector or curvilinear transducers used for abdominal scanning have frequencies of 3 to 5 MHz. In early pregnancy, the 7- to 10-MHz cavitary transducers are used. Higher-frequency ultrasound waves will provide greater detailed images but have minimal tissue penetration. It is important to consider this limitation when choosing an imaging approach.[5]

IMAGING TECHNIQUE

The patient should be placed in the supine or semirecumbent position. The abdomen from the pubic symphysis to the xiphoid process should be exposed. For transvaginal examinations, the patient is placed in the lithotomy position. Ultrasound gel is necessary as a coupling agent between the transducer and the patient. Gel is placed on the skin for transabdominal scans and directly on the protected probe for a transvaginal approach. Gel is also an effective lubricant during the scanning process, improving patient comfort.[5]

The transabdominal, curvilinear ultrasound probe is held in the right hand with the mark or groove oriented to the patient's right for a transverse image. With this orientation, the patient's right will be

Table 12.1. Indications for Ultrasound in Pregnancy

- Identifying the location of the pregnancy (e.g., intrauterine or extrauterine)
- Confirming fetal viability (fetal cardiac activity or fetal death)
- Establishing gestational age and estimated date of delivery
- Evaluating placenta location (anterior, posterior, fundal, partial or complete previa)
- Evaluating fetal presentation
- Performing a biophysical profile and evaluating fetal well-being
- Following fetal growth
- Evaluating vaginal bleeding
- Assessing the amniotic fluid index

From Cunningham FG, Gant NF, Leveno KJ, Gilstrap LC III, Hauth JC, Wenstrom KD. Ultrasound and Doppler. In: Cunningham FG, Hauth JC, Wenstrom KD, et al. eds. Williams Obstetrics. 22nd ed. New York, NY: McGraw-Hill; 2001:1111–1139.

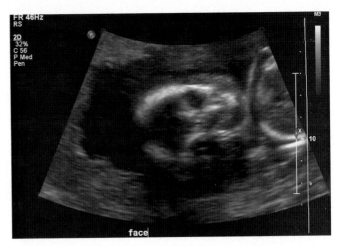

Figure 12.1. Facial bones on two-dimensional ultrasound.

(Figs. 12.1 and 12.2). Most modern ultrasound machines are equipped with an automatic save function that stores the last several seconds of images, allowing for the technician to scroll back to capture the best image.[5]

FIRST-TRIMESTER ULTRASOUND

Ultrasound can be an extremely useful tool in the evaluation of first-trimester bleeding by determining the presence of an intrauterine pregnancy, ruling out an ectopic pregnancy, and determining fetal viability by documenting cardiac activity. Cardiac activity is usually visible by transvaginal ultrasound at approximately 6.5 weeks' gestation. When pregnant patients are being evaluated in the office, the gestational age

displayed on the left side of the ultrasound imaging screen. The probe can be rotated in any direction to fully visualize the anatomic structure of interest. For transvaginal ultrasound, the probe is introduced into the vagina by the sonographer or by the patient. In many cases, it is more comfortable for the patient to insert the probe herself. The transvaginal probe is also marked, indicating the angle of sound wave propagation. The mark is generally oriented to the 12 o'clock position, resulting in the anterior pelvis being displayed on the left side of the ultrasound image.[5]

Scanning is generally initiated with a transabdominal approach. If the fetus is not identified or the gestation is suspected as early in the first trimester, the transvaginal approach may be indicated. Transabdominal scanning is performed by sliding the probe across the abdomen in both the horizontal and sagittal planes. It is best to identify the position of the baby (cephalic, breech, transverse right or left) at the onset of the procedure since this will affect the probe motions. It is also important to confirm cardiac activity early in the scanning process. The images are obtained by identifying an anatomic structure, pausing, and storing the image either in digital or hard-copy formats. Differences in image quality depend on both the probe and the machine's software and can be seen clearly between two-dimensional (2D) and 3D ultrasound

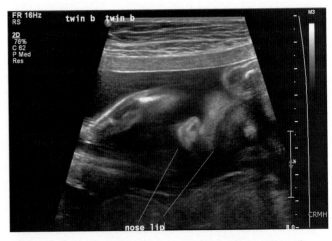

Figure 12.2. Facial features on three-dimensional ultrasound.

by the date of the last menstrual period should be determined. If the pregnancy is less than 12 weeks' gestation, the detection of the fetal heart rate by hand-held Doppler may be difficult. In this case, the use of transvaginal ultrasound may be of assistance in confirming viability and determining dates in those patients with unknown dates of last menses.

Bedside ultrasound in first-trimester bleeding can reduce morbidity and mortality by diagnosing an ectopic pregnancy prior to rupture. The best way to rule out an ectopic pregnancy is to determine the presence of an intrauterine pregnancy (IUP) by ultrasound. Although an IUP does not rule out an ectopic pregnancy, the incidence of a heterotopic pregnancy is rare, with an incidence of approximately 1 in 5,000 pregnancies. However, clinicians must recognize that in pregnancies achieved through advanced reproductive assistance, the incidence of heterotopic pregnancy can be as high as 1%. Therefore, a detailed obstetrics history is essential in addition to ultrasonography.[2]

When bedside ultrasound is used, it is essential to understand the discriminatory zone of the serum level of β-human chorionic gonadotropin (β-HCG). With a β-HCG level greater than 1,500 mIU/mL, an IUP should be seen on transvaginal ultrasound. A β-HCG level of 1,000 to 1,500 mIU/mL correlates with a gestation of approximately 4 to 5 weeks. Demonstrating a clearly defined yolk sac within the uterine cavity helps clinicians evaluate first-trimester bleeding and, importantly, helps to prevent a missed ectopic pregnancy, which, if left undiagnosed, may rupture, resulting in a life-threatening emergency (Fig. 12.3).[2]

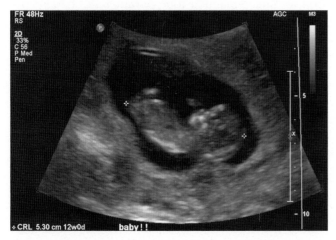

Figure 12.3. Early intrauterine pregnancy diagnosed by ultrasound.

It is also possible, though much less common, that an ectopic pregnancy itself may be identified on transvaginal ultrasound. However, only approximately 20% of ectopic pregnancies are definitively diagnosed with ultrasound. More often, an ectopic pregnancy diagnosis is suspected when there is an absence of an IUP on transvaginal ultrasound with a β-HCG level greater than 1,500 mIU/mL. Ultrasound images suggestive of an ectopic pregnancy include an adnexal mass or echogenic fluid present in the cul-de-sac. These findings combined with an empty uterus and a β-HCG level greater than 1,500 mIU/mL are highly suspicious for an ectopic pregnancy. In cases where no adnexal mass, cul-de-sac fluid, or an IUP is visualized, the ultrasound findings are classified as indeterminate. These patients require close monitoring and follow-up with serial β-HCG levels and clinical evaluation and examination.[2]

When an IUP and fetal cardiac activity are identified, and the first-trimester bleeding is minimal, the patient can be reassured. In cases of an indeterminate ultrasound or an ectopic pregnancy, an obstetrician should be consulted for ongoing management and follow-up. All pregnant women should be tested for the presence or absence of D antigen on their erythrocytes. If the patient's Rh status is unknown when she presents with bleeding early in pregnancy, a type and screen to assess the Rh status is warranted. Rh-negative patients with a negative antibody screen who experience bleeding in pregnancy should receive Rh$_o$(D) immune globulin to prevent Rh sensitization in subsequent pregnancies.[4]

When a screening ultrasound is performed early in the gestation or an evaluation for vaginal bleeding is undertaken, the identification of a nonviable IUP may be encountered. Without the use of ultrasound, this diagnosis is difficult or impossible to make early in the presentation. Additional information can be obtained with a first-trimester ultrasound, including an assessment for fetal number to rule out a multigestational pregnancy.[6] Ultrasound evaluation also can diagnose the presence of a complete hydatidiform mole. These patients often present with first-trimester bleeding, a uterine size greater than suspected gestational age, and hyperemesis. The β-HCG level is greater than 100,000 mIU/mL. Ultrasonography demonstrates no fetus or fetal pole within the uterus. Instead, the uterus is filled with cystic placental tissue with the classic appearance of a "snowstorm." Patients with a partial molar pregnancy also usually present with vaginal bleeding. Again, an elevated β-HCG level and an abnormal ultrasonographic appearance suggest a molar pregnancy. Partial molar pregnancies have an associated fetal pole, but usually these will be nonviable pregnancies with no cardiac activity. In either case, after finding an elevated β-HCG level and ultrasound findings not revealing a viable IUP, consultation from an obstetrician is essential.[7]

In addition to the important use of ultrasound in the first trimester, especially in evaluating bleeding, ultrasound has other uses in all trimesters.

While the most accurate method to assess gestational age is the first-trimester measurement, patients may present for prenatal care or emergent needs beyond the first trimester and, in fact, may not know how advanced the pregnancy is or be able to report a date of the last menstrual period. Therefore, the gestational age is unknown. Ultrasound can assist in determining a gestational age beyond the first trimester through measurements such as a biparietal diameter (BPD), abdominal circumference, and femur length.[6]

The BPD is most accurate between 12 and 28 weeks of gestation and is best measured at the level of the thalami from the outer edge of the proximal skull to the inner edge of the distal skull. Head circumference is measured at this same level.[8] The femur length, originally used to diagnose dwarfism, can be measured beginning at 10 weeks. Measurements are obtained from the femur origin to the distal end of the shaft but exclude the femoral head and distal ephiphysis.[8] The abdominal circumference is very sensitive to variations in fetal growth and is used in addition to other biometric parameters to establish an estimated fetal weight and diagnose intrauterine growth restriction and fetal macrosomia. Measurements are obtained at the level of the junction of the umbilical vein, portal sinus, and fetal stomach when visible.[6,8]

Other factors that should be assessed during an obstetric ultrasound include fetal viability at any gestational age, fetal number (Fig. 12.4), adnexal structures, and placental location and appearance.[6] Amniotic fluid volume and fetal well-being are assessed by the biophysical profile (BPP).

In some scenarios, identification of the presenting part in the vagina during the labor process is difficult because of the patients' body habitus or the advanced stage of labor. The use of ultrasound to determine the presenting part such as a vertex or breech would make a difference in the management of the patient, as currently most physicians will deliver breech presentations by cesarean section to minimize trauma during delivery.

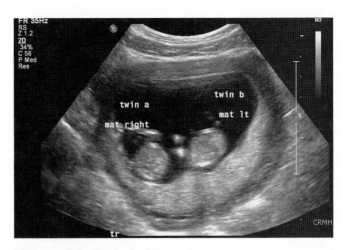

Figure 12.4. Twin pregnancy.

BIOPHYSICAL PROFILE

The BPP is a tool for providing antepartum fetal surveillance and is designed to evaluate the integrity of the fetal central nervous system with a goal of identifying a compromised fetus. The BPP was originally described by Manning et al and uses five parameters[9,10]: (1) nonstress test, (2) fetal movement, (3) fetal tone, (4) fetal breathing, and (5) amniotic fluid measurement (Table 12.2; Fig. 12.5 [see also color insert]). The nonstress test involves fetal heart rate monitoring for a period of 20 to 40 minutes. During this test, the fetal heart rate on fetuses with a gestational age greater than 32 weeks must increase by 15 beats per minute over baseline and last for 15 seconds to be called acceleration. Two accelerations are needed within a 20-minute time frame to qualify as a reactive nonstress test (Fig. 12.6). Ultrasound is performed to look for the remaining four parameters. Two points are given for each parameter met, and no points are given when the criteria for each parameter are not observed. The study is stopped when all four parameters are seen or 30 minutes pass. A composite score of 8 or 10 is considered normal with a low risk for chronic fetal asphyxia. A score of 6 is considered equivocal and requires repeat testing in 4 to 6 hours if gestational age is less than of 36 weeks. For pregnancies of 36 weeks' or more gestation, delivery is usually indicated. Scores of 0 or 4 are considered abnormal and suspicious for chronic asphyxia. Management of these patients depends on the gestational age. However, a fetus that persistently scores 4 or less should be delivered, regardless of gestational age.[11]

A Cochrane systematic review from 2007 provided insufficient evidence from randomized trials to support

Table 12.2. Biophysical Profile Parameters

Parameter	Normal = 2 Points	Pathophysiology
Nonstress test	Reactive	A fetus who is not acidotic, with an intact autonomic nervous system, should have increases in heart rate associated with movement.
Fetal movement	Three or more discrete fetal body/limb movements	Movement is navigated by a complex neurologic pathway.
Fetal tone	One or more movements of active extension with return to flexion or fetal limb/trunk, or opening and closing of hand	This is the last parameter to be lost with worsening asphyxia.
Fetal breathing movement	Downward movement of diaphragm and inward movement of chest for at least 30 continuous seconds	When present, movement reflects an intact neurologic system. It is seen more often in fetal rapid eye movement sleep and during maternal hyperglycemia. Maternal smoking and narcotic use is associated with decreased fetal breathing movement.
Amniotic fluid volume	At least one vertical fluid pocket measuring 2 cm	Amniotic fluid is mostly composed of fetal urine, and a low fluid level suggests chronic hypoxia.

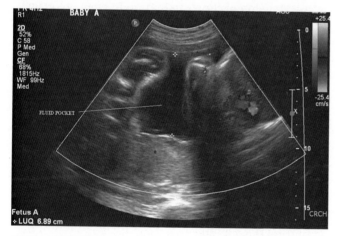

Figure 12.5. Measurement of amniotic fluid pocket. (See color insert.)

the use of the BPP as a test of fetal well-being.[12] However, antepartum fetal surveillance such as the BPP is frequently used to monitor high-risk pregnancies.

PLACENTAL EVALUATION

Evaluation of the placenta is an important part of every second- and third-trimester ultrasound. The placental location should be documented as anterior, posterior, fundal, low lying, or previa (Fig. 12.7). A low-lying placenta does not cover the opening of the cervix (cervical os) but is close. Typically, a vaginal delivery can take place if the placental edge is greater than or equal to 3 cm from the cervical os. Placenta previa is defined as implantation of the placenta over

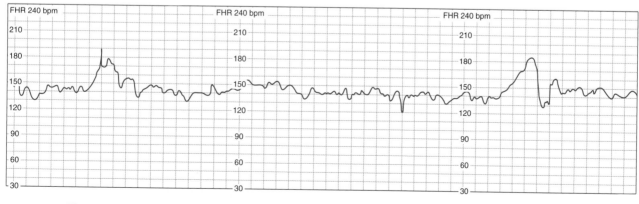

Figure 12.6. A fetal monitor tracing with two accelerations.

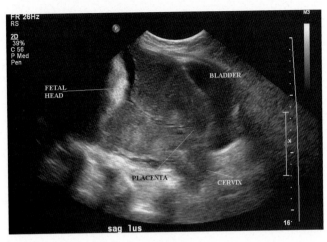

Figure 12.7. Placenta previa.

Table 12.3. Placental Implantation Abnormalities

Abnormality	Description
Placentation	Depth of uterine invasion
Placenta accreta	Invades endometrium and contacts myometrium
Placenta increta	Invades myometrium
Placenta percreta	Invades entire myometrium and uterine serosa and can enter other organs such as the bladder

the cervical os. In the second trimester, placenta previa can be seen in up to 15% of patients. However, secondary to the development of the lower uterine segment in the third trimester, only 1 in 200 live births is complicated by placenta previa.

A normal placenta will easily detach from the endometrium after delivery. If a placenta is abnormally implanted (Table 12.3), it can cause a life-threatening postpartum hemorrhage. Risk factors for abnormal placentation include prior cesarean or other uterine surgery including dilation and curettage, maternal age older than 35, and multiple previous pregnancies.

Ultrasound can be used to diagnose placental implantation abnormalities. Findings such as the loss of a normal hypoechoic rim of myometrial tissue beneath the placental surface or the presence of placental echo texture beyond the uterine serosa are suggestive of these abnormalities. If one of these placental abnormalities is suspected, magnetic resonance imaging may be used to better differentiate the placental planes. The clinician should perform a complete examination of the patient, but in those patients with unexplained vaginal bleeding in the second or third trimester, ultrasound should be used as an extension of the examination to evaluate placentation instead of performing a digital examination, if the patients' condition allows. The use of bedside ultrasound in the management of acute vaginal bleeding in the late pregnancy stages is recommended and should be encouraged.

ACKNOWLEDGEMENTS

The authors wish to acknowledge Dr. Thomas Stoecker for his contribution of ultrasound images as well as Lisa Smith for her endless assistance and work on putting this chapter together.

References

1. Routine prenatal ultrasonography as a screening tool. Available at: http://utdol.com/online/content/topic.do?topicKey=antenatl/18078&selectedTitle=1~150&source=search_result. Accessed August 2009.

2. Jang T, Chen J. Bedside ultrasonography first-trimester pregnancy. Available at: http://medscape.com. Accessed September 2009.

3. Physics and safety of diagnostic ultrasound in obstetrics and gynecology. Available at: http://utdol.com/online/content/topic.do?topicKey=antenatl/15779&selectedTitle=1~150&source=search_result. Accessed.

4. Cunningham FG, Gant NF, Leveno KJ, Gilstrap LC III, Hauth JC, Wenstrom KD. Ultrasound and Doppler. In: Cunningham FG , Hauth JC, Wenstrom KD, et al. eds. *Williams Obstetrics*. 22nd ed. New York, NY: McGraw-Hill; 2001:1111–1139.

5. Ultrasound examination in obstetrics and gynecology. Available at: http://utdol.com/online/content/topic.do?topicKey=obstetri/4473&selectedTitle=1~150&source=search_result. Accessed September 2009.

6. American College of Obstetricians and Gynecologists. ACOG practice bulletin no. 56. *Obstet Gynecol*. 2004;104:869–883.

7. Schorge JO, Goldstein DP, Bernstein MR, Berkowitz RS. What is new in the management of gestational trophoblastic disease. In: Ransom SB, Dombrowski MP, Evans MI, Ginsburg KA, eds. *Contemporary Therapy in Obstetrics and Gynecology*. Philadelphia, PA: WB Saunders Company; 2002:477–480.

8. Jeanty P. Fetal biometry. In: Fleisher AC, Romero R, Manning FA, Jeanty P, James EA Jr, eds. *The Principles and Practice of Ultrasonography in Obstetrics and Gynecology*. East Norwalk, CT: Appleton; 1991:101–103.

9. Manning F, Platt L, Sipos L. Antepartum fetal evaluation: development of a fetal biophysical profile. *Am J Obstet Gynecol*. 1980;136:787–795.

10. Manning FA, Harman CR, Morrison I, et al. Fetal assessment based on fetal biophysical profile scoring. *Am J Obstet Gynecol*. 1990;162:703–709.

11. Druzin ML, Gabbe SG, Reed KL. Antepartum fetal evaluation. In: Gabbe SG, Niebyl JR, Simpson JL, eds. *Obstetrics: Normal and Problem Pregnancies*. 4th ed. Philadelphia, PA: Churchill Livingstone; 2002:313–349.

12. Lalor J, Fawole B, Alfirevic D, Devane D. Biophysical profile for fetal assessment in high risk pregnancy Cochrane Database Systematic Review 2008, Issue 1. CD000038.

CHAPTER 13

Renal and Genitourinary Ultrasound

Yefim R. Sheynkin, MD, FACS

INTRODUCTION

Formal urologic ultrasound is a detailed examination of the genitourinary organs performed by a radiologist or radiology technician. Recent advances in technology have made ultrasound equipment readily available for internal medical practice. The development of versatile portable and hand-carried ultrasound machines has significantly improved its utility and clinical accuracy. Many clinicians without formal radiologic training have acquired sufficient skill to perform limited, focused examinations. While portable or office-based sonography is not a preferred tool for a comprehensive examination, it is a powerful and inexpensive modality particularly well-suited for quick and efficient evaluation. Ultrasound has become a valuable tool to supplement the information obtained through routine history, physical examination, and laboratory studies.

Easy accessibility of major organs of the urinary system makes ultrasound a commonly performed test. Genitourinary sonography has multiple applications including initial evaluation of patients with flank pain, hematuria, complicated urinary tract infection, decreased or absent urinary output, lower urinary tract syndrome, urolithiasis, and enlarged painful and painless scrotum, as well as monitoring of known pathology. In addition, many abnormalities may be found incidentally during sonographic evaluation. While they may not have an impact on immediate treatment decisions, physicians should be able to recognize them and provide appropriate care if necessary. While many of the genitourinary diseases require urologic intervention, a sonographic study may provide an internist with the diagnosis and guidance for rapid decision making necessary for treatment.

Finally, a level of genitourinary sonographic evaluation depends on the training and experience of the physician performing the examination. Attendance of widely and frequently offered ultrasound teaching courses will significantly improve diagnostic abilities and help to avoid common mistakes.

ULTRASOUND TERMINOLOGY

Sonographic images are generated by sound waves, which are sent by a transducer into the human body and are reflected back by different tissues (echo effect). Echogenicity is the ability to create an echo (i.e., return a signal in ultrasound examinations). Knowledge of sonographic terminology is essential for the diagnostic evaluation of different organs.

- **Hyperechoic:** bright and white (more echoes than surrounding tissue)
- **Hypoechoic:** dark (fewer echoes than surrounding tissue)
- **Isoechoic:** the same as a reference echogenicity (e.g., liver or paired organs such as the testes)
- **Anechoic:** black (absence of echo)
- **Homogenous:** uniform echogenicity (dark or bright)
- **Heterogenous:** mixed echogenicity (dark and bright)
- **Acoustic shadowing:** the presence of a uniform dark band behind an object (e.g., kidney stone)

SONOGRAPHIC ANATOMY OF THE URINARY TRACT

The normal adult kidney is a bean-shaped structure surrounded by a well-defined smooth echogenic capsule representing Gerota fascia and perinephric fat. The kidneys have a convex lateral edge and a concave medial edge called the hilum. The lower pole is located more laterally and anteriorly than the upper pole. The sonographically measured normal adult kidney is between 9 and 12 cm in length and about 4 to 5 cm wide.

The kidney parenchyma surrounds a centrally located hyperechoic fatty renal sinus, which contains the renal pelvis, calyces, major branches of the renal artery and vein, and lymphatic vessels. Parenchyma corresponds to the area between the renal sinus and outer renal surface and has two main components: a more echogenic peripherally located cortex and a centrally located hypoechoic medulla, which contains renal pyramids. A normal renal parenchyma is 1.0 to 1.8 cm thick. A visible distinction between the cortex and medulla is a sign of a normal kidney. While this is easily recognized in children and younger patients, it may not always be detectable in the elderly.

Parenchymal homogeneity is determined in comparison with that of the adjacent liver and spleen. Normally, a renal cortex is hypoechoic or isoechoic to the liver (right kidney) and hypoechoic to the spleen (left kidney).

A collecting system of a kidney is not usually visible with ultrasound since the calyces and pelvis are collapsed within the renal sinus.

The normal ureters measure about 8 mm wide and are difficult to evaluate sonographically. However, proximal or distal ends of a significantly dilated ureter (hydroureter) can be seen.

The shape and appearance of a normal bladder depend on the degree of distention. When empty, the bladder lies behind the symphysis pubis. On longitudinal transabdominal view, the full bladder has a teardrop-shaped anechoic appearance with a distinct wall, while on the transverse view it appears rectangular. Bladder wall thickness varies with a degree of bladder filling. When mildly distended or empty, the bladder wall is thick and irregular. With full distension, the normal bladder wall is thin and smooth and does not exceed 4 to 5 mm in thickness. Prostate imaging can occur through the distended bladder on a transverse bladder scan by directing the transducer more caudally toward the symphysis pubis. However, a transrectal approach provides the most detailed sonographic examination.

COLOR DOPPLER ULTRASOUND

Color Doppler ultrasound (CDU) is an imaging technique that demonstrates color blood flow images over real-time B-mode images. Red is allocated for blood flow toward the transducer and blue is allocated for blood flow away from the transducer. Color flow and spectral Doppler study are able to provide noninvasive indirect assessment of renal and testicular blood flow and patency of the ureters.

Renal Color Doppler Ultrasound

The Doppler spectral tracing reflects a low vascular resistance and classically has a ski slope appearance. From the many different indices introduced to quantify blood flow, the most commonly used single parameter is the resistive index (RI), a ratio between the end-diastolic velocity and peak systolic velocities. RI is a physiologic parameter reflecting a degree of renal vascular resistance. Normal renal blood flow has a low resistance pattern with a flow maintained throughout diastole. The normal RI values are 0.58 ± 0.10. Values greater than 0.70 are considered abnormal and may be due to lower arterial patency, although major clinical significance is observed for values greater than 0.80. Doppler signals are commonly obtained from the renal artery or interlobar/arcuate arteries at a corticomedullary junction and a border of medullary pyramids. The test is routinely performed to evaluate a transplanted kidney.

The RI has been proposed for the differential diagnosis between obstructive and nonobstructive hydronephrosis or the diagnosis of acute obstruction when dilatation has not yet developed. A minority of patients with obstructive renal failure may not show hydronephrosis due to dehydration or decompression caused by rupture of the calyceal fornix. High intrarenal pressure and changing renal hemodynamics due to release of vasoactive substances and vasoconstriction secondary to obstruction cause increases in intrarenal arterial resistance measured by a higher RI. While diagnostic accuracy of the RI still remains controversial because of a wide range of results, a normal RI may still be helpful in arguing against the presence of obstruction.

Scrotal Color Doppler Ultrasound

Scrotal CDU is presently performed in all examinations of the adult scrotum. Testicular CDU is the most useful and rapid technique to evaluate testicular blood flow and differentiate between testicular torsion and epididymo-orchitis. In torsion, blood flow is absent or significantly reduced in the affected testis compared with the normal contralateral testis. In epididymitis/epididymo-orchitis, CDU usually demonstrates increased blood flow in the epididymis or testis.

Bladder Color Doppler Ultrasound

Color flow Doppler ultrasound is frequently performed for the evaluation of the patency of the ureter. Jet phenomena should be seen in the bladder when the urine bolus from the ureter is being propelled into the bladder cavity because of periodic peristalsis (1–12 jets per minute). Ureteral jets are usually identified during transverse bladder scanning as a color projecting into the bladder lumen from the lateral posterior border and coursing superiorly and medially.

RENAL ULTRASOUND

Imaging Technique

Sonographic examination of the kidneys offers a quick evaluation of their location, size, shape, and echogenicity (Fig. 13.1. [see also color insert]). In accordance with the American Institute of Ultrasound in Medicine (AIUM) practice guideline, the examination of the kidneys should include longitudinal and transverse views of the upper poles, midportions, and lower poles and assessment of the cortex and renal pelvis. When possible, renal echogenicity may be compared with echogenicity of the adjacent liver or spleen. Kidneys and perirenal regions should be assessed for abnormalities.

Commonly, a sector or curved array transducer (3–5 MHz) is used, while higher-frequency probes (5–7 MHz) with higher space resolution may be necessary to evaluate children, thin patients, and a transplanted kidney. Imaging of the urinary tract must always include evaluation of both kidneys and the bladder.

The right kidney is best examined in the supine or left lateral decubitus position through the liver, which serves as an acoustic window. The probe should be placed along the right lateral subcostal margin in the

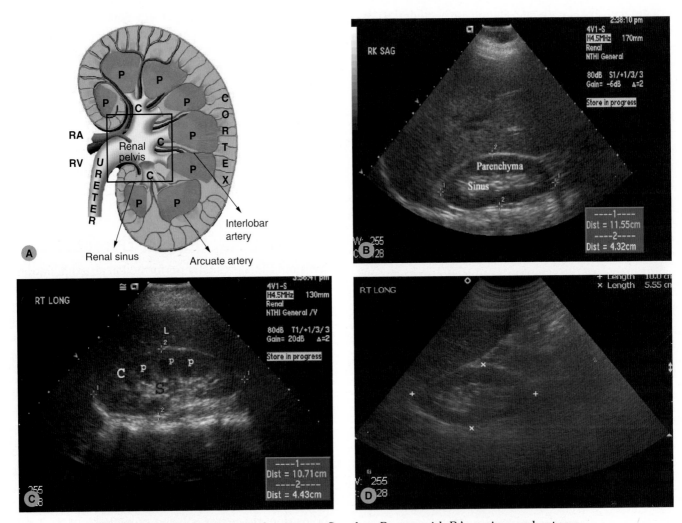

Figure 13.1. **(A)** Normal renal anatomy. C, calyx; P, pyramid; RA, main renal artery; RV, main renal vein. **(B)** Normal kidney. Longitudinal view of the kidney demonstrates peripheral hypoechoic universally thick parenchyma and a central hyperechoic renal sinus. Note the echogenic white Gerota fascia. Parenchyma is less echogenic than liver (L). **(C)** The cortical echogenicity (C) is equal to that of the liver (L). Several slightly hypoechoic renal pyramids are seen. **(D)** Portable ultrasound of the normal right kidney. Note less contrast appearance, but the renal contour, parenchyma, and renal sinus are clearly identified. (See color insert.)

anterior axillary line, scanning through the liver to locate the right kidney. After visualization of the whole kidney, optimal longitudinal view is obtained by slowly adjusting the probe's position up and down or side to side. The kidney is traditionally measured in the longest axis (length and width) since the longitudinal diameter has minor inter- and intraobserver variations. If needed, a transverse plane (short-axis view) can be obtained by rotating the probe 90° and evaluating the upper, mid-, and lower portions of the kidney separately.

The left kidney is typically less visible because of its location in a more superior position, the lack of the sonographic window generated by the liver, and the overlying small bowel and gastric gas. If possible, placing the patient in the right lateral decubitus position with the probe positioned in the posterior axillary line or left costovertebral angle may improve visualization. If bowel gas obscures the kidney (especially the left) and reflects ultrasound waves, the transducer can be positioned in the mid- or posterior axillary line.

Common Kidney Ultrasound Findings

Frequent clinical indications for a renal ultrasound include flank pain, hematuria, renal insufficiency, persistent obstructive voiding symptoms, and persistent urinary tract infection/urosepsis. Renal sonography provides an accurate but not a definitive diagnosis of many urologic diseases (e.g., benign versus malignant mass, cause of obstructive uropathy, ureteral stone, etc.). While additional diagnostic modalities will be necessary to establish the proper therapeutic approach, simple and fast ultrasound evaluation will put a patient on a fast track to timely specialized treatment.

Obstructive Uropathy (Hydronephrosis)

Obstructive uropathy remains the most important finding that requires urgent treatment since it is likely to be reversible. Sonography can usually diagnose obstruction quickly and simply with a sensitivity of approximately 95%. Dilatation of a renal collecting system (hydronephrosis) is the most important sonographic feature of obstructive uropathy. Renal pelvis and calyceal dilation are characterized by effacement of the renal sinus fat by an anechoic branched structure with through-transmission. Hydronephrosis is most commonly characterized as mild, moderate, or severe. The degree of renal damage can be quantified on the basis of parenchymal thickness reduction. Mild hydronephrosis (grade I) refers to minimal dilatation of the collecting system, known as splaying. Moderate hydronephrosis (grade II) shows rounding of the

calyces with obliteration of the papillae. Cortical thinning is minimal in moderate hydronephrosis. Severe hydronephrosis (grade III) refers to massive dilatation of the renal pelvis and calyces associated with cortical thinning (Fig. 13.2A–C, D, G). Analysis of ureteral jets by CDU may help to diagnose ureteral obstruction. Absence of ureteral jets does not correspond to the degree of hydronephrosis but is highly significant as an indication of obstruction.

Pyonephrosis

Pyonephrosis must be suspected in patients with hydronephrosis, urinary tract infection, and ultrasound findings of low-level echoes with occasional layering in the dependent position of the dilated collecting system. It represents pus in the obstructed and infected collecting system and requires immediate surgical treatment for renal drainage (Fig. 13.2F).

The American College of Radiology Appropriateness Criteria suggest ultrasound as a primary imaging technique in acute renal failure, which rapidly provides useful information about kidneys independent of renal function. About 5% of patients with acute renal failure suffer from obstructive uropathy (hydronephrosis). Postrenal acute renal failure can be efficiently corrected if promptly diagnosed. It is more common in patients with certain predisposing factors including urolithiasis, retroperitoneal cancer, or solitary kidney. In patients with no risk for urinary obstruction, only around 1% will have sonographically detected hydronephrosis. Nevertheless, knowing that obstruction is not present is as important as finding and treating obstruction.

Chronic Renal Failure

Chronic renal failure may be associated with small (5–8 cm in length) contracted kidneys with increased echogenicity. Renal sinus echoes are still visible. The parenchyma may show evidence of focal losses (Fig. 13.3A).

Nephrolithiasis

Nephrolithiasis is one of the most common kidney problems. Kidney stones are intensely hyperechoic linear or arching foci with posterior acoustic shadowing (Fig. 13.3B). They can be of different sizes and locations within the kidney. Ultrasound may detect with relative confidence stones greater than or equal to 5 mm. Smaller stones may not exhibit acoustic shadowing, making definitive diagnosis more difficult. Obstructing stones occasionally can be seen in patients with hydronephrosis and a dilated proximal or distal ureter. Nonobstructing kidney stones do not require urgent treatment.

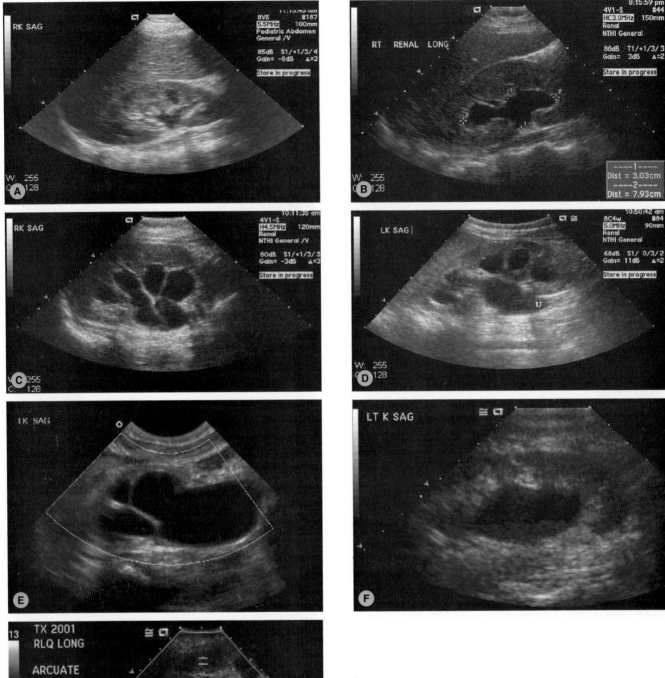

Figure 13.2. (A) Mild hydronephrosis with slight widening of the renal collecting system. **(B)** Moderate hydronephrosis. **(C)** Moderate hydronephrosis without loss of renal parenchymal thickness. **(D)** Hydronephrosis and proximal hydroureter (U). **(E)** Severe hydronephrosis with thinning of renal parenchyma. **(F)** Pyonephrosis. Moderate to severe hydronephrosis with fine debris in the renal collecting system. **(G)** Color Doppler study shows elevated resistive index of the arcuate arteries in hydronephrosis.

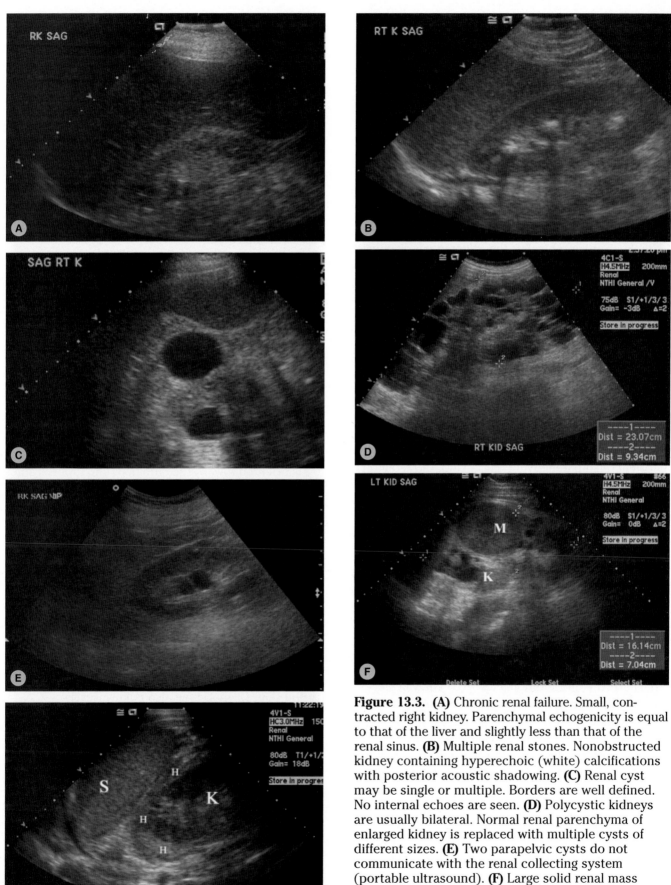

Figure 13.3. **(A)** Chronic renal failure. Small, contracted right kidney. Parenchymal echogenicity is equal to that of the liver and slightly less than that of the renal sinus. **(B)** Multiple renal stones. Nonobstructed kidney containing hyperechoic (white) calcifications with posterior acoustic shadowing. **(C)** Renal cyst may be single or multiple. Borders are well defined. No internal echoes are seen. **(D)** Polycystic kidneys are usually bilateral. Normal renal parenchyma of enlarged kidney is replaced with multiple cysts of different sizes. **(E)** Two parapelvic cysts do not communicate with the renal collecting system (portable ultrasound). **(F)** Large solid renal mass (M) distorting renal collecting system (K). **(G)** Perirenal hematoma in patient with left renal laceration. H, hematoma; K, kidney; S, spleen.

Renal Cysts

Renal cysts are the most commonly found renal masses. Sonographic features of the simple cyst include a spherical appearance, an anechoic lumen without internal echoes, a well-defined back wall, clear wall demarcation, no measurable wall thickness, and acoustic enhancement posterior to the cyst. Single or multiple cysts may be located anywhere in the kidney. A renal sinus cyst is called parapelvic and accounts for 6% of renal cysts. A parapelvic cyst does not communicate with the renal pelvis and calyces. Unlike the cauliflower appearance of the dilated pelvis, the parapelvic cyst is rounder, with good through-transmission (Fig. 13.3C–E). Sonographically, the differential diagnosis between hydronephrosis and a parapelvic cyst may be difficult, especially if the cysts are bilateral. Complex cysts do not meet the sonographic criteria of simple cysts. They may be septated and multilocular. While ultrasound diagnosis of simple cysts is very accurate, complex cysts may require additional imaging studies (e.g., computed tomography [CT] or magnetic resonance imaging) to rule out malignancy.

Solid Renal Masses

Solid renal masses are a heterogeneous, isoechoic or hypoechoic lesion of variable dimensions adjacent to a normal renal parenchyma (Fig. 13.3F). Ultrasound is used primarily to differentiate a solid mass from simple cysts. All solid renal masses in adults should be considered malignant until proven otherwise. Further evaluation with a CT scan is required for appropriate diagnosis.

Renal Intraparenchymal Abscesses

Renal intraparenchymal abscesses appear as complex hypoechoic masses with thick, irregular walls and occasional fluid-debris levels. A perinephric abscess will result in a heterogeneous, crescent-shaped fluid collection surrounding the kidney, which may deform the renal cortex. While additional tests (CT) may be necessary to differentiate between an abscess and renal cancer, ultrasound can be a valuable tool to monitor the diagnosed abscess during medical treatment.

Ultrasound presently is not advocated as a first-line imaging modality in renal trauma since its sensitivity in diagnosis and grading of renal injury remains low. It cannot provide crucial differentiation between blood, extravasated urine, and other types of free fluid. However, ultrasound is a very useful tool for bedside monitoring of the resolution or expansion of hematoma since recent management of even severe isolated renal injuries is mostly conservative (Fig. 13.3G).

BLADDER ULTRASOUND

Bladder ultrasound is usually performed together with renal ultrasound since bladder abnormalities may cause changes in the upper urinary tract (e.g., urinary retention may cause hydronephrosis). Limited bladder ultrasound is commonly used to evaluate postvoid residual urine volume in patients with lower urinary tract syndrome.

In accordance with the AIUM practice guideline, transverse and longitudinal images of the bladder should be obtained and abnormalities of the bladder lumen or wall noted. Postvoid residual urine volume may be quantitated.

Imaging Technique

The bladder can be examined only when it is distended. The average adult bladder comfortably holds about 500 mL. Sonographic evaluation is usually performed transabdominally with the patient in the supine position. A probe is placed 1 cm above the symphysis and angled laterally, inferiorly, and superiorly. Most commonly, a transverse scan is obtained first. The normal bladder is located midline and appears symmetric and smooth, without irregularities of the inner surface. On the longitudinal scan the bladder is oriented toward the umbilicus and tapered anteriorly. Transverse and longitudinal scans provide a fairly accurate calculation of bladder volume by measuring the horizontal and vertical dimensions of the bladder on transverse image and the maximum longitudinal dimension on longitudinal image and using the formula $0.52 \times$ length $\times$ width $\times$ height (this calculation is performed automatically by most current ultrasound machines). Sonographic estimation of the postvoid residual urine volume provides immediate diagnosis of urinary retention or incomplete bladder emptying in patients with decreased or absent urinary output without the need to attempt urethral catheterization (Fig. 13.4A–D [see also color insert]).

Common Bladder Ultrasound Findings

Bladder Stones

Bladder stones appear hyperechoic with posterior acoustic shadowing. They move with changes in a patient's position (Fig. 13.5F).

Superficial Transitional Cell Carcinoma

Superficial transitional cell carcinoma appears as a polypoid hyperechoic projection from the bladder

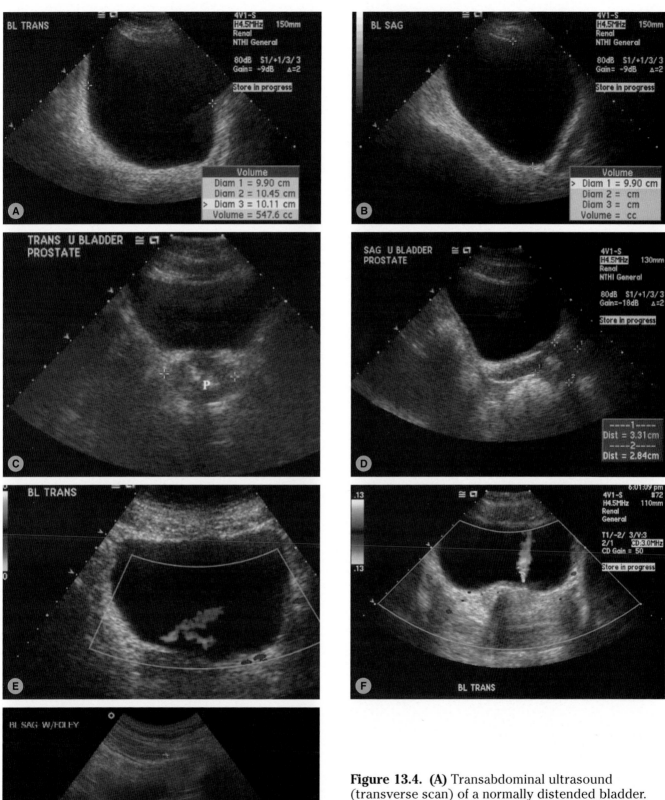

Figure 13.4. **(A)** Transabdominal ultrasound (transverse scan) of a normally distended bladder. **(B)** Longitudinal scan. **(C)** Transverse bladder scan and prostate measurements. **(D)** Longitudinal bladder scan and prostate measurements. **(E)** Color Doppler ultrasound of the urinary bladder shows crossing bilateral ureteral jets (see color insert.) **(F)** Loss of the right ureteral jet in patient with right obstructive hydronephrosis. **(G)** Foley catheter (F) in the collapsed bladder (portable ultrasound).

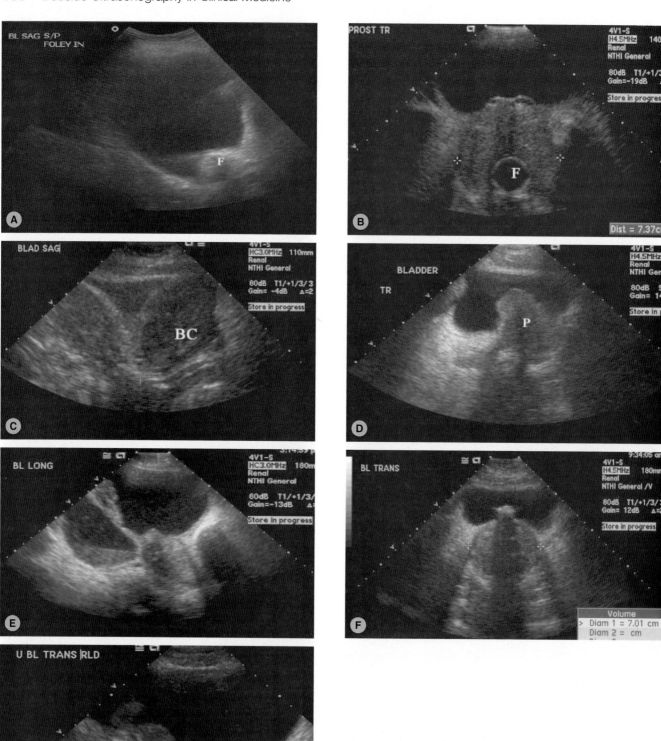

Figure 13.5. **(A)** Portable ultrasound. Distended bladder with obstructed Foley catheter (F). **(B)** Dislodged Foley catheter (F) in the prostatic urethra below the bladder. **(C)** A large blood clot (BC) in a patient with gross hematuria may simulate a bladder tumor. **(D)** Grossly enlarged prostate protruding into the bladder lumen. **(E)** Large bladder diverticulum. **(F)** Bladder stone. **(G)** Bladder tumor (BT).

wall. Although small lesions may not be well-appreciated, all tumors larger than 10 mm are detected. The sonographic appearance is nonspecific, and subsequent cystoscopy and biopsy are necessary for diagnosis (Fig. 13.5G).

Blood Clots

Blood clots may be visualized in patients with gross hematuria as mobile masses of increased echogenicity (Fig. 13.5C).

Diverticulum

Diverticulum presents sonographically as a sonolucent mass adjacent to the bladder. A large bladder diverticulum does not always empty and may be visible on postvoid scans (Fig. 13.5E).

Dislodged or Obstructed Foley Catheters

A dislodged or obstructed Foley catheter is a common cause of "anuria" in critical care patients. Bladder ultrasound may promptly visualize a distended bladder and locate the Foley catheter balloon within or outside a full bladder (Figs. 13.4G and 12.5A, B).

Prostate Enlargement

A grossly enlarged prostate may be seen as a round or polypoid mass protrusion at the bottom of the bladder (Fig. 13.5D).

Ureteral Obstruction

Color Doppler ultrasound detection of ureteral jets reflects urine flow from the ureteral orifice, and the absence of jets suggests ureteral obstruction (Fig. 13.4E, F).

SCROTAL ULTRASOUND

Anatomy

The scrotum is divided by a midline septum into two compartments, each containing a testis and associated structures. The normal ovoid-shaped adult testis is approximately 3 to 5 cm long, 2 to 4 cm wide, and 2 to 3 cm in anterior-posterior dimension. Sonographically, it has a smooth surface and homogenous echogenicity. It is surrounded by a fibrous capsule, the tunica albuginea, which appears as a thin, circumferential, more hyperechoic layer. The mediastinum testis corresponds to an exit and entry for testicular vessels and ducts and appears as a linear bright echogenic line in longitudinal testis imaging.

The epididymis is about 6 to 7 cm long and composed of a head, body, and tail. The most easily visible head of the epididymis sonographically is a 10- to 12-mm nodule capping an upper pole of the testis with a relatively coarser echotexture. The normal narrow body of the epididymis is isoechoic or slightly more echogenic than the testis and lies along its posterior aspect.

Imaging Technique

In accordance with the AIUM practice guideline, longitudinal and transverse images of each testis including superior, mid-, and inferior portions should be obtained. The size and echogenicity of each testis and epididymis should always be compared with its opposite side, when possible. A palpable abnormality must be directly imaged. Doppler sonography should be considered in all examinations of the adult scrotum.

The examination is performed in a warm room with the patient in a supine position and his legs placed together to provide necessary scrotal support. The penis is positioned over the suprapubic region and covered with a towel or drape. The optimal scanning is performed with the high-frequency linear array transducer (7.5–15 MHz).

A longitudinal scan provides initial information about the testis and paratesticular structures and measurements of the long axis and anteroposterior testicular size. The standard orientation of the testicular image should be with the upper pole to the left and the lower pole to the right of the screen. If the whole testis cannot be seen because of a small transducer size, superior and inferior portions of the testis should be scanned separately. A transverse scan is performed by rotating the transducer 90° so that the width of the testis can be measured (Fig. 13.6 [see also color insert]).

Targeted images including the area of concern should be obtained in patients referred for palpable scrotal lesions by putting the probe directly on the palpated lesion.

Common Ultrasound Findings

Frequent indications for the use of scrotal sonography are scrotal pain, palpable scrotal abnormalities (masses, scrotal enlargement, and asymmetry), follow-up of patients with prior testicular malignancies or incidentally found scrotal abnormalities that do not require immediate treatment, and acute scrotal pain with scrotal enlargement.

Epididymitis

Epididymitis is the most common cause of painful scrotal swelling in men older than 18 years of age. Although the epididymis is diffusely involved, limited focal involvement may affect up to one-third of patients. Ultrasound findings include hypoechoic enlargement primarily of the epididymal head and a

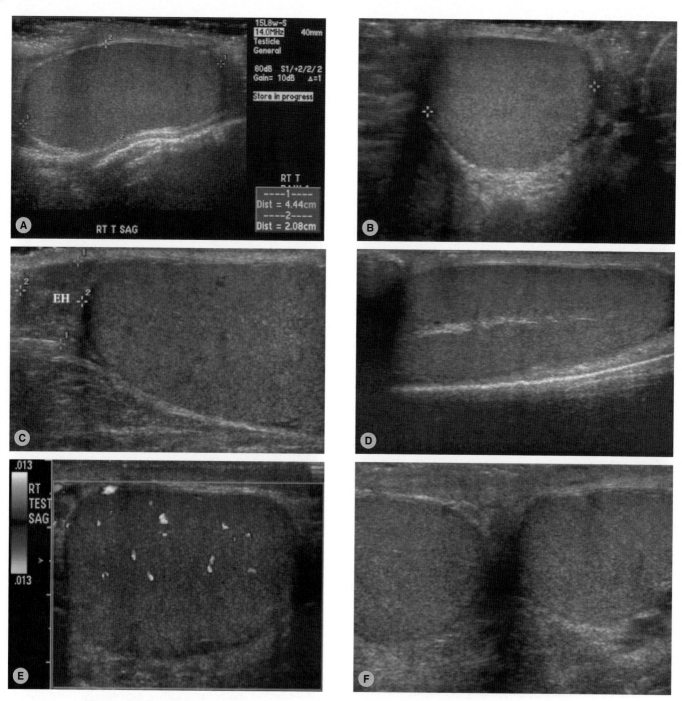

Figure 13.6. **(A)** Longitudinal ultrasound image of normal testis with homogenous parenchyma. **(B)** Transverse scan of the normal testis. **(C)** Epididymal head (EH) next to the upper pole of the testis. Compared to the normal testicle, the epididymis is normally isoechoic or slightly more echogenic with a more coarse appearance. **(D)** Longitudinal testicular scan demonstrates the mediastinum testis as a linear echogenic band. **(E)** Normal blood flow through the testis (blue, flow away from the transducer; red, flow toward the transducer [see color insert]). **(F)** Transverse scrotal scan to compare echogenicity of both testes.

reactive hydrocele. The testis becomes diffusely involved by direct spread of the infection in 20% to 40% of patients. Orchitis appears as an enlarged heterogeneous testis with hypoechoic areas. CDU usually shows asymmetrically increased blood flow in the epididymis or testis compared with the normal contralateral testis. Since testicular tumors may be masquerading as orchitis, follow-up ultrasound after treatment is recommended (Fig. 13.7C, D [see also color insert]).

Testicular Torsion

Testicular torsion is a rotation of the testis in the longitudinal axis of the spermatic cord with the interruption of testicular blood supply. It is a urologic emergency since the testicular salvage rate is time dependent and varies from between 80% and 100% if surgery is performed within 5 to 6 hours of the onset of pain to only 20% after 12 hours. It is most common in adolescent boys but also can be seen in young adults. Physical examination and prompt sonographic evaluation significantly reduce the time before necessary surgical intervention.

The testis becomes enlarged and inhomogeneous within the first 6 hours and more heterogeneous later. While these sonographic findings are nonspecific, CDU is instrumental in differentiating torsion from other causes of acute scrotal pain. Unilaterally absent or greatly diminished testicular blood flow is the most accurate sign of torsion with a sensitivity of 80% to 98% and specificity of 97% to 100% (Fig. 13.7A, B [see also color insert]). However, if CDU results are equivocal, clinical correlation is extremely important for timely diagnosis and treatment of testicular torsion.

Testicular Tumors

The usual clinical manifestation of testicular tumors is painless enlargement of the testis. The most common tumor types are seminomas and nonseminomatous germ cell tumors (NSGCTs). Seminomas usually present as homogenous hypoechoic masses, while NSGCTs are irregular heterogeneous with both solid and cystic components (Fig. 13.7E–G [see also color insert]). However, such sonographic features are nonspecific and cannot always differentiate malignant tumor from certain benign conditions (e.g., hematoma, infarction, or inflammation). Ultrasound has near 100% sensitivity for detecting testicular tumors but its specificity is low (44.4%), and therefore all testicular masses are malignant until proven otherwise. Clinical correlation and a high index of suspicion for possible testicular malignancy are necessary for correct diagnosis and prompt treatment.

Hydrocele

Hydrocele is an abnormal collection of fluid within the scrotum and a common cause of scrotal enlargement. It appears as anechoic regions surrounding the testis. Internal echoes within the hydrocele may indicate a hematocele, or blood collection within the scrotum, frequently seen in patients with scrotal trauma. Septated hydrocele and hydrocele with debris may suggest infection (Fig. 13.8A [see also color insert]).

Testicular Microlithiasis

Bilateral or unilateral testicular microlithiasis (TM) is an uncommon incidental finding. Microliths are small, calcified particles 1 to 2 mm in size. Histologically, these are laminated calcium deposits in the seminiferous tubules. The classic sonographic picture of TM is a diffuse speckled pattern with innumerable small bright echogenic foci without shadowing. Limited TM is determined as less than five microcalcifications per sonographic image of the testis (Fig. 13.9E, F). A wide variation is seen in the reported prevalence of testicular microlithiasis, ranging from 0.68% to 18.1%. The possible association of TM with the future development of testicular tumors remains controversial. Some authors recommend regular 6- to 12-month follow-up ultrasounds, especially in patents with a history of undescended testis, infertility, or contralateral testicular tumor.

Intratesticular Masses

Nonpalpable intratesticular masses are usually found incidentally. They are mostly benign. In one study, only 22% of nonpalpable testicular masses were malignant. However, risk of malignancy is higher in patients with a history of cryptorchidism, infertility, and contralateral testicular cancer. Sonographic findings are nonspecific and cannot differentiate between benign and malignant tumors. Treatment recommendations include a wide range of approaches including radical orchiectomy, excision of the tumor with intraoperative frozen section, and interval follow-up for masses less than 1 cm in size (Fig. 13.9A–D).

Intratesticular Cysts

Intratesticular cysts occur in up to 4% of patients. Benign cysts are usually single and unilocular and located near the margin of the testis (Fig. 13.8B).

Extratesticular Masses

The most common extratesticular scrotal masses are epididymal cysts and varicoceles. Epididymal cysts appear as anechoic, circumscribed lesions with no

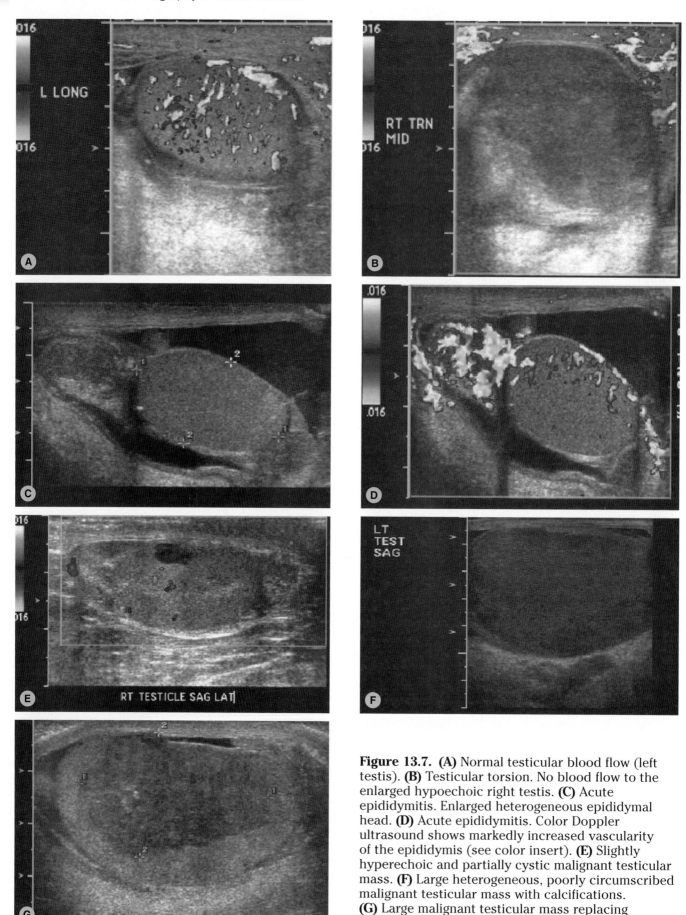

Figure 13.7. **(A)** Normal testicular blood flow (left testis). **(B)** Testicular torsion. No blood flow to the enlarged hypoechoic right testis. **(C)** Acute epididymitis. Enlarged heterogeneous epididymal head. **(D)** Acute epididymitis. Color Doppler ultrasound shows markedly increased vascularity of the epididymis (see color insert). **(E)** Slightly hyperechoic and partially cystic malignant testicular mass. **(F)** Large heterogeneous, poorly circumscribed malignant testicular mass with calcifications. **(G)** Large malignant testicular mass replacing entire testicular parenchyma.

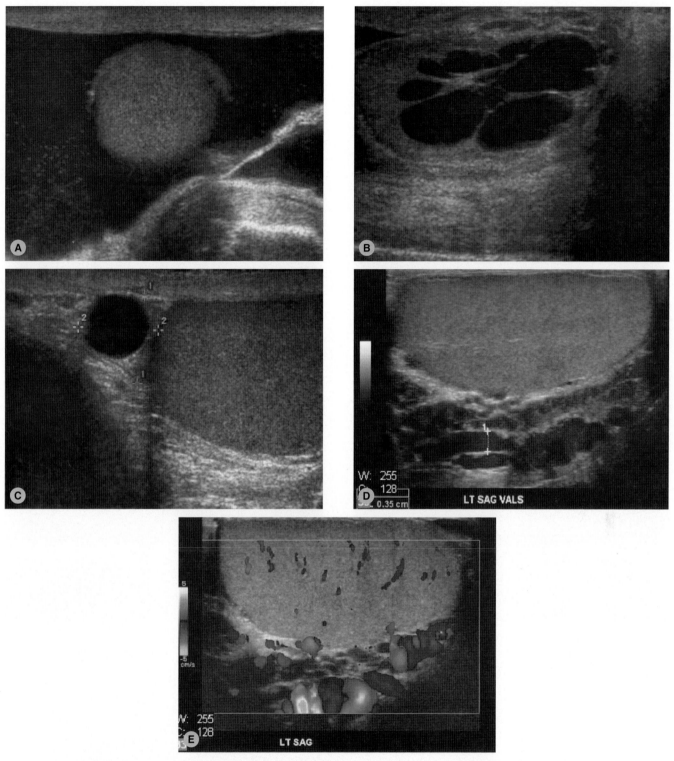

Figure 13.8. **(A)** Large hydrocele. Transverse scan shows anechoic fluid collection with some debris and without septations. **(B)** Large, benign, anechoic, intratesticular cysts. **(C)** Large, anechoic cyst in the head of the epididymis. **(D)** Varicocele. Longitudinal scan shows tortuous, dilated, hypoechoic veins. **(E)** Color Doppler ultrasound with the Valsalva maneuver shows the blood flow in a varicocele with engorged veins (see color insert).

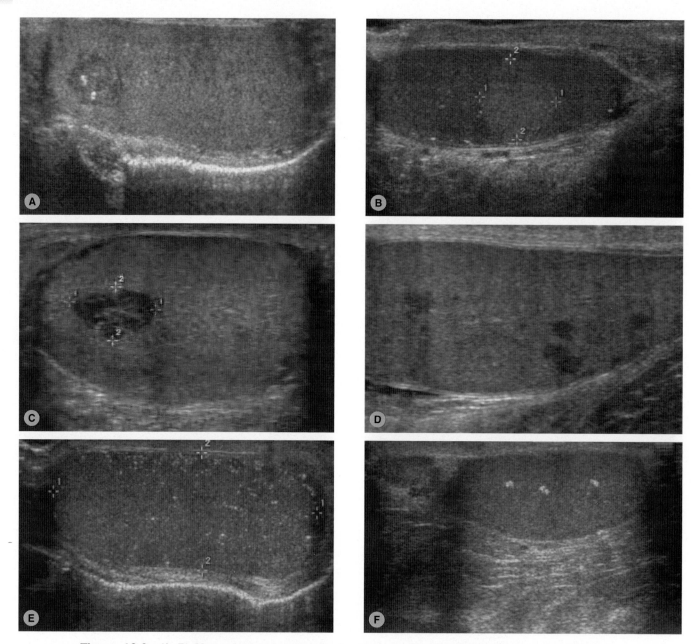

Figure 13.9. **(A–D)** Nonpalpable intratesticular tumors. **(E)** Classic testicular microlithiasis. Several small, nonshadowing, punctuate, hyperechoic foci scattered throughout the testicle. **(F)** Limited testicular microlithiasis with slightly large calcifications.

internal echoes. They are frequently located at the head of the epididymis but also can be found on the epididymal tail or body. A spermatocele is often larger and may be multilocular. It contains spermatozoa, whereas epididymal cysts contain clear fluid. The differentiation between these two entities is not necessary since they usually do not require treatment (Fig. 13.8C).

Varicocele

A varicocele is a dilatation of the pampiniform plexus, which is most commonly seen on the left side. Varicoceles have been found in up to 13% of asymptomatic, healthy men and in up to 40% in infertile men. Large varicoceles (grade III) are both palpable and visible through the scrotal skin. Sonographically, a varicocele appears as a serpentine, anechoic, tubular structure with diameters greater than 2 mm. Evaluation in the erect position or with a Valsalva maneuver is often required to observe additional distention of the veins. CDU confirms venous blood flow within tortuous veins (Fig. 13.8D, E [see also color insert]). A large or isolated right varicocele may occur secondary to the obstruction of the spermatic vein by retroperitoneal mass (e.g., renal cancer) or a hydronephrotic kidney, which requires further evaluation with renal ultrasound or CT scan.

DOCUMENTATION AND CODING EXAMPLES (TABLE 13.1)

Thorough documentation is a necessary part of the ultrasound examination. Interpretation of the test and appropriate images, properly labeled with patient and facility identification, examination date, and laterality (right or left side) of ultrasound examination, must be kept in the chart.

TABLE 13.1. Ultrasound Coding

Ultrasound Procedure	CPT Code
Measurement of postvoiding residual urine and/or bladder capacity	51798
Pelvis, limited or follow-up Transabdominal evaluation of the urinary bladder and/or prostate (not including kidneys)	76857
Retroperitoneum, limited examination (kidneys and bladder)	76775
Scrotum and contents	76870
Duplex scan of scrotal contents (real-time images with spectral or color flow Doppler imaging) integrating, limited study	93976

CPT, Current Procedural Terminology.

Suggested Readings

Gorman B, Carroll B. The scrotum. In: Rumack CM, Wilson SR, Charboneau JW, eds. *Diagnostic Ultrasound.* St. Louis, MO: Elsevier Mosby; 2005:849–883.

Hofer M. *Ultrasound Teaching Manual.* 2nd ed. Suttgart-New York: Thieme; 2005.

Lin EP, Bhatt S, Dogra VS, Rubens DI. Sonography of urolithiasis and hydronephrosis. *Ultrasound Clin.* 2007;2:1.

McAchran SE, Hartke DM, Nakamoto DA, Resnick MI. Ultrasound of the urinary bladder. *Ultrasound Clin.* 2007;2(1):17–26.

Noble VE, Brown DFM. Renal ultrasound. *Emerg Med Clin N Am.* 2004;22:641–659.

Ragheb D, Higgins J. Ultrasonography of the scrotum. Technique, anatomy, and pathologic entities. *J Ultrasound Med.* 2002;21:171–185.

Stengel J, Remer E. Sonography of the scrotum: case-based review. *AJR Am J Roentgenol.* 2008;190:S35–S41.

Thurston W, Wilson SR. The urinary tract. In: Rumack CM, Wilson SR, Charboneau JW, eds. *Diagnostic Ultrasound.* St. Louis, MO: Elsevier Mosby; 2005:321–417.

ULTRASOUND USE FOR THE EVALUATION OF ORGANS OF THE LIMBS AND MUSCULOSKELETAL SYSTEM

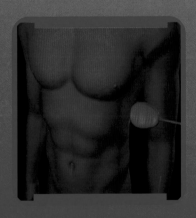

CHAPTER 14

Ultrasound Evaluation of the Musculoskeletal System

Apostolos P. Dallas, MD, FACP

INTRODUCTION

The advent of bedside ultrasound devices has revolutionized the imaging of musculoskeletal structures. In the past, simple x-rays, computed tomography (CT) scans, and magnetic resonance imaging (MRI) studies represented the mainstay of musculoskeletal imaging. Each modality had its limitations. X-rays could not image soft tissues well. CT scans and MRI provided more information but were costly, and all three provided static images only. Over the past several years, the number of publications describing the utility of ultrasound in musculoskeletal disorders has increased markedly. Newly developed imaging techniques and protocols have enhanced diagnostic accuracy and enabled physicians to make more timely decisions about their patients' care. While the majority of musculoskeletal ultrasound (MSKUS) previously had been performed by sonologists and sonographers, there has recently been an increase in ultrasound use by clinicians. Orthopedists, emergency and sports medicine physicians, rheumatologists, physiatrists, pain management specialists, and general internists have all recognized ultrasound's increasing applicability to their practices. As such, medical students, regardless of their choice of specialty, would be well-served by learning musculoskeletal ultrasound. Likewise, primary care physicians, often the first in line to address their patients' musculoskeletal concerns, are in a position to benefit their patients by acquiring the knowledge and skills in musculoskeletal ultrasound.

This chapter will concentrate on key normal findings in MSKUS. We envision the bedside ultrasound as a tool with which the clinician can augment his or her physical diagnostic skills. This approach will allow medical students and primary care physicians, with some practice, to develop some useful skills that they can apply in this area.

Several reasons make ultrasound attractive in the evaluation of the patient with musculoskeletal concerns. Ultrasound can be used dynamically. For example, a pop, creak, or pain with a certain shoulder motion can be imaged while the patient repeats that motion. Much pathology cannot be imaged with CT scans and MRI because of the static nature of those studies. In contrast, ultrasound imaging at the exact location of pain can often diagnose the pathology. Ultrasound does not use ionizing radiation, which can be harmful over time. Metal hardware around joints does not affect imaging with ultrasound as it does with CT scanning, and the limitations of MRI with metal and pacemakers is well known. Certain findings with ultrasound rival MRI at a fraction of the cost and surpass x-ray findings: erosion in small joints in rheumatoid arthritis is one example. Ultrasound can differentiate fluid-filled and solid masses, and ultrasound guidance for aspiration and joint injections can make these interventions increasingly accurate and successful while minimizing potential trauma to nearby nerves and vessels. Extended field-of-view imaging allows some structures—longer tendons, for instance—to be seen in their entirety.

While MSKUS image quality is operator dependent, the techniques can be learned relatively quickly. Currently, only a handful of medical schools provide ultrasound courses in their curriculum, but a modest investment in time and effort can have significant results in student skills. For the practicing physician, continuing medical education courses are increasingly available. Most concerns from learners revolve around attaining the image, identifying normal structures as they appear ultrasonographically, and interpreting pathology.

Attaining the image requires an acceptable bedside ultrasound machine. Many good ultrasound systems exist, and often, the choice has been made for the user by the hospital purchasing department. The smaller and more portable machines allow for easy transport from the patient examination room to the hospital room. Portability of different models must be measured against the price and image quality. A quick way to assess quality is for the user to test the ultrasound machine's imaging on his or her own wrist, looking for crisply detailed structures such as the median nerve.

As for the probe, the choice has been simplified. A broadband linear array probe, 5 to 12 MHz, should suffice for most musculoskeletal applications, although interrogating superficial structures such as the distal interphalangeal joints may require probes with smaller footprints (hockey stick) and higher frequencies up to 15 MHz. Imaging deeper structures such as the spine and hip joints may require 3 to 5 MHz probes with curved arrays. Each probe has a mark, notch, or reference point on one end. This will be important in the orientation of the image on the monitor.

Images should be obtained in two views, long-axis (longitudinal) and short-axis (transverse). This allows for cross-referencing, especially where it concerns pathology. Some structures may look pathologic, enlarged, or damaged in one view but normal in another. One view does not allow for conclusive diagnosis. In the long-axis views, the left side of the image is cephalad, provided the probe notch is also pointing cephalad. In the short-axis views, the left side of the image is to the patient's right, provided the probe notch is to the patient's right. As a test for orientation, the learner can use his or her finger on the right side of the probe and note the acoustic shadows on the left side of the image.

Normal appearances on images should be compared to the user's knowledge of normal anatomy. Bony structures are good starting points, and for each joint image the learner should remember the key bony landmarks, for example, the coracoid and humerus in the anterior views of the shoulder. Structures are referred to as hyperechoic, hypoechoic, and anechoic (see Chapter 3, Fig. 3.2). These are gradations of gray scale on ultrasound. Bones are hyperechoic, easy to recognize for beginners, and accompanied by the acoustic shadows below to them. Cartilage is either anechoic in the case of hyaline cartilage forming a small rim on the hyperechoic bony surface beneath it or slightly hyperechoic in the case of meniscal and fibrocartilage. Synovium is a midechoic tissue within the joint and usually can be highlighted by the anechoic synovial fluid. Fluid in general is anechoic but can contain debris, pathologically, which can add more gray to the image. Subcutaneous fat is midechoic, while peribursal fat is thicker and more echogenic. Muscle can have varying echo signals because of different muscle patterns (unipennate, bipennate) and fascia. Tendons have a fine fibrillar pattern. Changing the orientation of the probe can cause profound changes in the echogenicity of tendons (Fig. 14.1). This property, called anisotropy, is demonstrated ultrasonographically when the probe angle is not perpendicular to the tendon or other

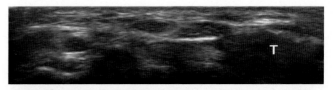
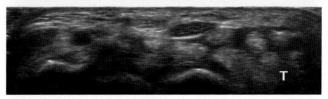

Figure 14.1. Anisotropy. Rocking motion of the probe makes tendons hyper- and hypoechoic. T, flexor tendons at the wrist.

structure being imaged. Anisotropy can be used to help differentiate tendons from other structures by using heel-toe probe maneuvers or rocking side to side (toggling). Ligaments are slightly less echoic than tendons and have inconsistent brightness because of fibrillar layering in varied directions. Nerves tend to be oval and coarser and give a starry night appearance (in the short-axis view) with slight changes in probe direction. Bursae are anechoic and can be compressed with probe pressure.

SHOULDER

The anatomy of the shoulder, amply covered in other texts, can be quickly reviewed (Fig. 14.2). Recall the associations of the humerus with the biceps tendon, the rotator cuff muscles and tendons, and the subscapularis, supraspinatus, infraspinatus, teres minor, and deltoid muscles. Review the anatomy of the glenoid with its anterior and posterior labrum, the acromioclavicular joint, and the associated key ligaments including the acromioclavicular with its effects on the rotator cuff. Also review the location of the subacromial-subdeltoid bursa.

The standard views of the shoulder begin with the transverse view of the biceps tendon (Fig. 14.3). The patient is seated perpendicular to the clinician with the monitor either across from the patient or to the clinician's left when he or she is examining the patient's right shoulder. Some sonologists will prefer scanning from behind. Either way, patient comfort, clinician access to the patient, acquisition of ultrasonographic views, and visualization of the monitor should be the key determinants in positioning of the patient and clinician. Physician handedness will also play a role.

The patient rests his or her hand palm upward on his or her thigh. The probe is positioned anterolaterally

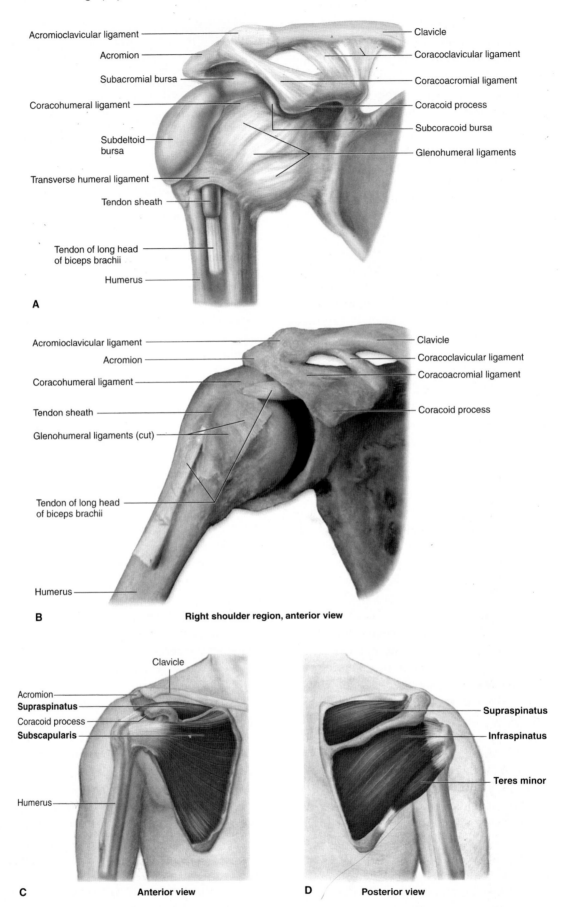

Acromioclavicular ligament —————— Clavicle

Acromion —————— Coracoclavicular ligament

Subacromial bursa —————— Coracoacromial ligament

Coracohumeral ligament —————— Coracoid process

—————— Subcoracoid bursa

Subdeltoid bursa —————— Glenohumeral ligaments

Transverse humeral ligament ——————

Tendon sheath ——————

Tendon of long head of biceps brachii ——————

Humerus ——————

A

Acromioclavicular ligament —————— Clavicle

Acromion —————— Coracoclavicular ligament

—————— Coracoacromial ligament

Coracohumeral ligament ——————

Tendon sheath —————— Coracoid process

Glenohumeral ligaments (cut) ——————

Tendon of long head of biceps brachii ——————

Humerus ——————

B　　　　**Right shoulder region, anterior view**

Clavicle

Acromion ——————

Supraspinatus ——————　　　　　**Supraspinatus**

Coracoid process ——————

Subscapularis ——————　　　　　**Infraspinatus**

　　　　　Teres minor

Humerus ——————

C　　　　**Anterior view**　　　　**D**　　　　**Posterior view**

Figure 14.2. Anatomy of the shoulder.

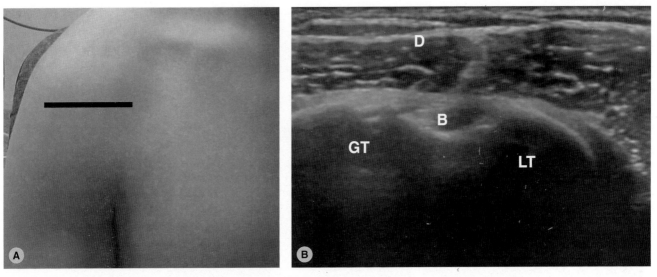

Figure 14.3. Transverse probe placement **(A)** and view **(B).** B, biceps tendon; D, deltoid muscle; GT, greater tuberosity; LT, lesser tuberosity.

and transversely on the shoulder, with the probe notch pointing toward the patient's right. This view enables the clinician to visualize the biceps tendon in the bicipital groove, the lesser tuberosity medially where the subscapularis inserts, and the greater tuberosity laterally where the supraspinatus inserts. Notice the anisotropy with heel-toe movements of the probe. The transverse humeral ligament holds the biceps tendon in place. The tendon is oval intra-articularly but rounder as it courses toward the musculotendinous junction. The normal biceps tendon is 3 to 7 mm in the transverse diameter.

The longitudinal view of the biceps tendon can be obtained by rotating the probe 90° in the same location (Fig. 14.4). The biceps tendon can now be seen longitudinally. The probe is then moved distally following the biceps tendon as it approaches the biceps muscle. The sagittal diameter of the biceps is 1 to 4 mm.

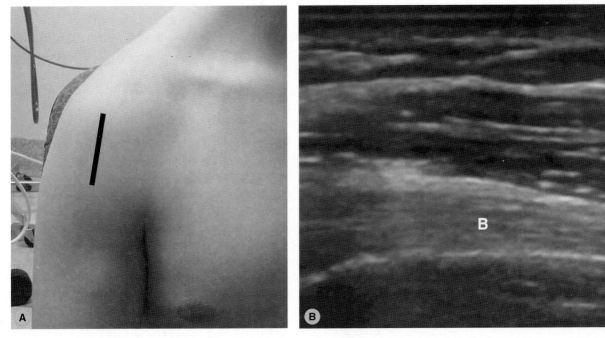

Figure 14.4. Longitudinal probe placement **(A)** and view **(B).** B, biceps tendon.

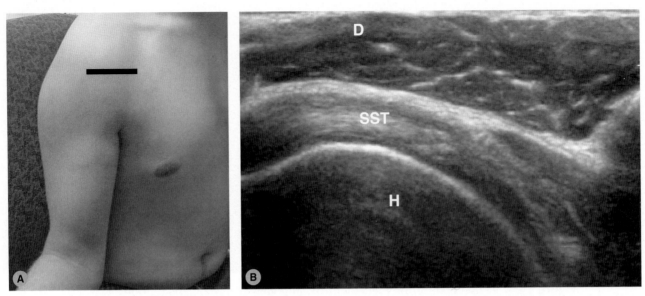

Figure 14.5. Anterior transverse probe placement **(A)** and view **(B)**. D, deltoid muscle; H, humerus; SST, subscapularis tendon.

The anterior transverse view is obtained by positioning the probe anteriorly on the shoulder, medial to the view just obtained with the biceps tendon view, with the patient's arm externally rotated (Fig. 14.5). This approach allows the subscapularis tendon to be viewed more fully. The clinician looks for any hypoechoic areas that may represent damage, and should be careful of some hypoechoic appearance at the myotendinous junction. The subscapularis muscle is a multipennate muscle and will look discontinuous when examined in cross section.

The anterior longitudinal view requires rotating the probe again 90° in the same location. The subscapularis tendon is now seen as a beaklike structure over the lesser tuberosity of the humerus. Moving the probe medially, one visualizes the coracoid and with internal and external rotation of the arm, one might see subcoracoid impingement of the subscapularis tendon. One can also visualize the subcoracoid bursa here.

A more lateral placement of the probe with the patient in the Crass position (maximal internal rotation, elbow flexed, and hand touching the opposite scapula) allows for visualization of the supraspinatus tendon, the tendon most likely to be involved in rotator cuff pathology. With the probe held transversely, the tendon is draped over the humerus, with a lucent subdeltoid bursa above it and a lucent cartilage below it. Superficial in this view is the deltoid muscle.

The lateral longitudinal view is obtained by turning the probe again 90° (Fig. 14.6). Again, a beaklike structure facing in the opposite direction of the subscapularis tendon is seen. The beak is attaching to the greater tuberosity. Ninety percent of rotator cuff pathology occurs in an area 1 cm proximal to this insertion. Notice the acromion. Having the patient attempt to kiss his or her elbow (internal rotation, flexed elbow, and abduction at shoulder) will make the supraspinatus tendon move under the acromioclavicular ligament. Any bunching of the muscle represents impingement.

The posterior oblique view can be obtained with the probe transversely oriented and the patient's arm crossed over the chest, resting on the opposite shoulder (Fig. 14.7). This view allows for visualization of the infraspinatus tendon and its broad insertion. The teres minor has a smaller tendon, but often it is difficult to differentiate the two. The teres minor has little pathology associated with it. Moving the probe further caudally, one can see the posterior labrum as a deep structure, hyperechoic and triangular (Fig. 14.8). The longitudinal view again is achieved by 90° rotation of the probe. Internal and external rotation can allow visualization of the humeral head.

The acromioclavicular joint view is obtained with the patient's arm resting by the side with the probe positioned above the joint in a position parallel to the clavicle (Fig. 14.9). The joint space is visualized. Acromioclavicular joint measurement allows for diagnosis of shoulder separation. This joint can be involved with any pathology that affects other synovial joints. Fluid in this joint can give the so-called geyser sign.

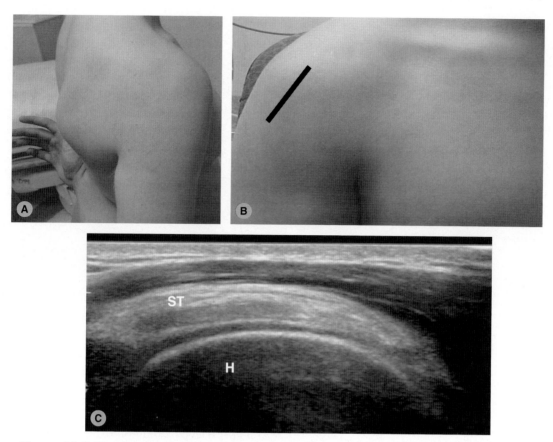

Figure 14.6. Longitudinal lateral patient **(A)** and probe position **(B)** and view **(C).** H, humerus; ST, supraspinatus tendon.

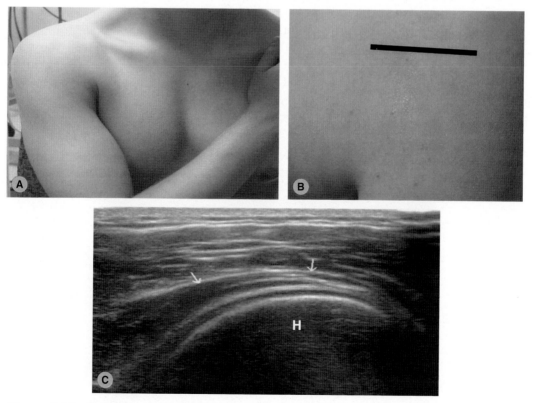

Figure 14.7. Posterior patient **(A)** and probe position **(B)** and view **(C).** The arrows indicate the infraspinatus tendon. H, humerus.

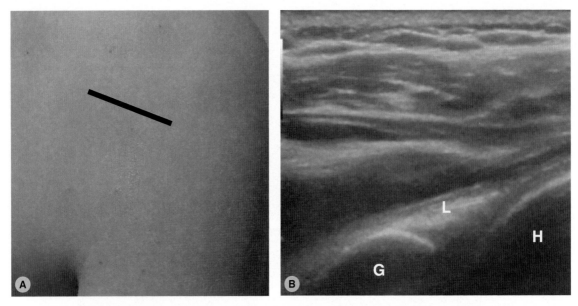

Figure 14.8. Posterior shoulder probe placement **(A)** and view **(B).** G, glenoid; H, humerus; L, labrum.

ELBOW

The elbow joint (Fig. 14.10) is a hinge-pivot joint composed of the ulnohumeral joint with the ulna trochlear notch articulating with the humeral trochlea, the radiocapitellar joint articulating with the radial articulation at the humeral capitellum, and the proximal radioulnar joint. Recall the olecranon in the humeral olecranon fossa. Major ligaments include the ulnar and radial collateral ligaments connecting the humerus with the ulna and radius bones, respectively. Tendons include the biceps, triceps, common extensor, and common flexor tendons. Key landmarks include the medial and lateral epicondyles. Important nerves that can be visualized at the elbow are the median, ulnar, and radial nerves. The brachial and ulnar arteries are key landmarks, as their proximity and ultrasonographic properties help in locating the median and ulnar nerves.

Standard views of the elbow include anterior, medial, lateral, and posterior views. The anterior transverse view is obtained with the patient's elbow extended and resting on a table or on his or her thigh

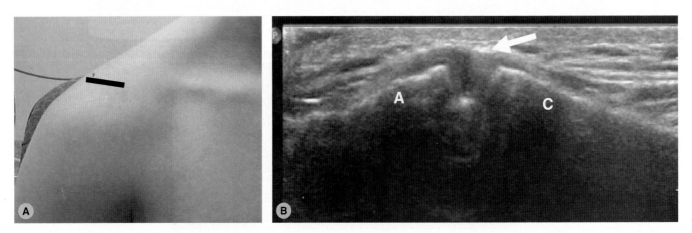

Figure 14.9. Acromioclavicular joint probe placement **(A)** and view **(B).** The arrow indicates the joint capsule. A, acromion; C, clavicle.

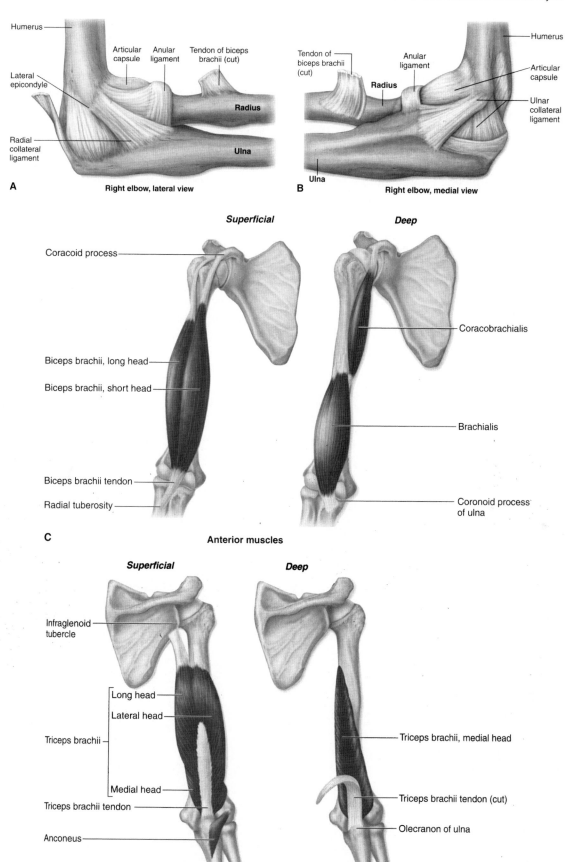

Figure 14.10. Anatomy of the elbow.

supported by a towel. Remember that the probe notch is facing to the patient's right. The left side of the image will be lateral. Scanning through the joint space, one sees the distal humerus with hypoechoic cartilage. Scanning medially (Fig. 14.11), one notices the pulsatile, noncompressible brachial artery. Medial to the brachial artery is the median nerve with its oval, starry-night appearance. More laterally in a longitudinal orientation, the biceps tendon and brachialis can be visualized, and the biceps tendon can be tracked distally to its insertion on the radial tuberosity, sometimes better seen on a posterior view.

The anterior longitudinal view is obtained by rotating the probe 90° and moving it medially and laterally to visualize the two primary joint spaces. The medial structures, the trochlea of the humerus, and the coronoid of the ulna are visualized. Notice the overlying brachialis and pronator teres. Laterally, the radial head

and humeral capitellum can be visualized (Fig. 14.12). Again, notice the hypoechoic hyaline cartilage and the overlying brachioradialis muscle.

The medial longitudinal view (Fig. 14.13) is obtained by first finding the medial epicondyle by palpation. The arm is extended. The common flexor tendon is seen superficial to the ulnar collateral ligament and attaches to the medial epicondyle. Injuries here are sometimes seen in golfers and in sports involving throwing. Look for calcifications, tears, and irregularities. Bony landmarks include the trochlea of the humerus and the trochlear notch of the ulna.

The lateral longitudinal view is best obtained with the patient's arms in the praying position (Fig. 14.14). Find the lateral epicondyle. The probe is positioned superior to the capitellum. The common extensor tendon inserts on the lateral epicondyle. The radial collateral ligament can be seen here. The structures of

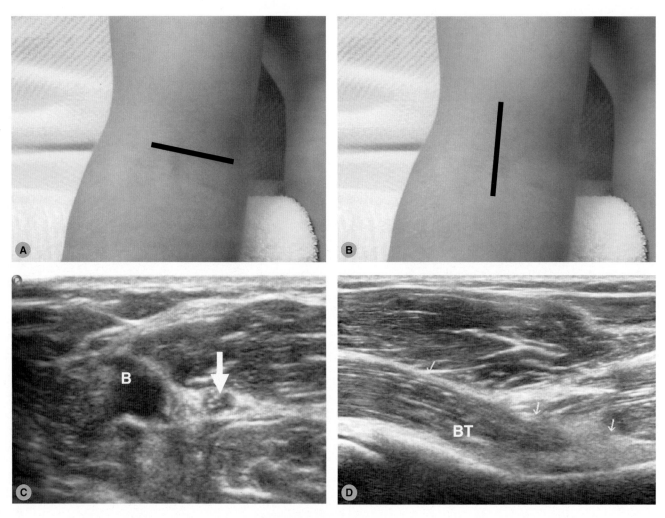

Figure 14.11. Anterior elbow probe placement **(A, B)** and views **(C, D)**. Arrow indicates the median nerve. B, brachial artery; BT, biceps tendon.

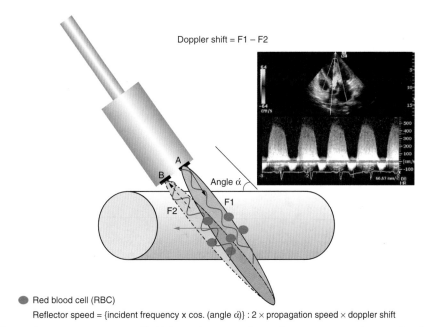

Doppler shift = F1 − F2

Angle α

A

B

F1

F2

● Red blood cell (RBC)

Reflector speed = {incident frequency x cos. (angle α)} : 2 × propagation speed × doppler shift

Figure 3.11. A continuous wave (CW) Doppler transducer has two piezoelectric (lead zirconium titanate) crystals. One constantly emits, and the other receives signals. Element A transmits continuous ultrasound waves with frequency F1. Element B receives frequency F (F1 − F2 = Doppler shift). Doppler shift is in the audible frequency range and can be presented to the operator in the form of sound. Backing material is not necessary because CW signals require no dampening. The large area of overlap between the incident beam and receiver beam results in an inability to assess where the sample is located, known as range ambiguity. The CW Doppler transducer can measure very high flow velocities. Knowing Doppler shift, reflector velocity (RBC) can be calculated. Flow velocity information can be presented in graphic form. Color flow Doppler is a pulsed mode demonstrating average flow velocity (speed and direction over the sample area). The colored map in the left upper corner is providing reference information to the direction and speed of the moving reflectors (blood = RBCs).

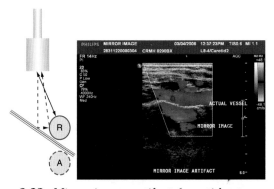

Figure 3.23. Mirror-image artifact (carotid artery duplication). The acoustic mirror (*triple black line*) reflects ultrasound toward the anatomic structure (R) (which takes longer to return to the transducer). The structure is therefore visualized twice directly (*solid black arrow*) and via the mirror reflection (*interrupted black arrow*). Since the indirect route takes longer, mirror-image artifact (A) is always positioned below the real structure.

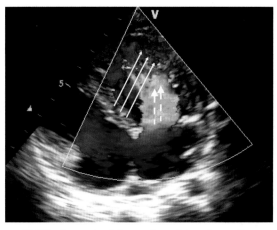

Figure 3.27. An apical four-chamber view of a noncompacted left ventricle with color flow into the noncompacted areas (*solid white arrows*). The central area within the color flow Doppler is an aliasing artifact (*interrupted white arrows*).

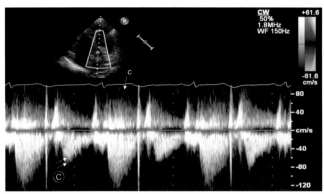

Figure 3.28. This image demonstrates the presence of cross-talk (C) artifact in a pulsed wave Doppler interrogation. It is seen both during systole (aortic flow, *single white arrow*) and diastole (mitral flow, *two white arrows*). Please note: True aortic flow is away from the transducer and should be below the baseline, while mitral flow is directed toward the transducer and should be above the baseline. (*Image courtesy of D. Adams, RDCS.*)

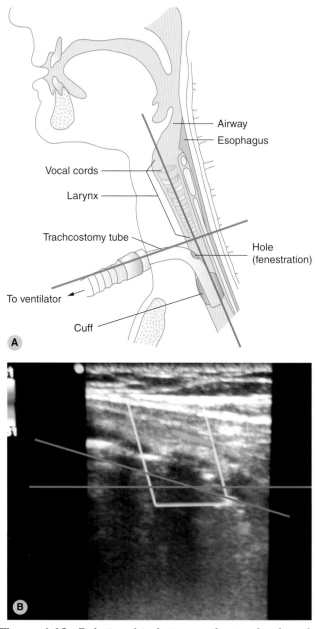

Figure 4.13. Relationship between the tracheal angle and tracheostomy tube angle.

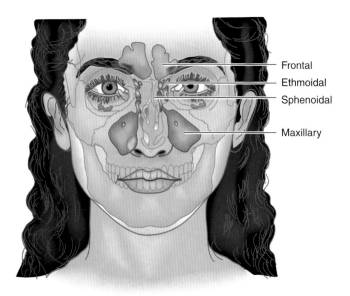

Figure 4.1. Anatomy of the paranasal sinuses.

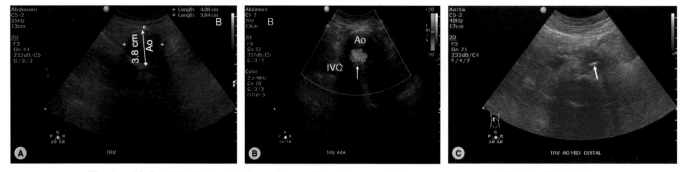

Figure 10.8. (A) Abdominal aortic spelling for consistency aneurysm (AAA). (B) AAA with thrombus (*solid white arrow*). (C) Short-axis view of abdominal aortic dissection (the arrow indicates an intimal flap within the aortic lumen). Ao, aorta; IVC, inferior vena cava.

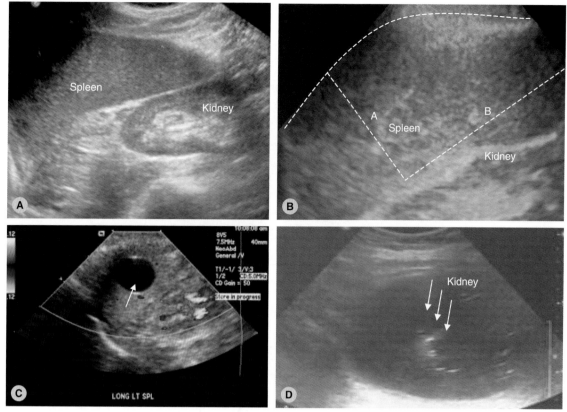

Figure 10.15. Spleen. **(A)** Normal spleen. **(B)** Splenomegaly noted in both transverse (A) and longitudinal (B) dimensions. **(C)** Splenic cyst. Note the anechoic appearance. **(D)** Splenic abscess. Note the internal acoustic signals within the abscess cavity and increased echogenicity, when compared to the cyst.

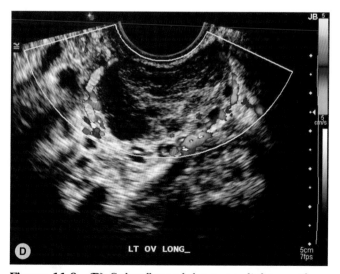

Figure 11.8. **(D)** Color flow of the ovary lights up the vasculature in the periphery of the ovary, which is sometimes referred to as the "ring of fire." The hues seen are indicative of the direction of vasculature flow relative to the probe. This can be remembered with the mnemonic "BART": blue away, red toward.

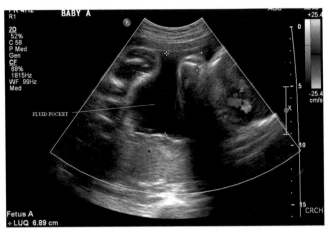

Figure 12.5. Measurement of amniotic fluid pocket.

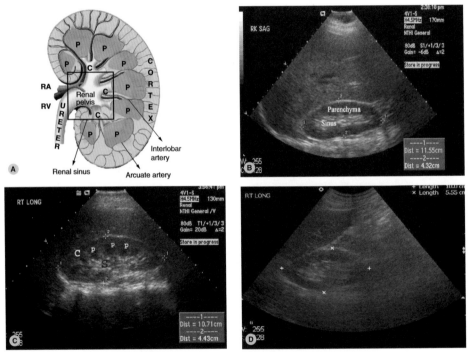

Figure 13.1. **(A)** Normal renal anatomy. C, calyx; P, pyramid; RA, main renal artery; RV, main renal vein. **(B)** Normal kidney. Longitudinal view of the kidney demonstrates peripheral hypoechoic universally thick parenchyma and a central hyperechoic renal sinus. Note the echogenic white Gerota fascia. Parenchyma is less echogenic than liver (L). **(C)** The cortical echogenicity (C) is equal to that of the liver (L). Several slightly hypoechoic renal pyramids are seen. **(D)** Portable ultrasound of the normal right kidney. Note less contrast appearance, but the renal contour, parenchyma, and renal sinus are clearly identified.

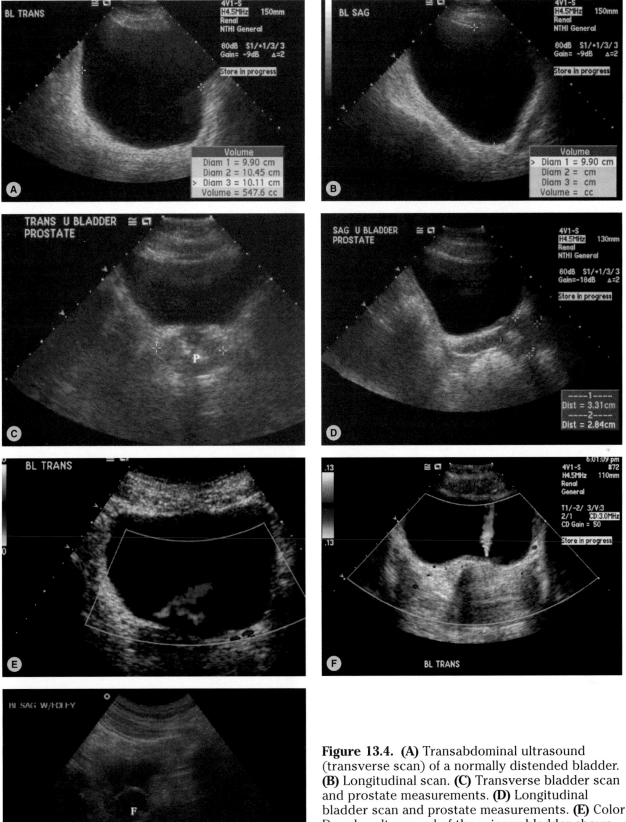

Figure 13.4. (A) Transabdominal ultrasound (transverse scan) of a normally distended bladder. **(B)** Longitudinal scan. **(C)** Transverse bladder scan and prostate measurements. **(D)** Longitudinal bladder scan and prostate measurements. **(E)** Color Doppler ultrasound of the urinary bladder shows crossing bilateral ureteral jets **(F)** Loss of the right ureteral jet in patient with right obstructive hydronephrosis. **(G)** Foley catheter (F) in the collapsed bladder (portable ultrasound).

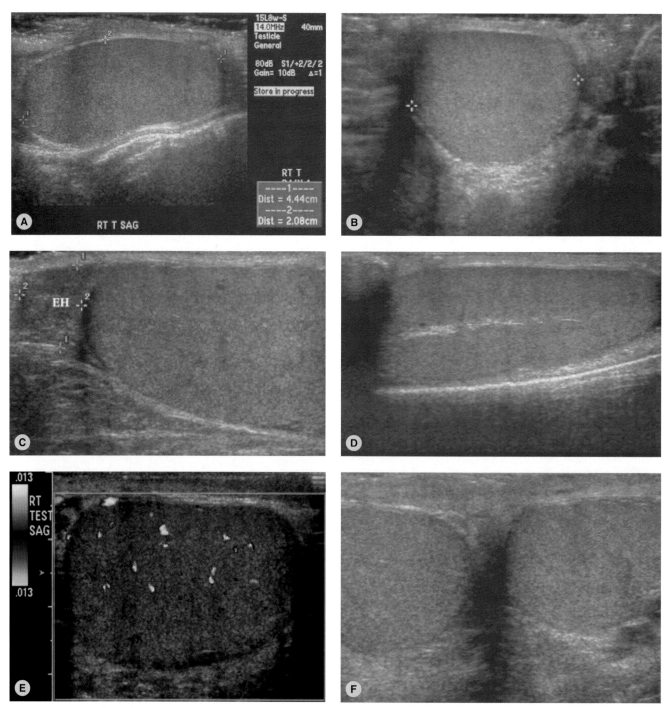

Figure 13.6. **(A)** Longitudinal ultrasound image of normal testis with homogenous parenchyma. **(B)** Transverse scan of the normal testis. **(C)** Epididymal head (EH) next to the upper pole of the testis. Compared to the normal testicle, the epididymis is normally isoechoic or slightly more echogenic with a more coarse appearance. **(D)** Longitudinal testicular scan demonstrates the mediastinum testis as a linear echogenic band. **(E)** Normal blood flow through the testis (blue, flow away from the transducer; red, flow toward the transducer). **(F)** Transverse scrotal scan to compare echogenicity of both testes.

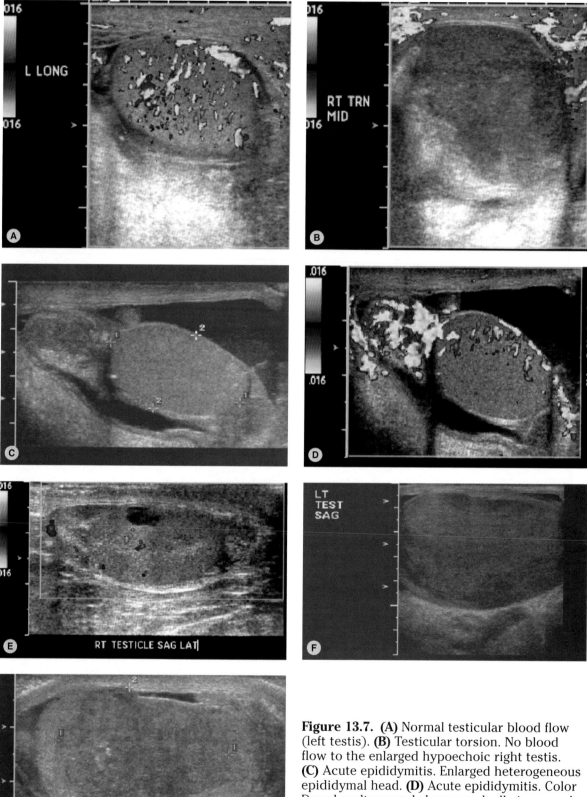

Figure 13.7. (A) Normal testicular blood flow (left testis). **(B)** Testicular torsion. No blood flow to the enlarged hypoechoic right testis. **(C)** Acute epididymitis. Enlarged heterogeneous epididymal head. **(D)** Acute epididymitis. Color Doppler ultrasound shows markedly increased vascularity of the epididymis. **(E)** Slightly hyperechoic and partially cystic malignant testicular mass. **(F)** Large heterogeneous, poorly circumscribed malignant testicular mass with calcifications. **(G)** Large malignant testicular mass replacing entire testicular parenchyma.

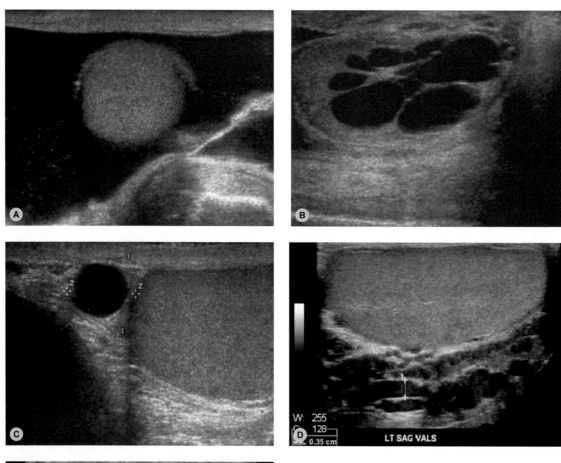

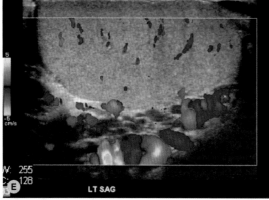

Figure 13.8. **(A)** Large hydrocele. Transverse scan shows anechoic fluid collection with some debris and without septations. **(B)** Large, benign, anechoic, intratesticular cysts. **(C)** Large, anechoic cyst in the head of the epididymis. **(D)** Varicocele. Longitudinal scan shows tortuous, dilated, hypoechoic veins. **(E)** Color Doppler ultrasound with the Valsalva maneuver shows the blood flow in a varicocele with engorged veins.

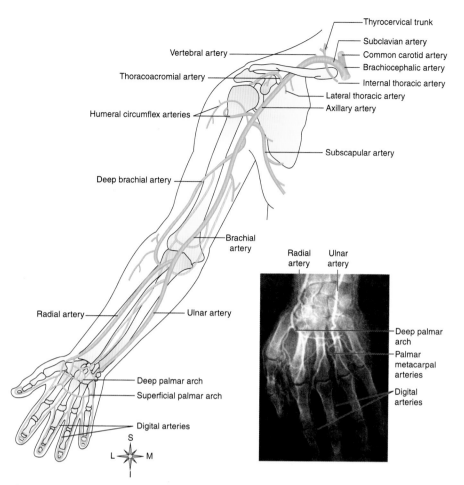

Figure 15.1. Upper extremity arteries. *(From Patton KT, Thibodeau GA, Anatomy and Physiology. 7th ed. St. Louis, MO: Mosby Elsevier; 2010:637.)*

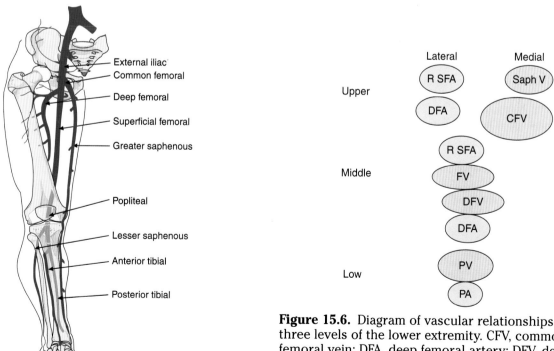

Figure 15.4. Lower extremity veins.

Figure 15.6. Diagram of vascular relationships at three levels of the lower extremity. CFV, common femoral vein; DFA, deep femoral artery; DFV, deep femoral vein; FV, femoral vein; PA, pulmonary artery; PV, pulmonary vein; R SFA, right superficial femoral artery; Saph V, saphenous vein.

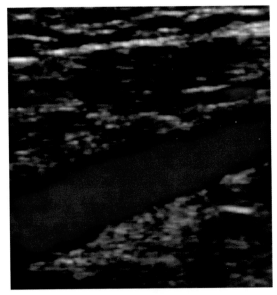

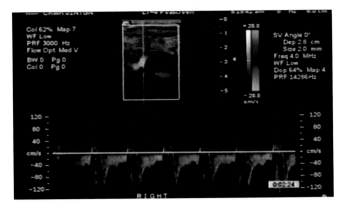

Figure 15.11. Normal color flow image of the common femoral vein. The common femoral vein when imaged without color provides limited information. When color is added the normal flow is identified.

Figure 15.14. Turbulent flow showing aliasing in the color flow image and the Doppler waveform.

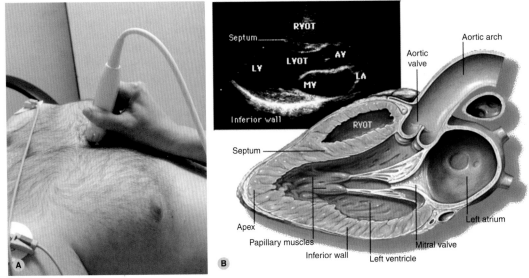

Figure 17.4. Parasternal long-axis echocardiographic view. (*Images and illustrations reproduced from FEEL-UK with permission*)

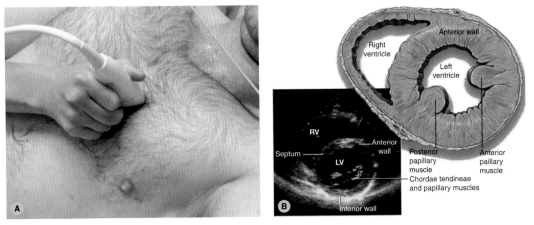

Figure 17.6. Parasternal short-axis echocardiographic view. LV, left ventricle; RV, right ventricle. (*Images and illustrations reproduced from FEEL-UK with permission*)

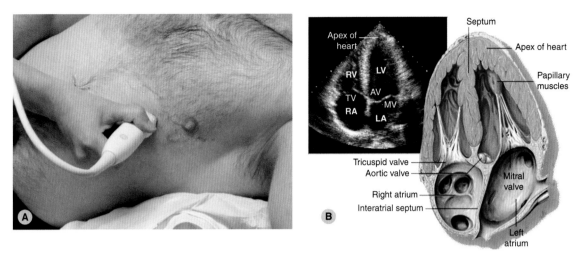

Figure 17.9. Apical four-chamber echocardiographic view. AV, aortic valve; LA, left atrium; LV, left ventricle; MV, mitral valve; RA, right atrium; RV, right ventricle; TV, tricuspid valve. *(Images and illustrations reproduced from FEEL-UK with permission)*

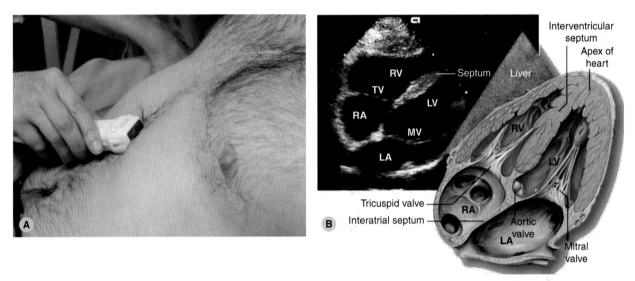

Figure 17.11. Subcostal echocardiographic view. LA, left atrium; LV, left ventricle; MV, mitral valve; RA, right atrium; RV, right ventricle; TV, tricuspid valve. *(Images and illustrations reproduced from FEEL-UK with permission)*

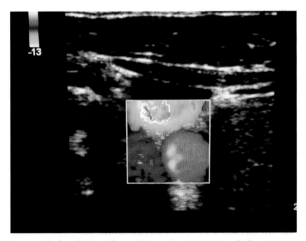

Figure 18.2. Color flow Doppler image of the internal jugular vein *(top)* and carotid artery *(bottom)*.

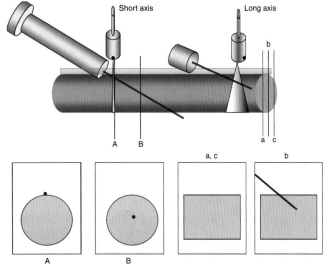

Figure 18.21. Diagram comparing transverse and longitudinal approach, illustrating the need for for the visualization of the needle tip. In plane B needle appears in the center of the vessel while the tip has penetrated the posterior wall. (*Adapted with permission*)

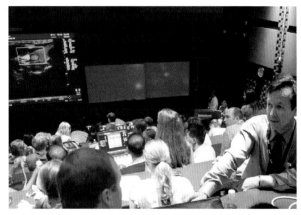

Figure 21.1. Demonstration of bedside ultrasound techniques to a group of medical students at Wayne State University School of Medicine in Detroit, Michigan (2006).

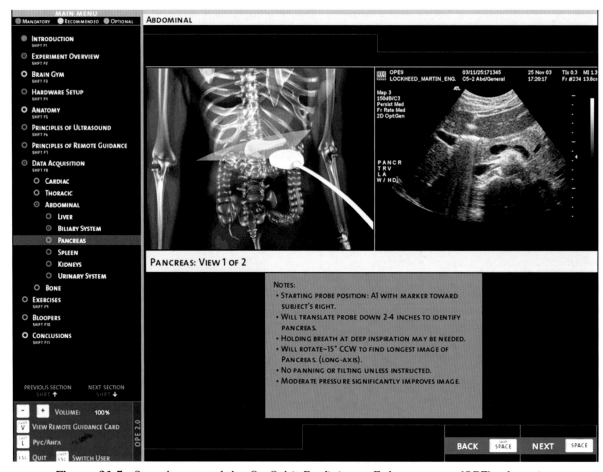

Figure 21.5. Sample page of the On-Orbit Proficiency Enhancement (OPE) e-learning tool. Note the menu prescription with mandatory, recommended, and optional items to best prepare the operator for a specific imaging session. (Advanced Diagnostic Ultrasound in Microgravity Investigation.)

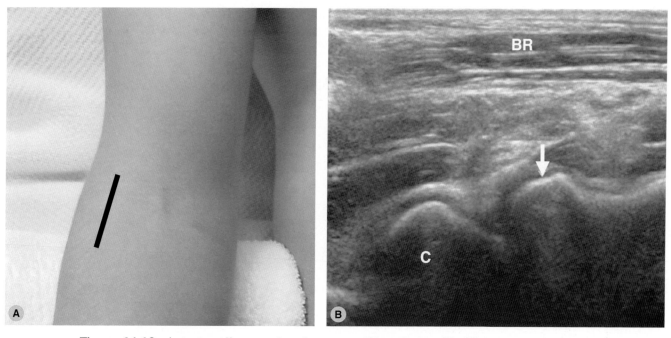

Figure 14.12. Anterior elbow probe placement **(A)** and view **(B).** The arrow indicates the radial head. BR, brachioradialis muscle; C, capitellum.

this site are sometimes injured with gripping motions as in tennis (tennis elbow). Asking the patient to pronate and supinate, one notices the motion of the radius against the capitellum of the humerus.

The posterior view of the elbow is obtained by having the patient rest his or her hand on the hip in the crab position (Fig. 14.15). Longitudinally, the trochlear nerve can be visualized proximally and the olecranon distally. Further distal is the olecranon bursa. Probe pressure should be applied gently to avoid compressing the bursa. The triceps tendon can then be seen. A transverse posterior view should be obtained to visualize the triceps tendon and muscles as well.

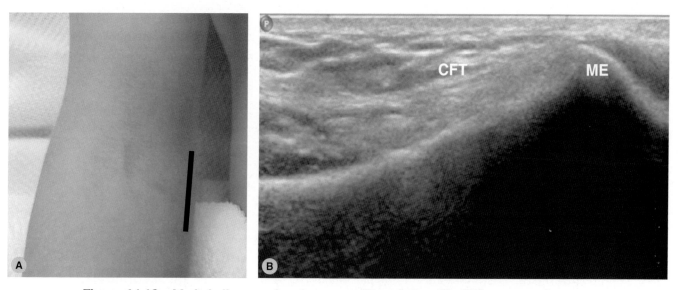

Figure 14.13. Medial elbow probe placement **(A)** and view **(B).** CFT, common flexor tendon; ME, medial epicondyle.

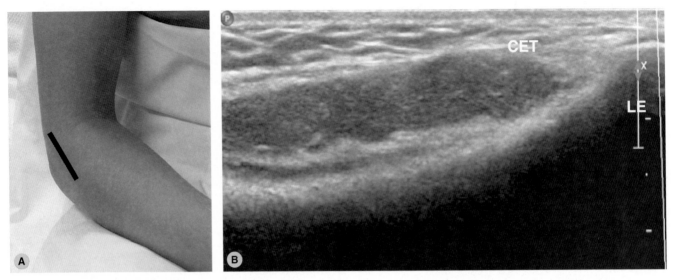

Figure 14.14. Lateral longitudinal probe placement **(A)** and view **(B)**. CET, common extensor tendon; LE, lateral epicondyle.

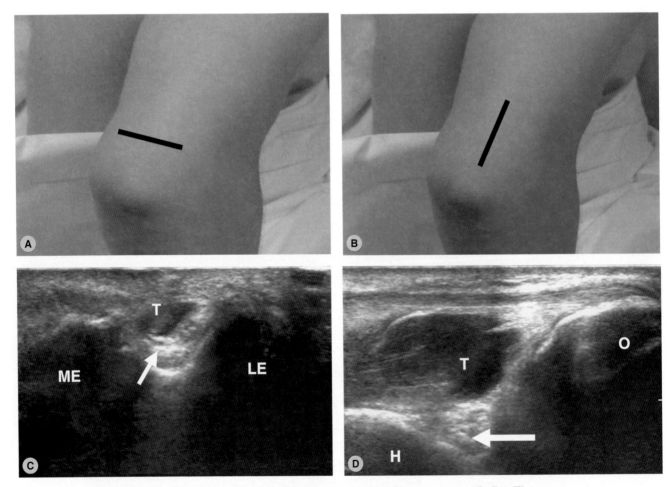

Figure 14.15. Posterior elbow probe placement **(A, B)** and views **(C, D)**. The arrow indicates a fat pad. H, humerus; LE, lateral epicondyle; ME, medial epicondyle; O, olecranon; T, triceps tendon.

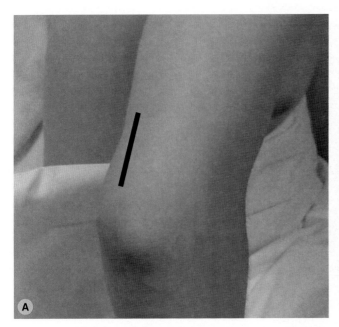 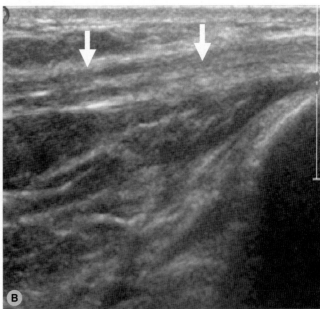

Figure 14.16. Medial longitudinal probe placement **(A)** and view **(B).** The arrows indicate the ulnar nerve.

A longitudinal posterior medial view, with the patient in the same position, allows for visualization of the ulnar nerve right next to the medial epicondyle in the cubital tunnel (Fig. 14.16). Flexion and extension of the elbow may cause subluxation of the ulnar nerve, while nerve impingement may also be seen here.

WRIST AND HAND

Examining the wrist and hand ultrasonographically requires a brief review of key landmarks (Fig. 14.17). The bony surfaces include the radius and ulna with the Lister tubercle on the dorsal surface of the radius as an important starting point. The proximal carpal bones, scaphoid, lunate, and triquetrum with pisiform and, distal row, carpal row, trapezium, trapezoid, capitate, and hamate form the two rows of carpal bones (see Fig. 14.17A). Remember that in surface anatomy the proximal transverse crease at the wrist is the location of the wrist joint, whereas the distal crease lies over the proximal flexor retinaculum. The key muscles consist of the extensors, including the radial and ulnar, as well as the digit flexors and the abductors of the thumb in the six dorsal compartments. Review the anatomic snuff box with its base composed of the radial styloid and scaphoid, its lateral edge formed by the extensor pollicis longus, and its medial edge formed by the extensor pollicis brevis and abductor pollicis longus.

Remember that the Guyon canal houses the ulnar nerve and artery. The triangular fibrocartilage is located at the intersection of the ulna, triquetrum, radius, and lunate. In the palmar aspect, the median nerve and radial and ulnar arteries represent important structures. Recall the metacarpal phalangeal joints with the A1 (anular) pulley structures and the ulnar and radial collateral ligaments of the various joints as well as the proximal interphalangeal and distal interphalangeal joints.

The superficial and smaller structures of the wrist and hand are visualized best with a high-frequency linear array probe, 9 to 15 MHz. A small hockey-stick probe can be used if available. The patient's hand should be resting comfortably in a neutral position. Dynamic movements will include flexion, extension, radial motion, and ulnar motion and maybe dynamic stressing of joints to bring out laxity.

The transverse palmar view allows visualization of the median nerve (Fig. 14.18). The starry-night structure, when involved in carpal tunnel syndrome, will enlarge proximally (>10 mm^2) and flatten at the site of compression. The median nerve is superficial to the flexor tendons and stays relatively stationary on the images, while the tendons move when the patient flexes the fingers. More medially, the pisiform can be identified with the ulnar nerve and artery in the Guyon canal. Arteries are pulsatile structures, better seen in real time. Structures seen in transverse view should also be imaged in longitudinal view.

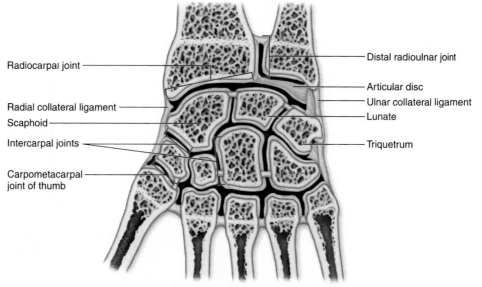

A   **Right radiocarpal joint, coronal section**

Radiocarpal joint

Radial collateral ligament

Scaphoid

Intercarpal joints

Carpometacarpal joint of thumb

Distal radioulnar joint

Articular disc

Ulnar collateral ligament

Lunate

Triquetrum

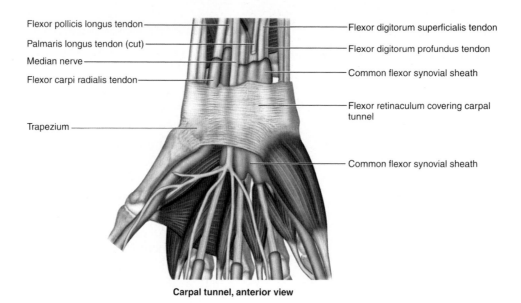

B   **Carpal tunnel, anterior view**

Flexor pollicis longus tendon

Palmaris longus tendon (cut)

Median nerve

Flexor carpi radialis tendon

Trapezium

Flexor digitorum superficialis tendon

Flexor digitorum profundus tendon

Common flexor synovial sheath

Flexor retinaculum covering carpal tunnel

Common flexor synovial sheath

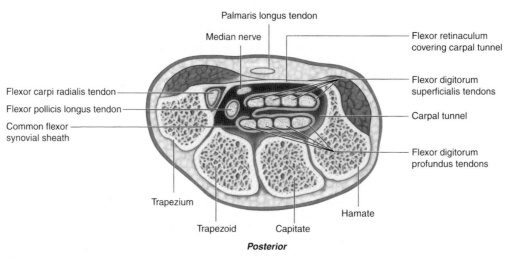

C   **Carpal tunnel, transverse section**

Anterior

Palmaris longus tendon

Median nerve

Flexor carpi radialis tendon

Flexor pollicis longus tendon

Common flexor synovial sheath

Flexor retinaculum covering carpal tunnel

Flexor digitorum superficialis tendons

Carpal tunnel

Flexor digitorum profundus tendons

Trapezium

Trapezoid

Capitate

Hamate

Posterior

Figure 14.17. Anatomy of the wrist and hand.

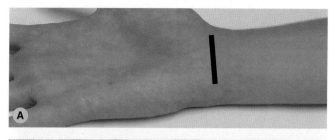

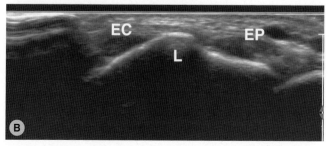

Figure 14.18. Transverse palmar probe position **(A)** and view of the wrist **(B).** M, median nerve; R, radial artery; T, flexor tendons.

The dorsal wrist view should utilize the Lister tubercle of the dorsal radius as the main landmark (Fig. 14.19). The six compartments from radial to ulnar include compartment 1 (extensor pollicis brevis and abductor pollicis, which are inflamed in De Quervain tenosynovitis), compartment 2 on the radial side of the Lister tubercle (extensor carpi radialis longus and brevis), compartment 3 on the ulnar side of the Lister tubercle (extensor pollicis longus), compartment 4

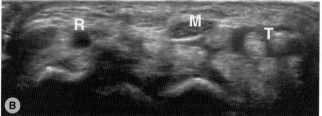

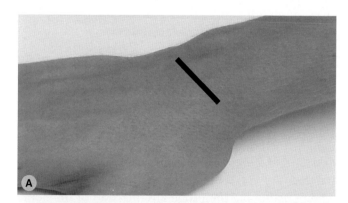

Figure 14.19. Dorsal transverse probe position **(A)** and view **(B).** EC, extensor carpi radialis brevis tendon; EP, extensor pollicis longus tendon; L, Lister tubercle.

(extensor digiti and indicis), compartment 5 (extensor digiti minimi), and compartment 6 (extensor carpi ulnaris) within the ulnar groove.

The fingers can be visualized in longitudinal views to evaluate the joints, usually from the dorsal surface looking for erosions and synovial thickening (Fig. 14.20). The thumb also can be imaged on the ulnar surface, as the ulnar collateral ligament is damaged in gamekeeper's and skier's thumb. Transverse views of the metacarpophalangeal (MCP), proximal interphalangeal (PIP), and distal interphalangeal (DIP) joints identify the annular pulleys, the flexor tendons, and the bony surfaces as well.

HIP

A review of the hip anatomy starts with surface landmarks (Fig. 14.21). The inguinal ligament stretches between the anterior superior iliac spine and the pubic tubercle, both felt as bony protuberances. The femoral artery can be felt at the midpoint of the inguinal ligament. The femoral nerve lies lateral to the artery and the femoral vein medially in the femoral triangle. The hip joint itself is composed of the head of the femur in the acetabulum. Key elements of the femur include the head, the neck, the greater and lesser trochanters, and the intertrochanteric ridge. Key muscles include anteriorly the sartorius and quadriceps; medially the iliopsoas, gracilis, pectineus, and adductors; laterally the glutei, obturators, piriformis, gemelli, tensor fascia lata, and iliotibial tract; and posteriorly the hamstrings, biceps femoris, semimembranosus, and semitendinosus. The capsule of the hip joint extends from the acetabulum to the intertrochanteric line. Three ligaments, the iliofemoral, the ischiofemoral, and the pubofemoral, compose the capsule. The locations of the ligamentum teres and the transverse acetabular ligament should be reviewed. The anterior superior portion of the labrum is the only part of the labrum that can be visualized with ultrasound.

The trochanteric, ischial, gluteofemoral, and iliopsoas bursae are important to remember. The sciatic nerve lies in the greater sciatic notch just lateral to the ischial tuberosity.

Since the hip is a deeper structure, adequate visualization may require a probe with lower frequencies, typically 5 to 9 MHz. A larger patient may best be visualized with a curved array probe with even lower frequencies in the 2- to 5-MHz range. Scanning depth should be approximately 9 to 10 cm.

The first view is the anterior longitudinal image, obtained by placing the patient's leg in the neutral

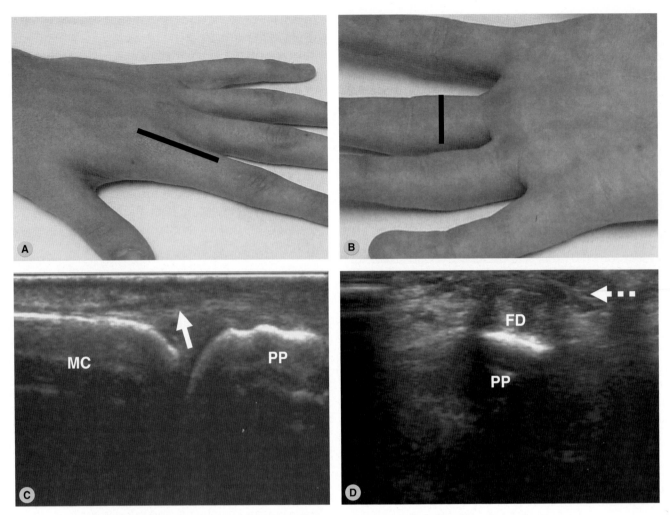

Figure 14.20. Dorsal metacarpal phalangeal joint long axis (**C**) view and volar transverse (**D**) view. Panels **A** and **B** demonstrate appropriate probe placement. Panels **C** and **D** demonstrate the respective views. The arrow indicates the extensor digitorum tendon, and the dashed arrow indicates the annular pulley. FD, flexor digitorum tendon; MC, metacarpal; PP, proximal phalanx.

position with the probe parallel to the femoral neck, slightly oblique, facing toward the femoral nerve inguinal ligament intersection (Fig. 14.22). Note the acetabulum, the hyperechoic iliofemoral ligament draping along the femoral head, and the femoral neck. The iliopsoas muscle lies superficial to these structures. A bursa lies over the capsule and deep to the muscle layer. The anterior superior labrum may also be visualized. The majority of symptomatic tears occur here.

Moving the probe laterally over the greater trochanter, one visualizes the greater trochanter, the trochanteric bursa, and the two glutei that insert here, the minimus more proximal and deeper and the medius more distal and superficial on the image (Fig. 14.23). With the probe in the transverse image, the iliotibial tract can be visualized as a hyperechoic structure above the gluteus minimus and gluteus medius.

KNEE

Anatomic landmarks in ultrasonography of the knee include the bony structures, the femur with its medial and lateral condyles, the tibia, the fibula, and the patella (Fig. 14.24). The key landmarks to identify when positioning the probe are the head of the fibula posterolaterally where the biceps femoris and lateral collateral ligament insert; the Gerdy tubercle of the tibia more medially where the iliotibial band inserts; and the insertion of the patellar tendon on the tibial tuberosity. Key ligaments in the knee include the medial collateral ligament composed of three layers, the innermost attaching to the medial meniscus and the first to tear with injury; the lateral collateral ligament; and the anterior and posterior cruciate ligaments. Muscles include the quadriceps inserting on the superior portion of the patella; the sartorius,

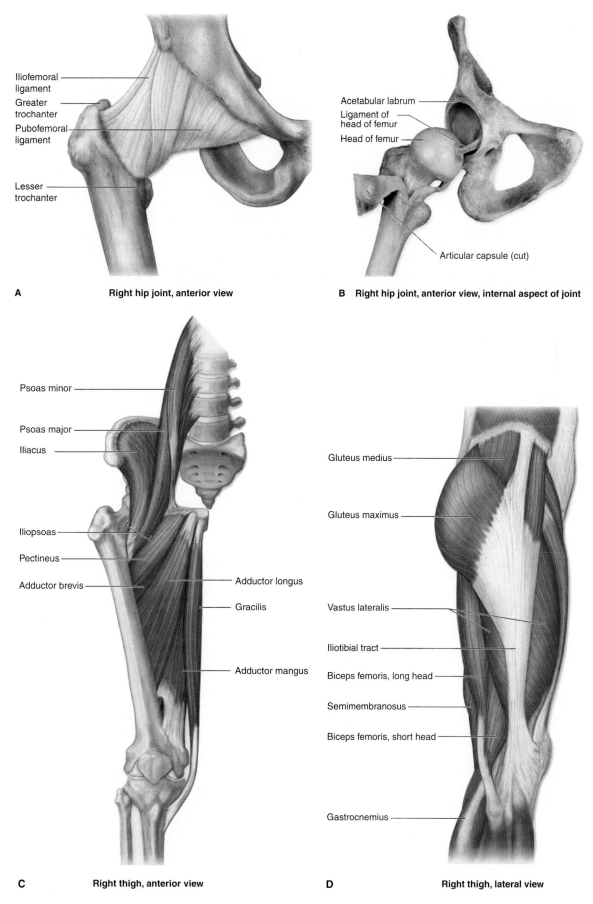

A   **Right hip joint, anterior view**

Iliofemoral ligament
Greater trochanter
Pubofemoral ligament
Lesser trochanter

B   **Right hip joint, anterior view, internal aspect of joint**

Acetabular labrum
Ligament of head of femur
Head of femur
Articular capsule (cut)

C   **Right thigh, anterior view**

Psoas minor
Psoas major
Iliacus
Iliopsoas
Pectineus
Adductor brevis
Adductor longus
Gracilis
Adductor mangus

D   **Right thigh, lateral view**

Gluteus medius
Gluteus maximus
Vastus lateralis
Iliotibial tract
Biceps femoris, long head
Semimembranosus
Biceps femoris, short head
Gastrocnemius

Figure 14.21. Anatomy of the hip.

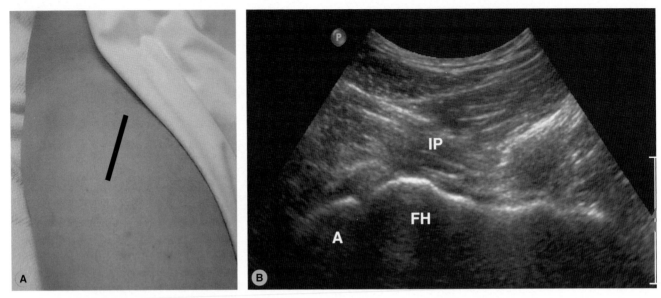

Figure 14.22. Anterior probe placement **(A)** and view of hip **(B)**. A, acetabulum; FH, femoral head; IP, iliopsoas muscle.

gracilis, and semitendinosus inserting on the tibia as the pes anserinus; the adductor magnus inserting on the adductor tubercle of the medial condyle of the femur; and the popliteus tendon in the sulcus of the lateral condyle. Posteriorly, the medial and lateral gastrocnemius muscles lie on either side of the popliteal artery, and the semimembranosus and semitendinosus lie medial to the medial gastrocnemius. The soleus lies deep to the gastrocnemii. The cartilaginous structures include the medial and lateral menisci, fibrocartilage visualized medially, laterally, and posteriorly ultrasonographically. Bursae include the medial gastrocnemius-semimembranosus (Baker cyst), superficial and deep infrapatellar, pes anserine, medial collateral

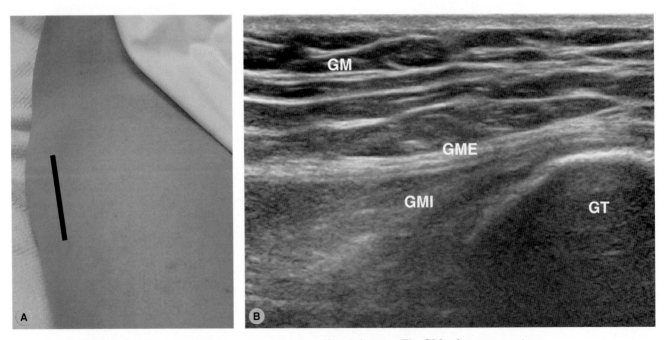

Figure 14.23. Lateral hip probe position **(A)** and view **(B)**. GM, gluteus maximus muscle; GME, gluteus medius tendon; GMI, gluteus minimus tendon; GT, greater trochanter.

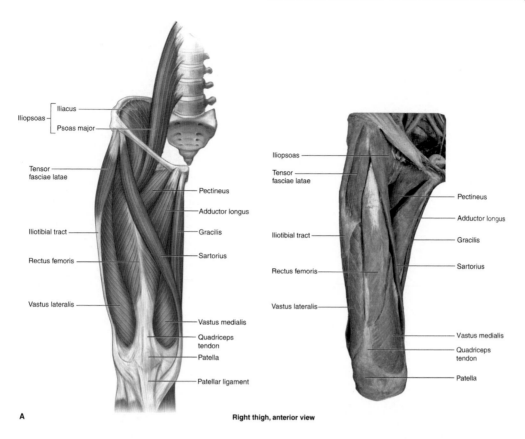

A

Right thigh, anterior view

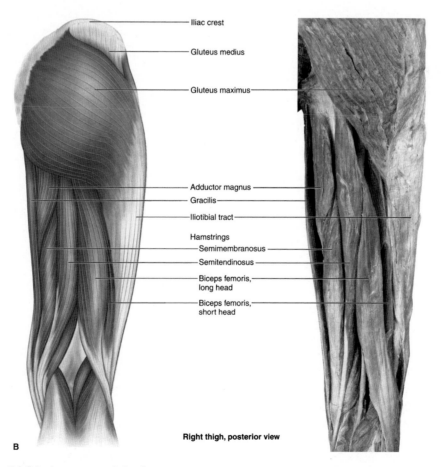

B

Right thigh, posterior view

Figure 14.24. Anatomy of the knee.

(*Continued*)

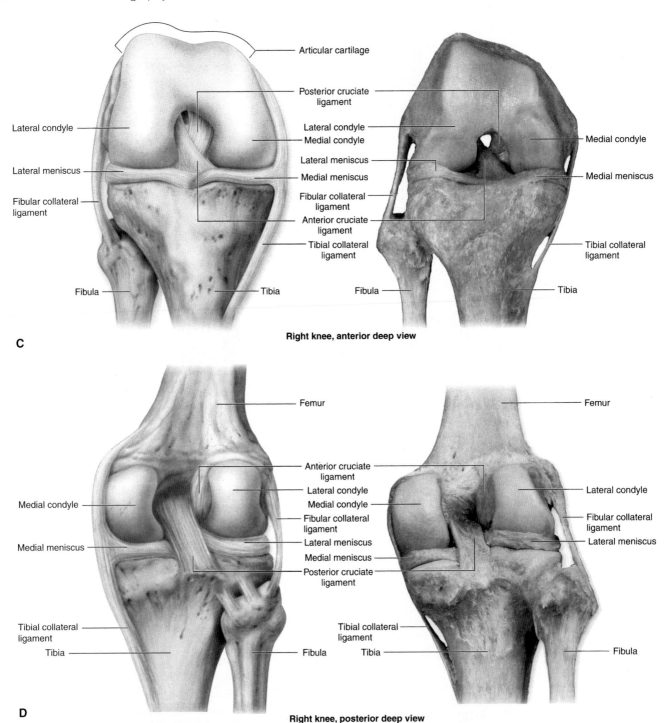

C

Right knee, anterior deep view

D

Right knee, posterior deep view

Figure 14.24. (*Continued*)

ligament, prepatellar, medial and lateral gastrocnemius, and semimembranosus-tibial collateral ligament bursae. The sciatic nerve divides into the tibial nerve, continuing into the popliteal fossa with the popliteal artery and vein and the common peroneal nerve, which continues laterally around the fibula with its branches, the anterior tibial and superficial peroneal nerves.

The anterior knee is examined ultrasonographically with the knee slightly flexed with a rolled towel underneath it for support. Longitudinal views superior to the patella may be employed to view the quadriceps tendon and the smooth patella cortex (Fig. 14.25) and inferior to the patella to view the patellar tendon. Remember the Hoffa fat pad deep to the patellar tendon. Transverse views should also be obtained, which allow visualization

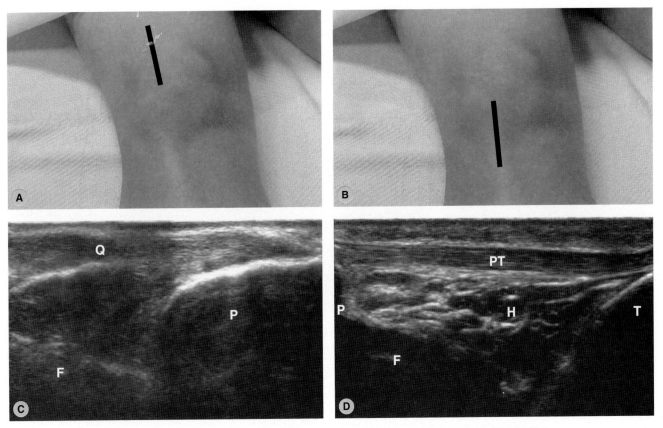

Figure 14.25. Anterior probe placement **(A, B)** and views of the knee **(C, D).** F, femur; H, Hoffa fat pad; P, patella; PT, patellar tendon; Q, quadriceps tendon; T, tibia.

of the medial and lateral patellar retinaculum. Suprapatellar transverse placement of the probe allows visualization of the femoral condyles and the thick hypoechoic hyaline cartilage overlying the femur.

At the medial knee with the probe positioned over the tibia and medial femoral condyle, one can visualize the medial collateral ligament with its two deepest layers (meniscofemoral and meniscotibial ligaments), the innermost one attaching to the medial meniscus, a hyperechoic fibrocartilage (Fig. 14.26).

At the lateral knee, with the probe over the lateral condyle, one can see the sulcus of the lateral condyle with the popliteal tendon coursing through it (popliteal groove) (Fig. 14.27). A plane stretching to the Gerdy tubercle from here allows visualization of the iliotibial band.

Over the popliteal groove lies the lateral collateral ligament, which attaches to the fibular head. The biceps femoris can also be picked up here by pivoting on the fibular head and angling the proximal probe more laterally. Just lateral to this is the common peroneal nerve.

At the posterior knee, transversely, one can visualize the medial and lateral gastrocnemius muscles (Fig. 14.28). Following the medial gastrocnemius proximally to a space between the medial and lateral femoral condyles, one can visualize the anisotropic semimembranosus tendon medially. The space between these two structures is the location of Baker cysts. Deep to the semimembranosus is the space where the semimembranosus bursa is seen and deep, and medial to the medial gastrocnemius is the location of the gastrocnemius tendon, between the muscles and the medial femoral condyle. The popliteal artery can be seen lateral to the medial gastrocnemius. Longitudinal views laterally and medially allow visualization of the posterior horns of the lateral and medial menisci, respectively. Laterally, a sesamoid bone in the lateral gastrocnemius tendon can sometimes be seen (fabella).

ANKLE AND FOOT

The anatomy of the ankle and foot includes key palpable surface structures, the medial and lateral malleoli,

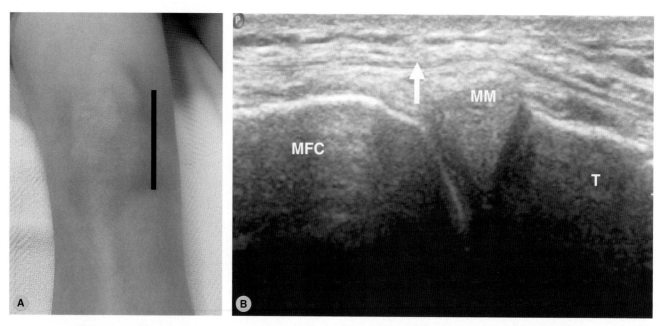

Figure 14.26. Medial knee probe placement **(A)** and view **(B).** The arrow indicates the medial collateral ligament. MFC, medial femoral condyle; MM, medial meniscus; T, tibia.

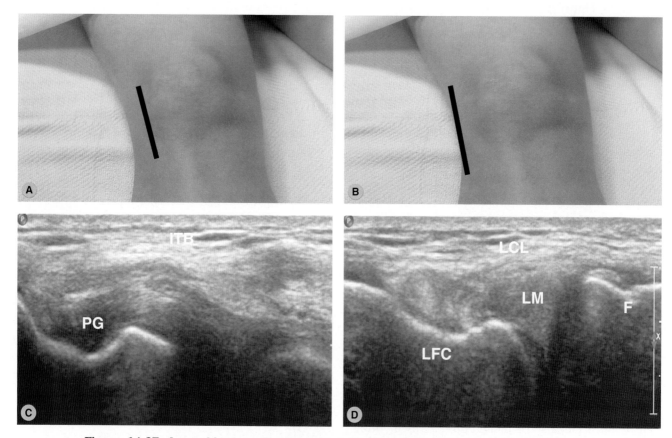

Figure 14.27. Lateral knee probe placement **(A, B)** and views **(C, D).** F, fibula; ITB, iliotibial band; LCL, lateral collateral ligament; LFC, lateral femoral condyle; LM, lateral meniscus; PG, popliteal groove.

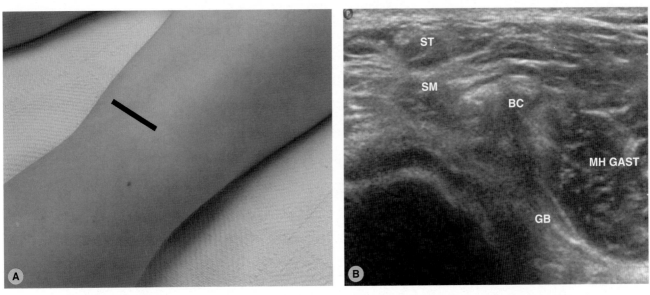

Figure 14.28. Posterior knee probe placement **(A)** and view **(B).** BC, area of potential Baker cyst; GB, area of potential gastrocnemius bursa; MH GAST, medial head of gastrocnemius; SM, semimembranosus tendon; ST, semitendinosus tendon.

the calcaneus, and the Achilles tendon (Fig. 14.29). A complete examination would include a review of the bony structures: the tibia, fibula, tarsal bones, calcaneus, and talus proximally; the cuboid, lateral, intermediate, and medial cuneiform distally; and the metatarsals and the phalanges. The navicular lies medially and separately from the other tarsal bones. The ankle joint, a hinged synovial joint, is formed by the tibia and talar dome. The tendons are separated into anterior (medial to lateral: the tibialis anterior, extensor

hallucis longus, extensor digitorum longus, and peroneus tertius), posteromedial (anteromedial to posteromedial: tibialis posterior, flexor digitorum longus, flexor hallucis longus), posterolateral (peroneus longus and brevis), and posterior groups (Achilles and plantaris). In the sole of the foot the plantar fascia often is involved pathologically at its insertion site on the calcaneus medially. Key ligaments include the often injured anterior talofibular, the anterior-inferior tibiofibular, the calcaneofibular, and the medial deltoid composed of

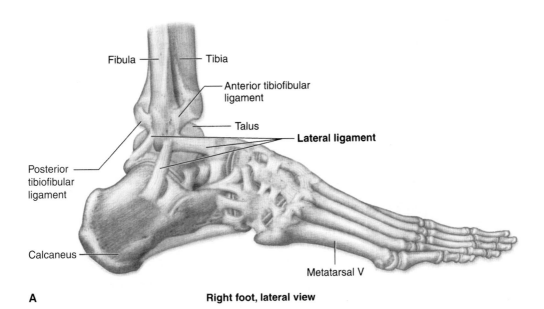

A   **Right foot, lateral view**

Figure 14.29. Anatomy of the ankle.

(Continued)

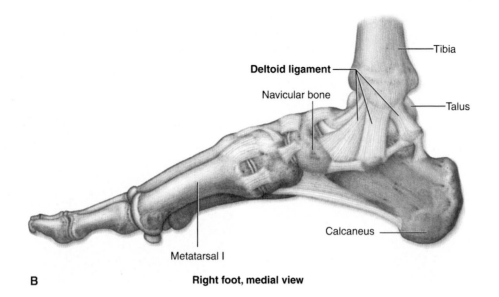

B   **Right foot, medial view**

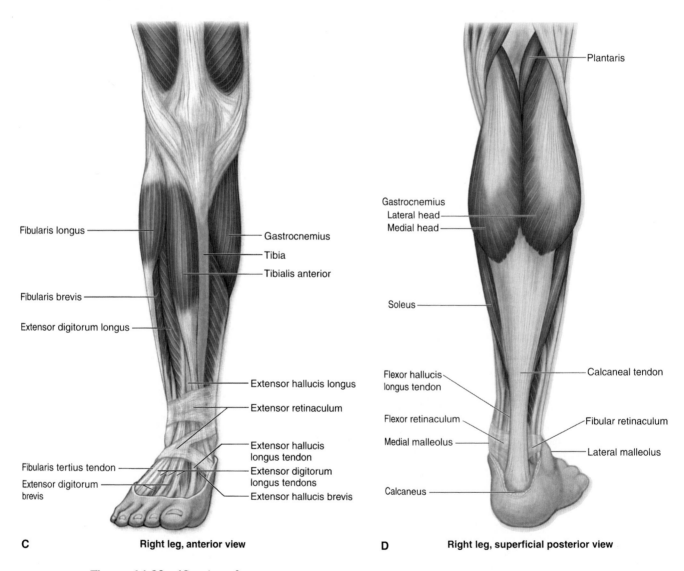

C   **Right leg, anterior view**   D   **Right leg, superficial posterior view**

Figure 14.29. (*Continued*)

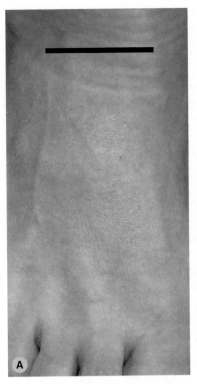
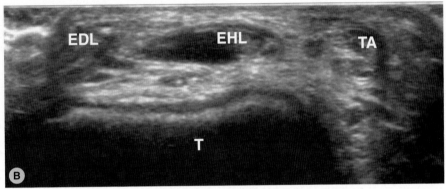

Figure 14.30. Anterior ankle probe position **(A)** and view **(B)**. EDL, extensor digitorum longus tendon; EHL, extensor hallucis longus tendon; T, tibia; TA, tibialis anterior tendon.

the tibiotalar, tibiocalcaneal, tibionavicular, and anterior tibiotalar. Vessels and nerves include the posterior tibial artery and nerve, the deep peroneal nerve, and the anterior tibial artery (distally becoming the dorsalis pedis). Bursae include the retrocalcaneal and retrocheilia bursae posteriorly.

The patient is positioned with the knee flexed and the foot flat on the examination table for the anterior views, lying on the side for medial and lateral views, or lying prone with the foot over the edge of the examination table for posterior views.

The anterior ankle view transversely allows examination of the tibialis anterior, extensor hallucis longus, and extensor digitorum longus, medial to lateral (Fig. 14.30). Superficial to these tendons is the superior extensor retinaculum above the level of the malleoli, attached anteriorly to the tibia and fibula. The inferior extensor retinaculum is a Y-shaped structure originating on the anterolateral calcaneus and splitting medially to end at the medial malleolus and plantar aponeurosis. The clinician visualizes the tibiotalar joint longitudinally with its hypoechoic hyaline cartilage. Tendons can be visualized dynamically with first-toe extension. More proximally, with anterolateral transverse and longitudinal probe placement, one can examine the anterior tibiofibular ligament, which is involved in high ankle sprains.

The posteromedial ankle view transversely allows examination of the tibialis posterior, flexor digitorum longus, and the flexor hallucis longus (Fig. 14.31). The vascular bundle just superficial and medial to the posterior tibial nerve also can be well visualized. The mnemonic Tom (tibialis posterior), Dick (flexor digitorum longus) and (posterior tibial artery with two veins) Nervous (posterior tibial nerve) Harry (flexor hallucis longus) serves as an aid in remembering the locations. As always, the tendons should be evaluated in their longitudinal views to determine any pathology. Extending and flexing the great toe and the four lateral digits will allow one to identify the tendon motion dynamically as well.

The posterolateral view enables the clinician to examine the peroneus longus and brevis tendons (Fig. 14.32). The lateral malleolus is used as a guide in positioning the probe. The peroneal tubercle of the calcaneus separates these two tendons distally, with the peroneus brevis superiorly and the peroneus longus inferiorly. The peroneus brevis then inserts on the lateral fifth metatarsal, while the peroneus longus travels in a plantar direction and inserts on the medial cuneiform and first metatarsal. Applying eversion stress can visualize tears in these tendons.

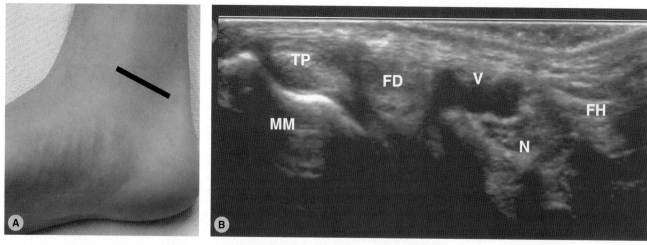

Figure 14.31. Posteromedial probe position **(A)** and view **(B)**. FD, flexor digitorum longus tendon; FH, flexor hallucis longus tendon; MM, medial malleolus; N, posterior tibial nerve; TP, tibialis posterior tendon; V, tibialis posterior artery and veins.

The posterior view in transverse and longitudinal views enables the clinician to visualize the Achilles tendon (Fig. 14.33). A thick structure, it should be kidney shaped in the transverse view. Round shaping and enlargement suggest pathology. In these views, one can also see the potential locations of the retrocalcaneal and retroachillean bursae. The common site for Achilles tendon tears is 6 to 7 cm proximal to its insertion in the calcaneus. The plantaris tendon is deep and medial to the Achilles tendon and superficial to the soleus muscle. The Kager fat pad is deep. Surrounding the tendon is the paratenon, a hypoechoic rim. The Achilles tendon does not have a synovial sheath.

The plantar view longitudinally allows for examination of the plantar fascia and its insertion into the medial calcaneus (Fig. 14.34). The probe is positioned with the distal end pointing to the first toe. Look for bone spurs on the calcaneus.

REIMBURSEMENT

While MSKUS reimbursement for radiology is generally well-established, billing for the clinical use of ultrasound remains to be fully defined or realized. The difference in clinical use and diagnostic use of ultrasound can be likened to the primary care physician reading a chest x-ray initially while the radiologist reads the film formally. Usually the primary care physician reading the film does not generate a bill for either the technical (performing the test) or professional (interpreting the test) portions

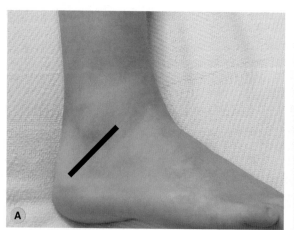

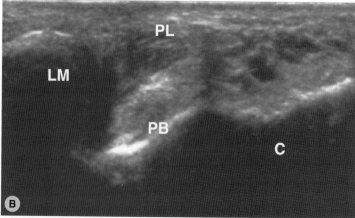

Figure 14.32. Lateral ankle probe position **(A)** and view **(B)**. C, calcaneus; LM, lateral malleolus; PB, peroneus brevis tendon; PL, peroneus longus tendon.

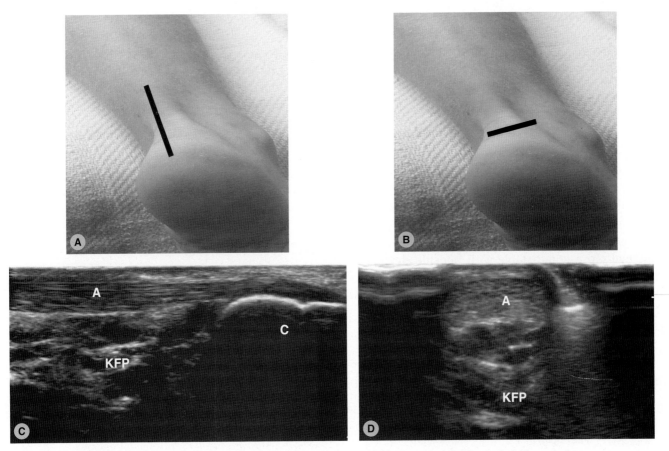

Figure 14.33. Posterior ankle probe placement **(A, B)** and views **(C, D).** A, Achilles tendon (note the anisotropy at the insertion to the calcaneus); C, calcaneus; KFP, Kager fat pad.

of the evaluation, but instead utilizes the information in that film to guide patient care prior to the formal radiologic reading. Reimbursement for MSKUS requires that formal identification, storage, and retrieval of information be available. In general, if those issues can be resolved in the primary care, rheumatology, or orthopedic settings, the *Current Procedural Terminology* (CPT) code

for diagnostic echography is 76800 and for therapeutic injections with ultrasound guidance is 76942. Insurance carriers interpret reimbursement differently, and clinicians should check with their carriers to ensure full compliance with billing criteria. As hand-held device use proliferates, reimbursement guidelines should change. Currently, clinical use of the stethoscope, the object of

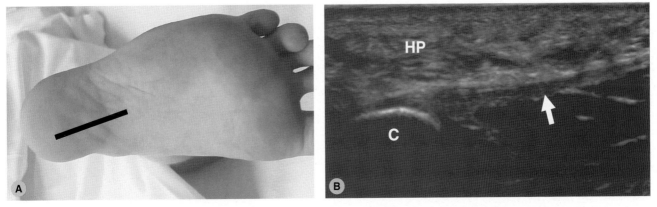

Figure 14.34. Plantar probe position **(A)** and view **(B).** The arrow indicates the plantar fascia. C, calcaneus; HP, fibrofatty heel pad.

expertise in obtaining and interpreting auscultatory findings, is figured in billing for the physical examination. We maintain that bedside ultrasound could eventually reach the same status.

FUTURE

MSKUS will no doubt find new applications. Refinement in technology has made some signs, for example, the cartilage interface sign, less helpful, while enhancing images make smaller structures clearer. Much fertile ground exists in pediatric use of MSKUS, in spinal imaging, in emergency medicine with acute musculoskeletal injuries, and in real-time sports. Rheumatologists now feel more comfortable with bedside devices in their offices, while sports medicine clinicians have begun including these devices in training rooms across the country. Even though resistance to ultrasound-assisted diagnostic and therapeutic joint and soft tissue injections exists, new data reveal that clinicians perform better with its use. Previously, clinicians questioned whether they could insert central venous catheters better with ultrasound guidance. This has now become the standard of care. Nerve blocks, previously performed by anatomic landmarks, now are more successful with ultrasound guidance. The use of MSKUS in medical schools will foster scientific inquiry that will doubtless generate new ways in which ultrasound will augment physical diagnosis for clinicians.

ACKNOWLEDGEMENT

The author wishes to acknowledge Dr. Thomas Stoecker for providing many of the images in this chapter.

Suggested Readings

Backhaus M, Burmester GR, Gerber T, et al. Guidelines for musculoskeletal ultrasound in rheumatology. *Ann Rheum Dis.* 2001;60:641–649.

Bruyn George AW, Schmidt Wolfang A. *Introductory Guide to Musculoskeletal Ultrasound for the Rheumatologist.* Houten, The Netherlands: Bohn Stafleu Van Loghum; 2006.

Harmon D, Frizell H, Sandhu N, Colreavy F, Griffin M. *Perioperative Diagnostic and Interventional Ultrasound.* Philadelphia, PA: Saunders Elsevier; 2008.

McNally E. *Practical Musculoskeletal Ultrasound.* St. Louis, MO: Elsevier-Churchill Livingstone; 2005.

O'Neil J. *Musculoskeletal Ultrasound Anatomy and Technique.* New York, NY: Springer; 2008.

Schmidt WA, Schmidt J, Schicke B, et al. Standard reference values for musculoskeletal ultrasonography. *Ann Rheum Dis.* 2004;63:988–994.

Van Hosbeeck MT, Introcaso J. *Musculoskeletal Ultrasound.* 2nd ed. St. Louis, MO: Mosby; 2001.

CHAPTER 15

Vascular System Ultrasound

James E. Foster, II, MD, FACS, RPVI

INTRODUCTION

Examination of the peripheral vascular system is an essential component of every thorough physical examination. Fortunately, the arterial and venous anatomy of the extremities is straightforward, allowing for relatively easy examination and documentation of peripheral pulses and signs of arterial insufficiency and venous congestion or insufficiency. Ultrasound examination of the peripheral arterial and venous systems has been refined to the point where bedside assessment of arterial waveforms and venous flow patterns should become part of every initial physical examination. It is particularly helpful when the history obtained from the patient suggests a possible component of vascular compromise. Abnormal findings can then direct more detailed duplex ultrasound examinations that can quantify the degree of impairment and the specific location of the abnormality. Duplex ultrasound has become the initial modality of choice for vascular diagnosis. Technical advances have improved the diagnostic accuracy such that treatment decisions previously based on angiographic studies can now be made based on noninvasive studies alone.

Figures 15.1 (see also color insert) through 15.4 (see also color insert) depict the complete anatomy of the arterial-venous system, while Figure 15.5 depicts the major arteries of the head and neck. Table 15.1 identifies the appropriate technology, patient position, and steps for various vascular studies.

ULTRASOUND EXAMINATION OF THE VENOUS SYSTEM (VIDEO 15.1)

When one is performing an ultrasound evaluation of the venous system, patient positioning, transducer selection, and technique are all important in achieving an optimal study.

Patient positioning is important to support patient comfort and allow direct and thorough access to vessels under examination. All patients receiving an upper or lower extremity study should be placed in the supine position. For an upper extremity examination, the patient should have the arm slightly abducted and supinated, while for a lower extremity examination, the patient should have the hip externally rotated and the knee flexed. A linear array high-frequency (7- to 10-MHz) transducer should be used, except when visualizing the deep veins, in which case a lower-frequency curved array transducer should be utilized.

Of importance, the technique needs to be systematic and organized. One must view the image in the transverse plane with high-resolution gray-scale imaging. If intraluminal echoes are identified, compression of the vein should be avoided as it represents venous thromboembolism. If the vein is clear, it should be compressed to demonstrate wall-to-wall apposition of the vein. This process should be repeated at 5-cm intervals along the length of the vein. Vascular relationships at three levels of the lower extremity are summarized in Figure 15.6 (see also color insert).

If intraluminal echogenic material is identified, the transducer should then be rotated 90° to assess the extent of the thrombus in the longitudinal plane. It is also important to evaluate the flow characteristics. The examiner must identify the common femoral vein in the transverse plane and rotate the transducer to the longitudinal plane. One should observe the Doppler signal for respiratory phasic changes (normal). The Valsalva maneuver and augmentation maneuvers can also be used to alter the flow characteristics.

Diagnostic criteria for identifying a deep venous thrombosis (DVT) can be divided into vessel characteristics and flow characteristics. The primary vessel characteristic is compressibility, the ability to demonstrate wall-to-wall apposition of the vein when adequate pressure is applied using the ultrasound transducer in the transverse plane. Adequate pressure is determined by noting mild deformation of the adjacent artery (Figs. 15.7 and 15.8, Video 15.2). Noncompressibility indicates that intraluminal thrombus is preventing the vessel walls from collapsing. It is important to remember that fresh, immature thrombus may not be echogenic since a newly formed clot has acoustic impedance similar to that of blood. The second vessel characteristic is identification of intraluminal echogenic material. This often can be seen on the initial survey of the venous system and should

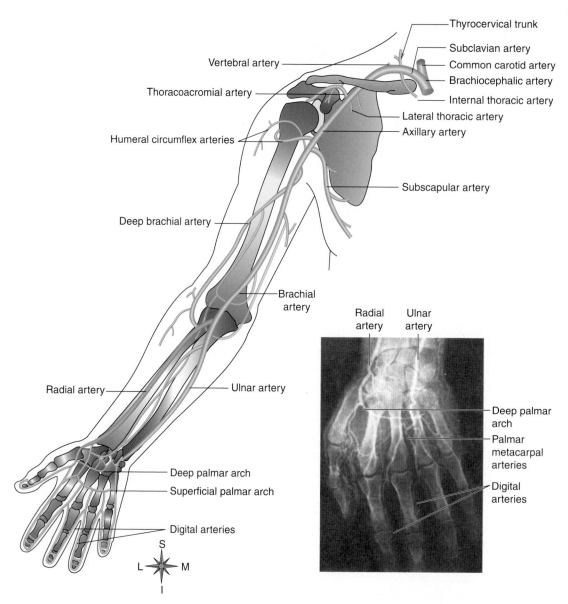

Figure 15.1. Upper extremity arteries. (See color insert.) *(From Patton KT, Thibodeau GA, Anatomy and Physiology. 7th ed. St. Louis, MO: Mosby Elsevier; 2010:637.)*

alert the clinician to the presence of thrombus. Intraluminal echogenic material should be confirmed in both imaging planes, and when thrombus is identified, compression should be limited because of the possibility of dislodging the clot. Longitudinal imaging provides the best view for determining the extent or length of thrombus and whether it is adherent to the vessel wall or may have a free-floating tip (Figs. 15.9 and 15.10, Video 15.3). A third vessel characteristic that may be helpful is the assessment of valve function. Occasionally, venous valves are visible in situations where higher-frequency transducers can be used (thin patients, children). Normal valves tend to open and close in conjunction with venous flow. However, since valve

cusps are often the site of thrombogenesis, an immobile valve cusp may be a clue to the presence of thrombus.

Venous blood flow characteristics are also important in assessing the presence of acute DVT. Normal venous flow patterns (Fig. 15.11 [see also color insert], Video 15.2) show a phasic characteristic that varies with respiration. Normal inspirations decrease intrathoracic pressures and cause an associated increase in venous flow. Similarly, expiration increases intrathoracic pressure and is reflected in a reduction in venous flow. A Valsalva maneuver increases intrathoracic pressure enough to completely interrupt venous flow. An augmentation in venous flow is noticed when the Valsalva maneuver is released. These changes are

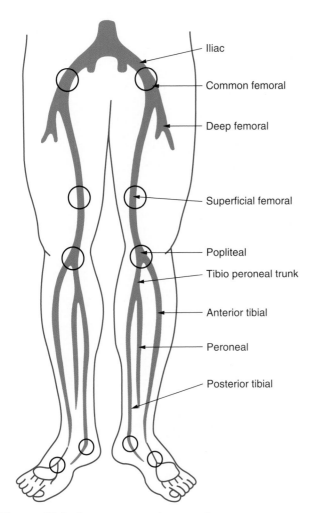

Figure 15.2. Lower extremity arteries.

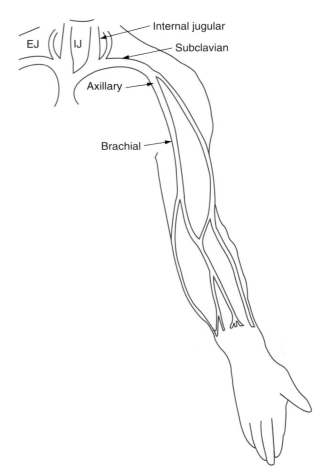

Figure 15.3. Upper extremity veins. EJ, external jugular; IJ, internal jugular.

easily identified by observing the Doppler waveform or by listening to flow patterns with a continuous wave Doppler unit. Any obstructive process between the thoracic cavity and the site of insonation of the lower extremity veins can alter the normal phasic changes associated with respiration. Absence of phasic changes with a continuous flow pattern or loss of augmentation with deep inspiration suggests obstruction of the venous system. Additional maneuvers to augment flow include compression of calf muscles and the distal thigh to demonstrate increased flow at the site of insonation. Loss of normal augmentation with compressions also suggests the presence of obstruction in the venous system. The assessment of both vessel characteristics and venous blood flow characteristics leads to highly accurate and reliable detection of DVT. Normal vessel and flow characteristics provide a very high negative predictive value for DVT as well. One should remember that bilateral symmetry allows comparison of both left and right extremities and can be very helpful in identifying abnormalities in a symptomatic limb.

ULTRASOUND EXAMINATION OF THE PERIPHERAL ARTERIES

The most common application of ultrasound in the evaluation of the arterial system is to assess the presence and degree of atherosclerotic peripheral disease. Atherosclerotic plaque and calcification of arterial walls are easily demonstrated by gray-scale imaging. Duplex imaging and Doppler waveform analysis provide reliable information related to flow characteristics and arterial stenosis. There are three basic steps for examining the peripheral arteries: (1) determine the ankle-brachial index (ABI), (2) evaluate arterial waveforms, and (3) identify the sites of turbulent flow (stenosis).

Ankle-Brachial Index

Again, patient positioning, transducer selection, and technique are all important in achieving optimal results. The patient is placed in either the supine or sitting position. A continuous wave or high-frequency pulse wave transducer should be chosen for this

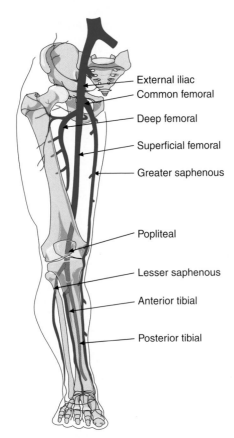

Figure 15.4. Lower extremity veins. (See color insert.)

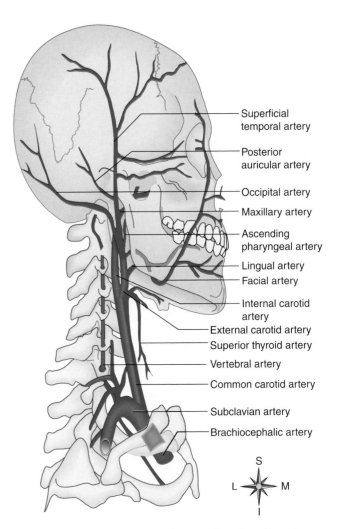

Figure 15.5. Major arteries of the head and neck. *(From Patton KT, Thibodeau GA,* Anatomy and Physiology. *7th ed. St. Louis, MO: Mosby Elsevier; 2010:633.)*

study. As for technique, one must first acquire bilateral brachial blood pressures. This is achieved by placing the blood pressure cuff above the ankle and identifying the ultrasound signal from the dorsalis pedis location. The blood pressure cuff is inflated until the signal is lost and then deflated until the signal is again heard and that pressure is recorded. This process must be repeated on the posterior tibial artery. The ABI is the higher of the two ankle pressures divided by the higher brachial pressure. This entire process must then be repeated for the opposite lower extremity. Table 15.2 provides a range of normal and abnormal values for the ABI.

Screening ultrasound examinations are most often directed to determining the presence or absence of flow and evidence of arterial injury such as arterial dissection, pseudoaneurysm, or arteriovenous fistula. The diagnosis of these problems is based on the accurate assessment of flow characteristics and requires a basic understanding of arterial anatomy, hemodynamics, and the fundamentals of pulsed Doppler ultrasound to optimize results. Because bedside arterial examinations may be technically challenging, suspected abnormalities are best confirmed by formal complete sonographic examination or by angiographic

modalities. Normal peripheral arterial hemodynamics are characterized by laminar flow in a high-resistance system that generates a characteristic triphasic waveform (Fig. 15.12). The initial forward flow is generated by ventricular systole (phase 1). The second phase is a short period of reversed flow, which occurs as the aortic valve closes. Phase 3 reflects forward flow generated by the elastic recoil of normal arterial walls. The normal triphasic waveform is easily recognized by Doppler spectral analysis or color flow imaging (Fig. 15.13). In addition, the characteristic auditory signal is easily recognized when continuous wave Doppler instruments without imaging capability are used.

Arterial Waveform Analysis

Again, the patient is placed in the supine position. If the upper extremity is being examined, there should

TABLE 15.1. Summary of Transducer Selection and Examination Steps

	Lower Venous	*Upper Venous*	*Lower Arterial*	*Carotid*
Transducer	Linear array (7–10 MHz)	Linear array (7–10 MHz)	Linear array (7–10 MHz)	Linear array (7–10 MHz)
Patient position	Supine; extremity externally rotated; knee flexed	Supine; head turned away from extremity; chin raised	Supine; extremity externally rotated; knee flexed	Supine; no pillow; head turned away from imaging side; chin raised
Examination preset	Venous	Venous	Arterial	Carotid
Step 1	Transverse compressions: CFV, SFV, Pop V	Transverse compressions: IJV, axillary vein, brachial vein	Gray scale of CFA, SFA, Pop A Transverse and long axis	Gray scale of CCA and ICA with and without color Doppler Transverse and long axis
Step 2	Long-axis color and spectral Doppler of CFV, SFV, Pop V	Long-axis color and spectral Doppler of IJV and subclavian vein	Long-axis color and spectral Doppler of CFA, SFA, Pop A	Long-axis spectral Doppler of CCA and ICA (proximal, mid, distal)

CCA, common carotid artery; CFA, common femoral artery; CFV, common femoral vein; ICA, internal carotid artery; IJV, internal jugular vein; Pop A, popliteal artery; Pop V, popliteal vein; SFA, superficial femoral artery; SFV, superficial femoral vein.

be a slight abduction, and if the lower extremity is being examined, there should be a slight external rotation, with the knee flexed. In these cases, a continuous wave- or 3- to 7-MHz linear transducer should be used with Doppler mode.

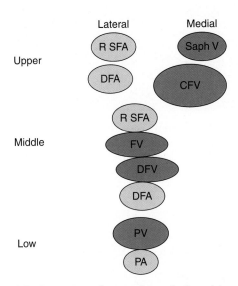

Figure 15.6. Diagram of vascular relationships at three levels of the lower extremity. (See also color insert.) CFV, common femoral vein; DFA, deep femoral artery; DFV, deep femoral vein; FV, femoral vein; PA, pulmonary artery; PV, pulmonary vein; R SFA, right superficial femoral artery; Saph V, saphenous vein.

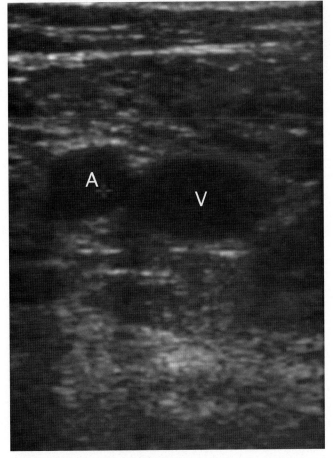

Figure 15.7. Normal right common femoral artery (A) and vein (V) (transverse plane).

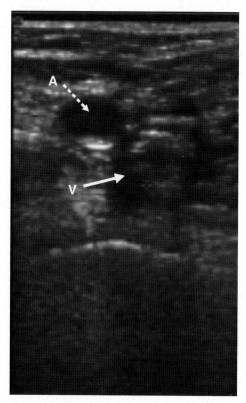

Figure 15.8. Right common femoral artery (A, *interrupted arrow*) with compressed femoral vein (V, *solid arrow*).

Abnormal findings for the ABI and waveform analysis indicate that an arterial stenosis is likely. Duplex scanning can locate arterial stenoses by recognizing areas of turbulent flow (Fig. 15.14 [see also color insert]). Turbulence corresponds to the audible bruit and is easily recognized by Doppler

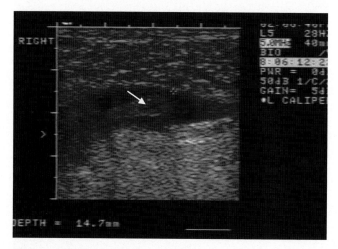

Figure 15.9. Acute thrombus in common femoral vein (longitudinal view, *arrow*).

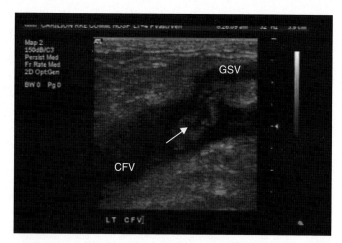

Figure 15.10. Thrombus *(arrow)* extending from the greater saphenous vein (GSV) into the common femoral vein (CFV).

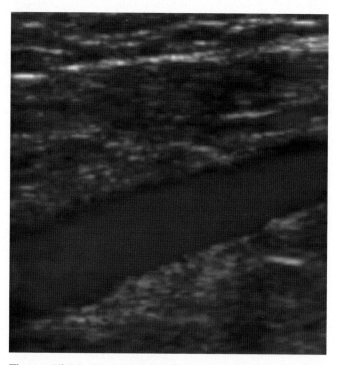

Figure 15.11. Normal color flow image of the common femoral vein. The common femoral vein when imaged without color provides limited information. When color is added (see color insert) the normal flow is identified.

TABLE 15.2. Ankle-Brachial Index Values and Correlation with Disease

Interpretation	Range
Normal	0.9–1.2
Mild disease	0.7–0.9
Claudication	<0.7
Severe disease	<0.4

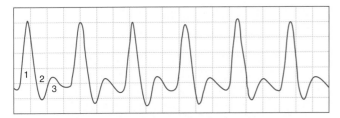

Figure 15.12. Normal triphasic peripheral arterial waveform.

ultrasound or color flow imaging. However, these studies are often time consuming and not always suited to the screening or initial examination setting.

Turbulent Flow

Turbulent flow is associated with spectral broadening and generates audible bruits. The ultrasound manifestation of high-grade stenosis is a Doppler artifact known as "aliasing." Aliasing occurs when the flow velocity exceeds the ability of the pulsed Doppler signal to accurately describe the flow rate. The duplex instrument falsely generates an opposite image or color map of the arterial flow. Aliasing is beneficial in quickly directing the sonographer to a point of maximal stenosis. When aliasing is identified, the sonographer should

change instrument settings to eliminate the artifact. Only after appropriate adjustments can accurate flow information be obtained. Critical degrees of arterial stenosis eventually lead to low flow states and occlusion, often as a result of thrombosis. Arterial occlusion is characterized by the absence of a Doppler signal (Fig. 15.15, Video 15.4) or color flow signal in the vessel distal to the point of obstruction.

ULTRASOUND EXAMINATION OF THE EXTRACRANIAL CAROTID ARTERY

There are four major steps in evaluating the extracranial carotid artery depicted in Figure. 15.5. One must first identify the carotid bifurcation; second, assess the degree of calcification; third, evaluate the arterial waveforms; and finally, identify any abnormal flow (stenosis or occlusion).

The screening evaluation of the carotid arteries is directed at determining the presence and degree of atherosclerosis and arterial calcification. This is easily recognized in gray-scale imaging by the recognition of highly echogenic areas in the vessel wall associated with acoustic shadowing. Primary interest is directed to the internal carotid artery since disease in this

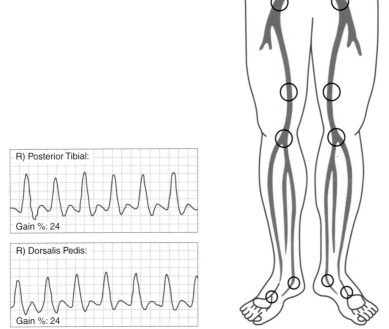

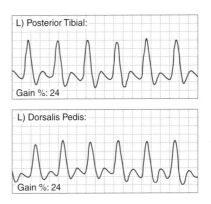

Figure 15.13. Normal lower extremity arterial waveforms on different levels.

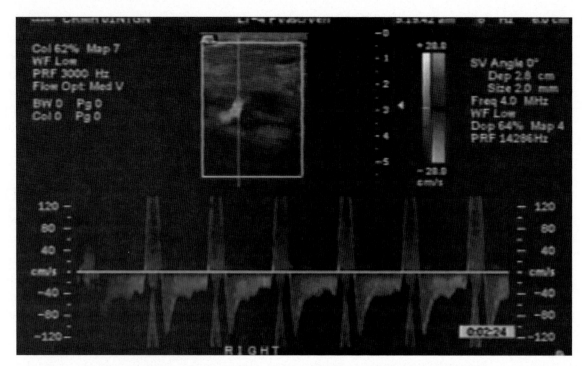

Figure 15.14. Turbulent flow showing aliasing in the color flow image and the Doppler waveform. (See color insert.)

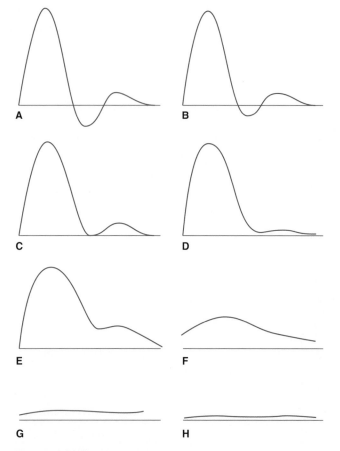

Figure 15.15. Arterial waveform changes from normal to total occlusion **(A–H).**

vessel predisposes the patient to transient ischemic attack and stroke. Dense atherosclerotic calcification can often obscure sites of arterial stenosis. The suspicion for stenosis is raised when arterial flow patterns change across an area of acoustic shadowing. Increased peak systolic velocities or evidence of spectral broadening of the Doppler waveform indicate possible stenosis and warrant further evaluation. Findings of turbulent flow often coincide with bruits detected by auscultation. The arterial waveform of the external carotid is similar to that of other peripheral arteries supplying high-resistance vascular beds, while the waveform in the internal carotid is a low-resistance pattern that maintains forward flow throughout the cardiac cycle. A decreased amplitude and loss of diastolic flow indicates downstream (intracranial) occlusion of the internal carotid artery and warrants further investigation for confirmation.

Carotid Duplex Examination

Ultrasound duplex examinations are well-suited for examining the external carotid. This examination will require an ultrasound system with high-resolution gray-scale imaging, color Doppler capability, and spectral analysis directional Doppler for velocity measurements. A linear array high-frequency transducer

(7–10 MHz) is generally appropriate, but the occasional use of a curved array transducer (3–5 MHz) may be required for deep vessels.

The patient is again placed in the supine position, with the head elevated slightly without a pillow. The head is turned away from the side of the examination, and the chin is raised slightly. This approach helps to extend the neck. The patient's head position can and should be altered during the examination to obtain the best image.

The examination consists of three stages: gray-scale imaging, color Doppler imaging, and spectral analysis. Gray-scale imaging will require the practitioner to first examine the carotid arteries in at least two long-axis views and one transverse view. Next he or she will need to identify the bifurcation of the common carotid into the internal and external carotid arteries. Last, he or she will need to document the extent and severity of plaque formation (location, characteristics, and luminal reduction).

The practitioner will then examine the carotid arteries in a transverse plane with color Doppler to demonstrate the patency of the vessels and to determine the flow disturbances caused by plaque formation or other abnormalities.

The last step is spectral analysis. The practitioner will need to obtain a velocity spectrum from the following locations: subclavian artery (high-resistance waveform), proximal and distal common carotid artery, proximal external carotid artery (high-resistance waveform), proximal internal carotid artery (low-resistance waveform), and vertebral artery, which is found by rotating the transducer laterally and identifying the vessel between the transverse processes of the cervical vertebrae. In conducting these studies, all velocity readings should be made with an angle of 60° or less, parallel to the vessel wall and in the center of the vessel where flow is highest. The practitioner should obtain a velocity spectrum at the level of any stenosis as well as immediately distal to the lesion to assess flow disturbance. The aliasing artifact can be very helpful at this time in identifying the areas of maximum flow velocity/stenosis.

CODING AND REIMBURSEMENT

As with all ultrasound examinations, vascular studies must be properly documented to support medical necessity and justify reimbursement. A written report should include the reason the study was performed, the equipment used, and the relevant findings. Generally, this includes recorded images (photographic or electronic) that confirm the written documentation. Local policies of third-party payers should be reviewed to ensure that appropriate diagnosis codes (International Classification of Diseases [ICD]-9) and procedure codes (*Current Procedural Terminology* [CPT]) are used to support the submitted billing forms. Table 15.3 provides a list of relevant CPT codes and their descriptions.

FUTURE

Current investigational work is being performed with ultrasound contrast agents consisting of stabilized microbubbles of various compositions. These agents resonate at frequencies different from the base carrier frequency and allow signal processing that significantly enhances signal-to-noise ratios and provides higher-quality duplex images. These agents are proposed for assisting ultrasound diagnosis of malignant tumors and small-vessel vascular disease and for evaluating solid organ injury. The development of high-frequency intravascular transducers may allow duplex evaluation of organs and tissues inaccessible to transcutaneous duplex examination. Combined with computer-aided three-dimensional imaging, ultrasound imaging can provide detailed anatomic information without exposing patients to the complications of radiologic imaging with intravenous contrast agents.

The availability of high-quality portable bedside duplex scanners has brought the ability to accurately

TABLE 15.3. Ultrasound Scan CPT Codes	
Procedure Description	*CPT*
Duplex scan of extremity veins, complete bilateral	93970
Duplex scan of extremity veins, unilateral or limited	93971
Lower extremity arterial examination, physiologic	93923
Lower extremity arterial duplex examination, complete	93925
Lower extremity arterial duplex examination, limited	93926
Bilateral carotid duplex examination	93880

CPT, Current Procedural Terminology.

diagnose acute DVT within the capability of every physician dealing with critically ill patients. The education and skills required to become comfortable with the techniques are an extension of physical examination skills. It is almost axiomatic that the individual who is best able to interpret the findings is the one who has daily responsibility for the care of the patient and who can correlate the results within the clinical context for that individual patient. A working knowledge of arterial anatomy and a basic understanding of arterial hemodynamics provide the bedside sonographer a solid foundation on which to perform and interpret the arterial duplex examination. Current portable duplex equipment provides high-quality information and puts this diagnostic modality within the skill set of every clinician willing to acquire the necessary experience.

CHAPTER 16

Nerve Ultrasound for Pain Control: Regional Anesthesia

Santhanam Suresh, MD, FAAP

INTRODUCTION

The proliferation of literature in the area of regional anesthesia with available ultrasound guidance workshops at major anesthesia meetings including the American Society of Regional Anesthesia, the American Society of Anesthesiologists, and the Society for Pediatric Anesthesia has emboldened more clinicians to use regional anesthesia techniques with the aid of ultrasound guidance. The impact of better anatomic visualization has allowed physicians to hasten and provide precise regional techniques with better pharmacodynamic modeling.[1,2] This chapter will deal with common peripheral nerve blocks that are now performed with ultrasound guidance with an evidence-based approach to the blocks. We will divide the chapter into several segments including central neuraxial blocks (epidural analgesia), upper and lower extremity blocks, and some truncal blocks that are now commonly used in practice. Images will be provided to facilitate understanding of the anatomic structures using ultrasound guidance.

CENTRAL NEURAXIAL BLOCKS

Anatomy and Application

The use of ultrasound guidance was introduced in the obstetric anesthesia practice as an aid to recognizing the distance to the epidural space from the skin.[3] This allows the clinician to visualize structures prior to puncture and potentially avoid a subarachnoid puncture. All images can be identified including the ligamentum flavum, the posterior dura mater, and the anterior complex (including the anterior dura mater and the posterior longitudinal ligament). The identification of the dura mater has allowed clinicians to determine the ideal position of the needle and the interspace at which to intervene. More recently, a technique employing a gas-powered needle was used to perform neuraxial blocks with ultrasound-aided guidance in adults.[4] Ultrasound-aided blocks are used in children, with an extra pair of hands holding on to the probe.[5]

Ultrasound Probe Selection

The choice of the probe is dependant on the depth of penetration needed for the blockade. Because of the varying depths, especially in the adult population, it may be prudent to use a low-frequency, curvilinear probe for localization of the epidural space. In children and infants, however, a linear high-frequency probe can be used with excellent visualization of structures. The probe is placed by using a paramedian midline approach. The spinous processes are identified, and between the two spinous processes, the epidural space is identified. All structures can be easily identified by using this approach (Fig. 16.1A). An axial view of the structures can also be used to identify the structures. This is especially useful in the case of purely identifying the depth of the epidural space for needle placement (Fig. 16.1B).

Evidence-based Data

A prospective, blinded pilot study of imaging in 32 infants found that use of the paramedian longitudinal plane by using a linear hockey-stick probe allowed the best delineation of the neuraxial structures, with the lumbar spine offering a more superior "acoustic window" than the thoracic spine.[5] Visibility was greater in neonates up to 3 months of age, with significant impairments in visibility, especially in the thoracic spine, in older children (e.g., 7 years of age). The visibility of the dura mater (which is more readily identifiable as a hyperechoic structure than the ligamentum flavum) correlated with both age and body weight. The authors commented that besides identifying the dura mater, ultrasound made it possible to confirm the epidermal space by the clear visibility of the pulsations of the surrounding vessels and the cauda equina. They speculated that ultrasound imaging could help confirm epidural catheter placement through visualization of the local anesthetic and direct identification of the catheter within the epidural space. However, because of accelerated

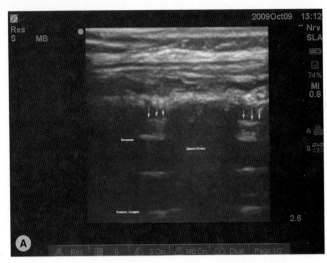
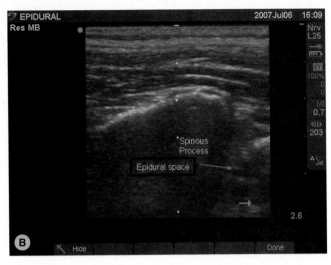

Figure 16-1. Epidural access. **A**: Longitudinal, **B**: Axial.

reductions in visibility in patients weighing more than 10 to 12 kg, this technique would be recommended only for small infants.

The earlier-mentioned relative visibility of the dura mater and ligamentum flavum was confirmed by Kil et al in their study evaluating the depth of the epidural space as measured by prepuncture ultrasound.[6] These authors found that the dura mater had "good" visibility in 170 of 180 infants and small children, while the view of the ligamentum flavum was "good" in only 91 of the 180 patients. This is a common experience that we also have encountered in our practice.

Coding the Reimbursement

There are no specific codes, except for an ultrasound modifier, to bill for the utilization of ultrasound guidance in these procedures.

Future Directions

With more training, central neuraxial block using ultrasound guidance could become the way to determine the depth of the epidural space prior to puncture. It can also be used in patients undergoing lumbar puncture for diagnostic procedures where a single needle placement can be performed without the need for multiple punctures.

PERIPHERAL NERVE BLOCKS

Common peripheral nerve blocks performed by using ultrasound guidance will be described in this section along with common approaches, local anesthetic solution used, and potential benefits and complications of these blocks (Table 16.1). It is important to understand the approach to the peripheral nerves while using ultrasound guidance. The common in-plane approach where a needle is inserted along the axis of

TABLE 16.1. Commonly Used Types of Blocks and Transducers Using an In-Plane Approach

Type of Block	Transducer Type
Interscalene/brachial plexus	Linear/high frequency
Supraclavicular/brachial plexus	Linear/high frequency
Axillary/brachial plexus	Linear/high frequency
Intercostal	Linear/high frequency
Transversus abdominis plane	Linear/high frequency
Ilioinguinal nerve	Linear/high frequency
Femoral nerve	Linear/high frequency
Sciatic	Linear/high frequency or curvilinear/low frequency

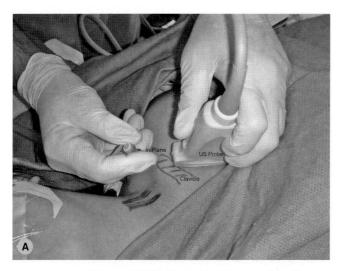

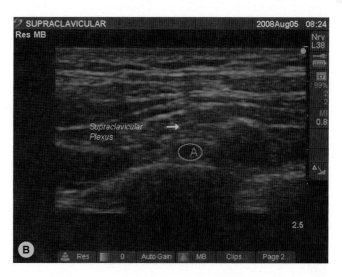

Figure 16-2. Peripheral nerve block.

the probe allows for greater visualization of the needle, while the out-of-plane approach allows immediate access to the structures but poorer visualization of the needle. In our practice we tend to use the in-plane approach most commonly to allow better visualization of the needle (Fig. 16.2A, B).

Brachial Plexus Blocks

The brachial plexus can be accessed at various levels as it comes off the cervical roots. The plexus can be blocked at the roots by using an interscalene approach, at the trunks and the divisions by using a supraclavicular approach, at the cords by using an infraclavicular approach, and at the branch level by using an axillary approach. We will discuss each one of these techniques, the use of the ultrasound probe, and the value for particular postoperative settings.

Interscalene Blocks

Anatomy

Ultrasound-guided interscalene blocks are commonly performed for shoulder surgery to provide analgesia after major reconstructive procedures.[7-9] The interscalene groove can easily be identified by using a high-frequency linear ultrasound probe. The roots are recognized as hypoechoic structures noted to be placed one on top of the other (Fig. 16.3).

Ultrasound Probe and Access

A linear probe is used most commonly to identify the superficial nature of the structures. Once a linear probe is placed on the neck over the posterior border of the sternocleidomastoid muscle at the level of cervical spine C6, the structures are seen placed one on

top of the other, described sometimes as a "snowman appearance." An in-plane approach is generally used for blocking this plexus at the interscalene level, although an out-of-plane technique can be used effectively for the blockade.

Local Anesthetic Solution

A solution of 0.25% bupivacaine or 0.2% ropivacaine can be used for blocking the brachial plexus at the interscalene area. Smaller volumes of local anesthetic solution can be used to produce similar results with ultrasound guidance after visualization of the spread of the local anesthetic solution around the plexus.[1] This may be one of the most important advantages of ultrasound guidance—pharmacodynamics of the local anesthetic solution, with dose reduction.

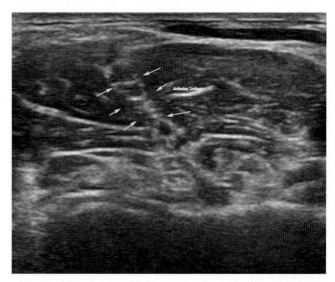

Figure 16-3. Interscalene block. Arrows demonstrate the cervical roots.

Evidence-based Ultrasound-guided Interscalene Blocks

The interscalene block was one of the earliest blocks that was mastered with ultrasound guidance. Several prospective studies comparing the use of ultrasound guidance with standard stimulation techniques have demonstrated the superiority of ultrasound guidance with respect to nerve stimulation.[7–10] In addition, this is a site of catheter placement for postoperative pain management.[11]

Interscalene Block: Pearls

High-frequency ultrasound probe

In-plane or out-of-plane approach

Volume of local anesthetic should surround the plexus

Usual recommended volume: 10 mL

Adverse effects: intravascular placement, diaphragmatic paresis, potential nerve root injury

---

Supraclavicular Brachial Plexus Block
Anatomy

The supraclavicular block is generally considered to be one of the easiest blocks when performed with ultrasound guidance. It is also one of the nerve blocks that could potentially lead to harm if it is performed by using conventional methods because of the close proximity to the pleura and the subclavian vessels. The supraclavicular approach to the brachial plexus entails blocking the divisions of the brachial plexus as they surround the subclavian artery. The plexus looks like a bunch of grapes surrounding the subclavian artery.[9,12] Immediately inferior to the artery is the pleura; hence, one must exercise caution while providing a block of the plexus at this level (Fig. 16.4). This provides analgesia for the upper extremity, and some data show that this also can be used for shoulder surgery. When performed, the block will lead to immediate motor blockade, and this is sometimes referred to as the spinal of the upper extremity.

Evidence-based Outcomes

In an audit of supraclavicular blocks performed using ultrasound guidance in a tertiary-care unit, 510 ultrasound-guided, supraclavicular blocks were performed (50 inpatients, 460 outpatients) by 47 different operators at different levels of training over a 24-month

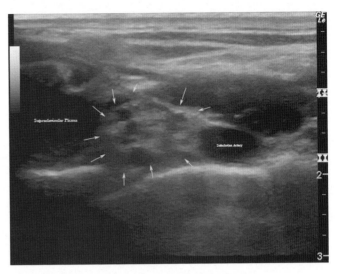

Figure 16-4. Supraclavicular block.

period. Successful surgical anesthesia was obtained after a single attempt in 94.6% of patients; 2.8% required supplemental blocks, and 2.6% received an unplanned general anesthetic intervention. Although the plexus is located close to the pleura, there were no incidences of pneumothorax.[13] Complications included symptomatic hemidiaphragmatic paresis (1%), Horner syndrome (1%), unintended vascular punctures (0.4%), and transient sensory deficits (0.4%).

Supraclavicular Blocks: Pearls

High-frequency ultrasound probe

In-plane or out-of-plane approach

Volume of local anesthetic should surround the plexus

Usual recommended volume: 5 to 10 mL

Adverse effects: intravascular placement, diaphragmatic paresis, pneumothorax

---

Axillary Block of the Brachial Plexus
Anatomy

The terminal branches of the brachial plexus are identified easily in the axilla by using ultrasound. The median nerve, ulnar nerve, and radial nerve are seen surrounding the axillary artery in the axilla, with the musculocutaneous nerve located between the coracobrachialis and the short head of the biceps. The nerves are located very superficially and easily can be

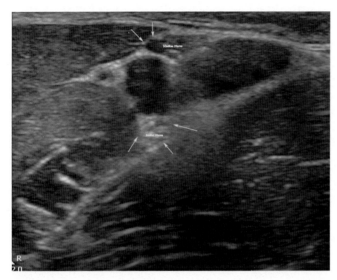

Figure 16-5. Axillary block. Arrows demonstrate the nerves.

blocked by using small quantities of local anesthetic solution (Fig. 16.5).

Evidence-based Outcomes

This is one of the nerve blocks that has become much easier to perform using ultrasound guidance. Although it can be performed by using nerve stimulation and surface landmarks, the technique using ultrasound guidance has greater potential for successful blockade of the individual nerves.[14] In a study by Chan et al, patients undergoing elective hand surgery were randomly assigned to one of three groups. Axillary blocks were performed by using three motor response endpoints in the nerve stimulator (NS) group, real-time ultrasound guidance in the ultrasound group, and combined ultrasound and nerve stimulation in the ultrasound-NS group. The need for local and general anesthesia supplementation and postblock adverse events were documented. One hundred and eighty-eight patients completed the study. The block success rate was higher in the ultrasound (82.8%) and ultrasound-NS (80.7%) groups than in the NS group (62.9%) ($P = 0.01$ and 0.03, respectively). Fewer patients in the US and ultrasound-NS groups required supplemental nerve blocks and/or general anesthesia. Postoperatively, axillary bruising and pain were reported more frequently in the NS group. There are some data to show that the volume required to produce a successful blockade could be decreased if ultrasound guidance was used. O'Donnell and Iohom demonstrated a successful blockade of the axillary plexus with 1 mL of 2% lidocaine per nerve.[15] This pharmacodynamic modeling would not be possible without the use of ultrasound guidance.

Axillary Block: Pearls
High-frequency ultrasound probe
In-plane approach
Volume of local anesthetic should surround each nerve
Usual recommended volume: 2 to 5 mL per nerve
Adverse effects: intravascular placement, nerve injury

TRUNCAL BLOCKS

Truncal blocks have in some ways made a significant comeback because of the use of ultrasound guidance. A variety of truncal blocks can now be performed because of the direct visualization of local anesthetic injection. This has introduced techniques that were otherwise not utilized in patients without complications.

Intercostal Blocks

Anatomy

Intercostal blocks are performed for a variety of procedures including chest tube placement, thoracotomy, and other chest wall procedures. The intercostal nerves run along the neurovascular bundle in a pocket between the inner intercostal and the innermost intercostal muscles (Fig. 16.6). This easily can be identified by ultrasound guidance. It is also easy to recognize the pleura. A dreaded complication of blind intercostal

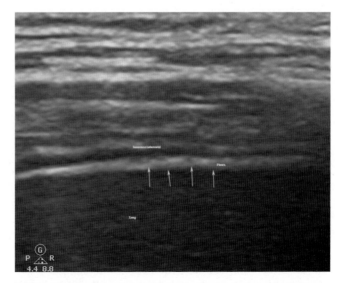

Figure 16-6. Intercostal block. Arrows demonstrate the nerves.

nerve blocks is piercing the pleura.[16] The use of ultrasound guidance certainly has reduced this incidence tremendously. Using a linear probe, the intercostal space is scanned: three layers of muscles, the external intercostals, the internal intercostals, and the innermost intercostals and the pleura are identified.[17] Using an in-plane approach, the innermost intercostal area is accessed, and local anesthetic solution is injected into the space. A volume of 2 to 3 mL can provide adequate blockade of the intercostal space.

Evidence-based Outcomes

This is a relatively newer block using ultrasound guidance. In our experience in the pain clinic, we have used this approach for patients with persistent chest wall pain and have had very good success using ultrasound guidance. The main complications with this block are (1) the potential for creation of a pneumothorax and (2) the potential for intravascular injection.

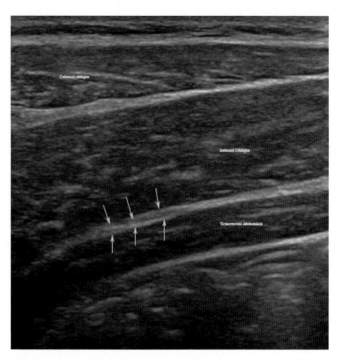

Figure 16-7. Transversus abdominus plane. Arrows indicate a muscle layer.

Intercostal Block: Pearls
High-frequency ultrasound probe
In-plane approach
Volume of local anesthetic should spread along the innermost intercostal muscle
Usual recommended volume: 2 to 5 mL per intercostal space
Adverse effects: intravascular placement, pneumothorax

Evidence-based Outcomes

This is one of the most common blocks that has become very popular in postoperative analgesia and for pain management.[19,20] The efficacy of the block has been compared to standard central neuraxial blocks and has been demonstrated to be just as effective in the surgical population. Future studies looking at pharmacokinetic data have to be carried out to determine the exact volume and efficacy of this block for pain control. The block has to be performed on either side to completely cover the entire anterior abdomen.

Transversus Abdominus Plane Block

Anatomy

The thoracolumbar nerve roots as they emerge from the lateral aspect of the trunk pass through a potential space that exists between the internal oblique muscle and the transversus abdominis muscle supplying the anterior abdominal wall. The thoracolumbar nerves can be blocked with ease by using an ultrasound-guided approach. The three muscle layers of the abdominal wall, the external oblique, the internal oblique, and the transversus abdominis, can be recognized by using a linear high-frequency ultrasound transducer[18] (Fig. 16.7). Once the plane is identified, 10 to 20 mL of local anesthetic solution is injected. This can provide analgesia for the entire anterior abdominal wall.

Transversus Abdominis Plane Block: Pearls
High-frequency ultrasound probe/curvilinear probe for larger patients with increased body mass index
In-plane approach
Volume of local anesthetic should spread along the plane between the internal oblique and the transversus abdominis
Usual recommended volume: 10 to 20 mL per side
Adverse effects: intravascular placement

LOWER EXTREMITY BLOCKS

The most commonly performed regional blocks for the lower extremity include the femoral nerve block and the sciatic nerve block. In this section, the femoral nerve block and the sciatic nerve block performed at the popliteal fossa will be described.

Femoral Nerve Block

Anatomy

This is perhaps one of the most common peripheral nerve blocks performed for managing pain after femoral fracture or after major surgery to the knee including an anterior cruciate ligament tear.[21-23] The femoral nerve is located lateral to the femoral artery in the femoral triangle. It is enveloped by the facia iliaca and is found to overlay the iliacus muscle. It can be easily identified by palpation of the femoral artery followed by the placement of a needle lateral to the pulsation. Although this is effective most times, there is the possibility that the needle may be placed, even with the aid of nerve stimulation, into the iliacus muscle or outside the facia iliaca compartment. The femoral nerve is noted to be elliptical and lateral to the femoral artery with ultrasound guidance (Fig. 16.8). By using an in-plane approach, the femoral nerve can easily be accessed in the femoral triangle. A dose of 10 to 15 mL of local anesthetic solution is injected to surround the femoral nerve.

Evidence-based Outcomes

The femoral nerve has been studied as a model for improving the blockade of the femoral nerve compared to neurostimulation.[22,24] In a large retrospective analysis of regional anesthesia using nerve stimulation versus ultrasound guidance, it was noted that the incidence of major complications including seizures, was offset by the use of ultrasound guidance, supporting its use in block placement.[25]

Femoral Nerve Block: Pearls

High-frequency ultrasound probe

In-plane approach

Volume of local anesthetic solution: approximately 10 to 15 mL

Additional neurostimulation: look for quadriceps contraction

Adverse effects: intravascular placement, intraneural injection

---

Sciatic Nerve Block

Anatomy

The sciatic nerve exits through the sciatic notch and continues its pathway through the popliteal fossa to supply the motor and sensory supply to the foot except for the medial aspect of the foot, which is supplied by the saphenous branch of the femoral nerve. The sciatic nerve can easily be identified in the popliteal fossa between the biceps femoris tendon and the semitendinosus and semimembranosus. A linear, high-frequency probe is placed in the posterior part of the knee at the popliteal crease. The popliteal artery is identified, followed by the popliteal vein, which is located superficial to the artery. The tibial nerve is located on top of the popliteal vein as a hyperechoic structure. When the ultrasound transducer is moved laterally, the common peroneal nerve is visualized. The transducer is then gently moved cephalad until the two hyperechoic structures merge into one large "honeycombed structure," the sciatic nerve prior to its bifurcation (Fig. 16.9). A local anesthetic volume of 15 to 20 mL is placed to surround the structure. This will provide a complete blockade of the sciatic nerve. One must exercise caution when discharging the patient, because a motor block will lead to difficulty in ambulation lasting for 20 hours in some cases.

Evidence-based Outcomes

The visualization of the sciatic nerve makes it an easy target for performing the nerve blockade.[22] There are

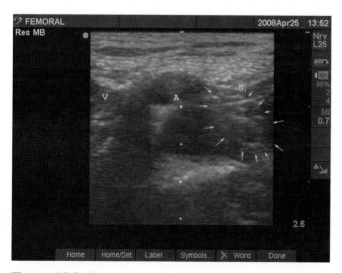

Figure 16-8. Femoral nerve block. Arrows highlight the femoral nerve.

fewer complications with an ultrasound-guided technique than with a neurostimulation technique. Future studies have to be performed particularly looking at volumes of local anesthetic solutions and selective blockade of the nerves. The performance time to blockade is certainly reduced with the use of ultrasound guidance, thereby improving patient satisfaction.

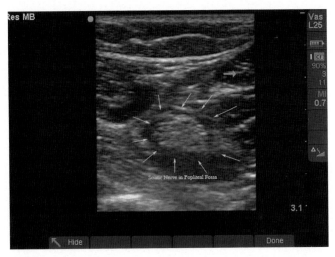

Figure 16-9. Popliteal fossa block. Arrows highlight the sciatic nerve.

Sciatic Nerve Block: Pearls
High-frequency ultrasound probe/curvilinear probe if patient is obese
In-plane approach/out-of-plane approach (for catheters)
Volume of local anesthetic solution: approximately 15 to 20 mL
Additional neurostimulation: look for ankle eversion
Adverse effects: intravascular placement, intraneural injection

CONCLUSIONS

The use of ultrasound guidance for nerve localization for pain management has become very popular in anesthesia practice. The introduction of ultrasound as a technical guide early on in training may allow the clinician to use it as part of his or her regular diagnostic armamentarium very similar to the stethoscope, which is used for listening to breath sounds or cardiac tones. Future training should include easy educational modules that can help clinicians navigate the already cumbersome world of technocratic medicine, which can easily steer them clear of technology that can benefit them tremendously in patient care. This chapter is meant to be a primer on the use of ultrasound guidance for nerve localization. As the research in this field continues, there will be a day when ultrasound guidance may be the only option for performing nerve blocks, similar to our turning on a switch for the light to go on versus using a candle at nighttime.

References

1. Riazi S, Carmichael N, Awad I, Holtby RM, McCartney CJ. Effect of local anaesthetic volume (20 vs 5 ml) on the efficacy and respiratory consequences of ultrasound-guided interscalene brachial plexus block. *Br J Anaesth.* 2008;101:549–556.

2. Willschke H, Bosenberg A, Marhofer P, et al. Ultrasonographic-guided ilioinguinal/iliohypogastric nerve block in pediatric anesthesia: what is the optimal volume? *Anesth Analg.* 2006;102:1680–1684.

3. Borges BC, Wieczoreck P, Balki M, Carvalho JC. Sonoanatomy of the lumbar spine of pregnant women at term. *Reg Anesth Pain Med.* 2009;34:581–585.

4. Karmakar MK, Li X, Ho AM, Kwok WH, Chui PT. Real-time ultrasound-guided paramedian epidural access: evaluation of a novel in-plane technique. *Br J Anaesth.* 2009;102: 845–854.

5. Willschke H, Bosenberg A, Marhofer P, et al. Epidural catheter placement in neonates: sonoanatomy and feasibility of ultrasonographic guidance in term and preterm neonates. *Reg Anesth Pain Med.* 2007;32:34–40.

6. Kil HK, Cho JE, Kim WO, Koo BN, Han SW, Kim JY. Prepuncture ultrasound-measured distance: an accurate reflection of epidural depth in infants and small children. *Reg Anesth Pain Med.* 2007;32:102–106.

7. Perlas A, Chan VW, Simons M. Brachial plexus examination and localization using ultrasound and electrical stimulation: a volunteer study. *Anesthesiology.* 2003;99:429–435.

8. Fredrickson MJ, Ball CM, Dalgleish AJ, Stewart AW, Short TG. A prospective randomized comparison of ultrasound and neurostimulation as needle end points for interscalene catheter placement. *Anesth Analg.* 2009; 108:1695–1700.

9. Klaastad O, Sauter AR, Dodgson MS. Brachial plexus block with or without ultrasound guidance. *Curr Opin Anaesthesiol.* 2009;22:655–660.

10. Naik VN, Perlas A, Chandra DB, Chung DY, Chan VW. An assessment tool for brachial plexus regional anesthesia performance: establishing construct validity and reliability. *Reg Anesth Pain Med.* 2007;32:41–45.

11. Clendenen SR, Riutort KT, Feinglass NG, Greengrass RA, Brull SJ. Real-time three-dimensional ultrasound for continuous interscalene brachial plexus blockade. *J Anesth.* 2009;23:466–468.

12. Marhofer P, Greher M, Kapral S. Ultrasound guidance in regional anaesthesia. *Br J Anaesth.* 2005;94:7–17.

13. Perlas A, Lobo G, Lo N, Brull R, Chan VW, Karkhanis R. Ultrasound-guided supraclavicular block: outcome of 510 consecutive cases. *Reg Anesth Pain Med.* 2009;34: 171–176.

14. Chan VW, Perlas A, McCartney CJ, Brull R, Xu D, Abbas S. Ultrasound guidance improves success rate of axillary brachial plexus block. *Can J Anaesth.* 2007;54:176–182.

15. O'Donnell BD, Iohom G. An estimation of the minimum effective anesthetic volume of 2% lidocaine in ultrasound-guided axillary brachial plexus block. *Anesthesiology.* 2009;111:25–29.

16. Moore DC. Intercostal nerve block for postoperative somatic pain following surgery of thorax and upper abdomen. *Br J Anaesth.* 1975;47(suppl):284–286.

17. Tsui B, Dillane D, Pillay J, Walji A. Ultrasound imaging in cadavers: training in imaging for regional blockade at the trunk. *Can J Anaesth.* 2008;55:105–111.

18. Suresh S, Chan VW. Ultrasound guided transversus abdominis plane block in infants, children and adolescents: a simple procedural guidance for their performance. *Paediatr Anaesth.* 2009;19:296–299.

19. Pak T, Mickelson J, Yerkes E, Suresh S. Transverse abdominis plane block: a new approach to the management of secondary hyperalgesia following major abdominal surgery. *Paediatr Anaesth.* 2009;19:54–56.

20. McDonnell JG, O'Donnell B, Curley G, Heffernan A, Power C, Laffey JG. The analgesic efficacy of transversus abdominis plane block after abdominal surgery: a prospective randomized controlled trial. *Anesth Analg.* 2007;104:193–197.

21. Edkin BS, McCarty EC, Spindler KP, Flanagan JF. Analgesia with femoral nerve block for anterior cruciate ligament reconstruction. *Clin Orthop Relat Res.* 1999; 289–295.

22. Oberndorfer U, Marhofer P, Bosenberg A, et al. Ultrasonographic guidance for sciatic and femoral nerve blocks in children. *Br J Anaesth.* 2007;98:797–801.

23. Tobias JD. Continuous femoral nerve block to provide analgesia following femur fracture in a paediatric ICU population. *Anaesth Intensive Care.* 1994;22:616–618.

24. Williams R, Saha B. Best evidence topic report. Ultrasound placement of needle in three-in-one nerve block. *Emerg Med J.* 2006;23:401–403.

25. Orebaugh SL, Williams BA, Vallejo M, Kentor ML. Adverse outcomes associated with stimulator-based peripheral nerve blocks with versus without ultrasound visualization. *Reg Anesth Pain Med.* 2009;34:251–255.

ULTRASOUND USE FOR THE EVALUATION OF CLINICAL PROCEDURES AND SPECIAL POPULATIONS

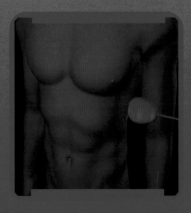

Focused Ultrasound in Cardiopulmonary Resuscitation and Advanced Cardiac Life Support

Shahana Uddin, MD, MB, BS, FCARCS(I), EDICM; Susanna Price, MB, BS, BSc, MRCP, EDICM, FESC, PhD; Holger Steiger, MD; Gabriele Via, MD; and Raoul Breitkreutz, MD, EDIC

INTRODUCTION

Currently, cardiac ultrasound (echocardiography) assessment is not mandatory in advanced cardiopulmonary life support guidelines, nor is it routinely performed in the assessment and diagnosis of critically ill or peri-arrest patients. There is, however, increasing evidence supporting the use of echocardiography in these situations.[1-4] Two-dimensional (2D) ultrasound imaging facilitates the exclusion or confirmation of life-threatening diagnoses, such as pericardial collections causing tamponade, in a rapid, noninvasive manner and enables more experienced users to assess other hemodynamic parameters in real time.

RELEVANT PROTOCOLS

Echocardiography is an ultrasound examination that looks at the anatomic structures and the physiologic function of the heart and therefore requires an understanding of cardiac anatomy and physiology. A comprehensive echocardiogram provides considerable information ranging from structural anatomy (including congenital heart disease) to in-depth detail regarding valve leaflets, the functioning of individual cardiac segments, cardiac chamber interactions, and the physiologic functioning of the heart. Echocardiography can be performed via several techniques. The transthoracic technique is most commonly used in the emergency setting. It is noninvasive, is easily achieved, and can be performed with small, portable machines, even using noncardiac probes if necessary. Transesophageal echocardiography does not interfere with cardiopulmonary resuscitation (CPR) but is invasive and requires specialized equipment and more complex training. If inadequate windows are obtained by transthoracic echocardiography, then transesophageal echocardiography may be considered in an intubated patient. Intracardiac ultrasound is used in the cardiac catheterization labatory but is beyond the scope of this text. Epicardial echocardiography is performed during cardiac surgery with an open chest.

Focused echocardiography refers to examinations following a structured protocol to investigate answers to a few simple questions. In the periresuscitation setting, this is used to identify reversible pathology, guide therapeutic interventions, and potentially reverse a patient's deterioration. In the intensive care unit, focused echocardiography may be used to evaluate the response to various interventions (e.g., a fluid bolus). When compared to other forms of cardiac monitoring, such as pulmonary artery catheterization, echocardiography has the advantage of providing potential diagnoses and the assessment of hemodynamic variables. The major limitation of focused echocardiography is that it is not a complete examination, and the information must always be considered in relation to the current clinical status of the patient (which may be in a state of flux).

Focused Echocardiographic Evaluation in Life Support

There are several protocols in use and under evaluation. The simplest of these is focused echocardiographic evaluation in life support (FEEL), which in the United Kingdom has been accepted as a basic entry-level certification suitable for nonspecialists who wish to use echocardiography for patient assessment in the peri-arrest setting.[3,5] Internationally, there are additional protocols that require a additional training and take slightly longer to perform, making them more useful in the critical care setting. These include Focused Assessment with Transthoracic Echocardiography assessed transthoracic echocardiography (FATE), bedside limited echocardiography by the emergency physician, goal-directed limited echocardiography, goal-oriented hand-held echocardiography, cardiovascular limited ultrasound examination, and focused cardiac ultrasound study.[6,7]

Focused echocardiography is ideally suited for periresuscitation care when a patient has suffered a cardiac arrest.[3,8] Echocardiography may help to diagnose potentially reversible causes of cardiac arrest or to identify fine ventricular fibrillation not visible from the surface electrocardiogram. Evidence-based medicine and recent guidelines from national and international resuscitation experts have suggested that continuous sustained periods of cardiac compressions with minimization of interruptions may result in improved flow and better patient outcomes. Thus, it is important that any echocardiographic study not interrupt chest compressions, and a clear protocol with appropriate training be assured. The current protocol for peri-resuscitation echo (FEEL) is shown in Figure 17.1.

Strict adherence to resuscitation guidelines is essential, and stored echocardiographic clips may be reviewed either in real time or played back while CPR is ongoing. The emphasis in FEEL is on advanced life

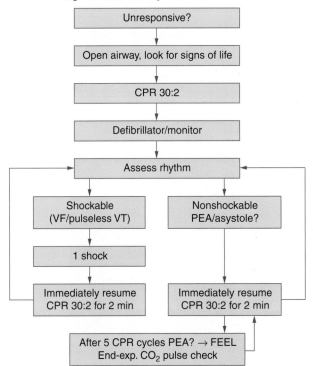

Integration of FEEL into the ALS algorithm to identify reversible causes

Figure 17.1. Current protocol for peri-resuscitation echocardiography (FEEL) is shown. ALS, advanced life support; CO_2, carbon dioxide; CPR, cardiopulmonary resuscitation; End-exp., end-expiratory; FEEL, focused echocardiography in emergency life support; PEA, pulseless electrical activity; VF, ventricular fibrillation; VT, ventricular tachycardia.

support (ALS) compliance, and although any or all of the standard echocardiographic views may be obtained and in any order (one at each interruption of chest compressions for pulse check), frequently only one view is required to make a diagnosis.[3] Thus, there is a strict time limit of 10 seconds for this echocardiographic examination to ensure ALS compliance during mechanical CPR. The potential findings and implications for patient management are described below.

1. The heart appears to be in fine ventricular fibrillation despite the electrocardiogram suggesting asystole: Defibrillation should be considered while continuing CPR according to ALS guidelines.

2. There is no palpable pulse and the electrocardiogram demonstrates a rhythm compatible with cardiac output: The diagnosis is pulseless electrical activity (PEA). During echocardiography, if the heart is not moving, this can be considered as true (primary) PEA. If the heart is moving, this can be considered as false (secondary) PEA. Current resuscitation guidelines require investigation for and management of reversible causes while continuing CPR in both situations. The echocardiographically demonstrable diagnoses are as follows:

   a. Empty left ventricle (= severe hypovolemia) → give volume (intravenous fluids).

   b. Pericardial collection (= tamponade) → consider pericardiocentesis.

   c. Dilated right heart ± clot in right heart (= ? pulmonary embolism) → consider thrombolysis.

   d. Severe left ventricular dysfunction (primary or secondary to arrest) → consider inotropic support/mechanical circulatory support/revascularization.

Although there is enthusiasm for the use of echocardiography in the intensive care unit and in the peri-resuscitation state,[2,4,9] to date, there are few data supporting the use of focused periresuscitation echocardiography in terms of outcomes following cardiac arrest. Until the evidence is available, echocardiography can be considered only as an addition to current guidelines and should not be used to terminate resuscitation efforts.

Focus Assessed Transthoracic Echocardiography (FATE)

FATE was developed so that echocardiography could be used in a manner analogous to the way a fixed ultrasound protocol (focused assessment with sonography for trauma [FAST] scanning) is used in trauma medicine. In addition to the findings noted in FEEL, FATE also assesses the pleural spaces bilaterally for pleural effusions, the lungs for a pneumothorax, the inferior vena cava for volume status and measurements of the left ventricular dimensions.[9] The FATE protocol can be applied within a few minutes and consists of the same four echocardiographic views performed in sequence with the following objectives:

1. To exclude obvious pathology

2. To assess wall thickness and chamber dimension

3. To assess ventricular contractility

4. To visualize the pleural spaces bilaterally

5. To relate the findings to the clinical context

The components of the FATE protocol are summarized and available in a pocket card (Fig. 17.2).

TRANSDUCER CHOICE AND MANIPULATION

The transducer used for transthoracic echocardiography is generally a phased array probe of frequency between 2.5 and 3.5 MHz, although in the periarrest situation, in which only very gross pathology is expected to be identified, almost any transducer will suffice.

The transthoracic echocardiography probe has a marker (dot, groove, or light, depending on the machine) to help orientate its position (left/right). In echocardiography this corresponds to the right of screen when viewing images, marked correspondingly with a colored indicator. This may not be the case if a noncardiac probe is being used because the marker or indicator corresponds to the left of the screen. In Figure 17.3A, the probe marker is a green light and is pointing toward the patient's right shoulder; in Figure 17.3B, the marker (V) is identified by the arrow on the right of the display. If the operator is uncertain of the left/right orientation of the probe, simply tapping one or the other side of the probe will cause a corresponding distortion on the corresponding side of the image on the screen.

Before starting to scan, the operator must ensure that the depth setting on the machine is set at 12 to 18 cm. The structures to be assessed should be centered on the screen by moving the probe laterally or medially or up/down an intercostal space. To achieve the correct view, the probe may be turned clockwise

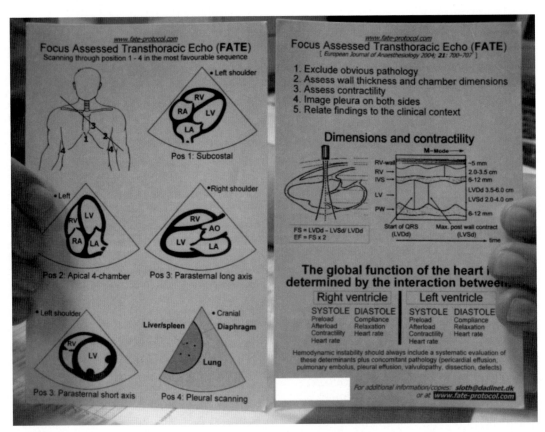

Figure 17.2. A handheld card demonstrating the focus assessed transthoracic echocardiography (FATE) protocol.

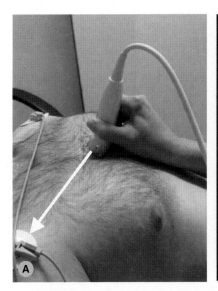
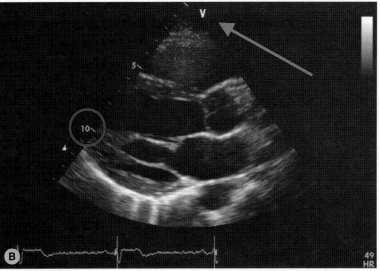

Figure 17.3. **(A)** Placement of the ultrasound probe using the probe marker (green light [*white arrow*]), which is pointing toward the patient's right shoulder. **(B)** The marker V is identified by a blue arrow on the right of the display. The circled area demonstrates the depth in centimeters marked to the left of the display.

or counterclockwise and tilted caudally or cranially to optimize the visualized structures. Each of the standard views in FEEL is described in detail, together with how they should be obtained.

ECHOCARDIOGRAPHY ANATOMY

Even in focused periresuscitation echocardiography, normal anatomic variants can be a major source of error in image interpretation. Since the heart is a 3-dimensional moving organ, familiarity with cardiac anatomy makes image acquisition and structure visualization much simpler. To standardize examination findings, an internationally agreed upon nomenclature is used to describe the views required to perform echocardiography.

The views are described using a combination of the location on the patient, the anatomy obtained, and the orientation (axis) through the heart.

Location on the patient

a. Parasternal | Second intercostal space, left sternal edge

b. Apical | Cardiac apex

c. Subcostal | Below the xiphoid process

Description of image obtained

a. Axis | Long or short

b. Chambers | Four- or five-chamber view

Parasternal Long-Axis (Figs. 17.4 [see also color insert] and 17.5)

Location: This view is achieved with the patient lying in a left lateral position or supine.

The probe is placed in the second left intercostal space.

The marker on the probe points toward the patient's **right** shoulder.

Depending on patient characteristics, it may help to move down an intercostal space.

Anatomy: This view is used to identify the left ventricle (LV).

The LV is bordered by the mitral valve and the aortic valve.

The left atrium (LA) drains into the LV via the mitral valve.

The interventricular septum separates the LV from the right ventricle (RV).

The RV lies just below the sternum and thus is closest to the probe at the top of the picture.

The aortic valve leads into the aorta.

Parasternal Short-Axis (Figs. 17.6 [see also color insert] and 17.7)

Location: This view is achieved with the patient lying in a left lateral position or supine.

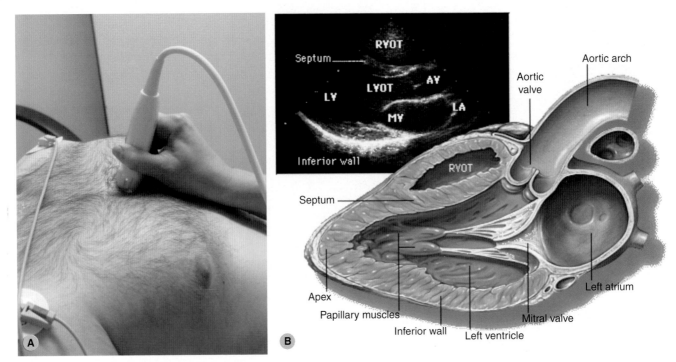

Figure 17.4. Parasternal long-axis echocardiographic view. AV, aortic valve; MV, mitral valve; LA, left atrium; LV, left ventricle; LVOT, left ventricular outflow tract; RVOT, right ventricular outflow tract. *(Images and illustrations reproduced from FEEL-UK with permission)*

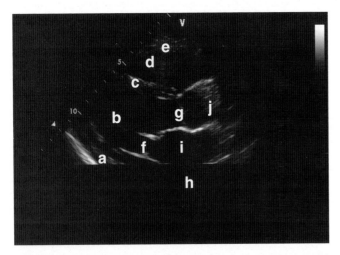

Figure 17.5. Parasternal long-axis view of a normal heart. The ultrasound sector image is represented as inverted, with the transducer at the top. The V marker to the right of the image confirms that the probe is in the correct orientation. The key structures are labeled: a, left ventricular posterior wall; b, left ventricular cavity; c, interventricular septum; d, right ventricular outflow tract; e, right ventricular free wall; f, mitral valve; g, aortic valve; h, descending aorta; i, left atrium; j, ascending aorta.

The probe is placed in the second left intercostal space.

The marker on the probe points toward the patient's **left** shoulder.

From the parasternal long-axis, the probe is turned 90° clockwise.

Depending on patient characteristics, it may help to move down an intercostal space.

Anatomy: This view is useful to identify the LV and LV walls.

Angling the probe on the chest demonstrates different short-axis slices through the LV.

The view here is at the level of the papillary muscles.

Tilting the probe up will bring the mitral valve into view, and further up, the aortic valve.

Tilting the probe down will examine the apex.

The RV is a thin-walled structure compared to the LV.

The RV is D-shaped and curves around the thick-muscled circular LV.

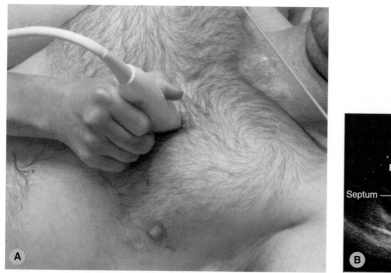

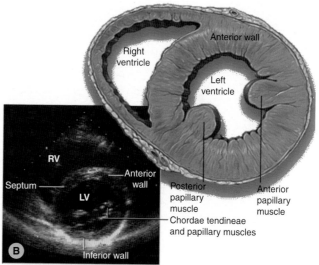

Figure 17.6. Parasternal short-axis echocardiographic view. (See color insert.) LV, left ventricle; RV, right ventricle. *(Images and illustrations reproduced from FEEL-UK with permission)*

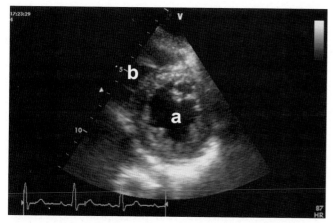

Figure 17.7. Parasternal short-axis view of a normal heart. The key structures are labeled: a, left ventricular cavity; b, right ventricular cavity. Separating the two chambers is the interventricular septum.

This is the only view that gives an indication of all coronary artery territories when considering ischemia/infarction.

The difference between parasternal long-axis and parasternal short-axis views is illustrated in Figure 17.8. Figure 17.8A shows a pear sliced in its long axis, and Figure 17.8B shows it in its short axis. The corresponding echocardiographic images are also shown. The cavity of the LV on the echo images is arrowed.

Apical Four-Chamber (Figs. 17.9 [see also color insert] and 17.10)

Location: This view is achieved with the patient lying in a left lateral position or supine.

The probe is placed over the patient's cardiac apex (as determined clinically).

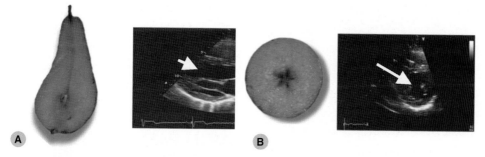

Figure 17.8. The difference between the parasternal long-axis and parasternal short-axis view is illustrated. **(A)** A pear is sliced in its long axis. **(B)** A pear is sliced in its short axis. The corresponding echocardiographic images are also shown. The cavity of the left ventricle on the echo images is arrowed. *(Images and illustrations reproduced from FEEL-UK with permission)*

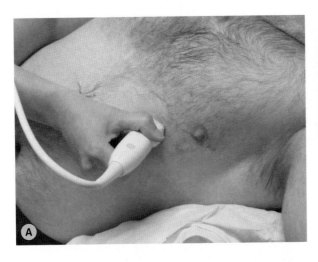

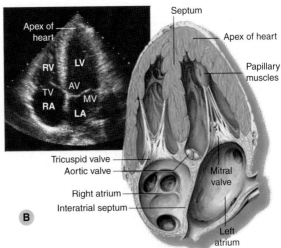

Figure 17.9. Apical four-chamber echocardiographic view. (See color insert.) AV, aortic valve; LA, left atrium; LV, left ventricle; MV, mitral valve; RA, right atrium; RV, right ventricle; TV, tricuspid valve. *(Images and illustrations reproduced from FEEL-UK with permission)*

The marker on the probe points toward the patient's left flank.

Anatomy: This view is useful to identify all four cardiac chambers: right atrium (RA), RV, LA, and LV.

Also seen are the mitral and tricuspid valves and the interventricular septum.

Turning the probe counterclockwise may open up the aortic valve five-chamber view.

The RV is a smaller, thin-walled structure compared to the LV.

The RV is D-shaped and curves around the thick-muscled LV.

Subcostal (Figs. 17.11 [see also color insert] and 17.12)

Location: This view is achieved with the patient lying in a supine position.

The probe is placed under the xiphoid process almost flat on the patient's abdomen.

The marker on the probe points toward the patient's **left** flank.

The probe should be angled slightly to point toward the heart.

Anatomy: This view is useful to identify all four cardiac chambers: RA, RV, LA, and LV.

Also seen are the mitral and tricuspid valves and the interventricular septum.

The overlying liver improves the echocardiographic window, unlike the lungs in the other views.

Figure 17.10. Apical four-chamber view of a normal heart. The key structures are labeled: a, left ventricular cavity; b, mitral valve; c, left atrium; d, pulmonary veins; e, right ventricular cavity; f, tricuspid valve; g, right atrium; h, interventricular septum; i, apex; j, left ventricular free wall; k, right ventricular free wall.

COMMON PATHOLOGY IN PERIRESUSCITATION: MINI-ATLAS

In this section, a number of images that demonstrate pathologic conditions are shown, with additional text to aid diagnoses.

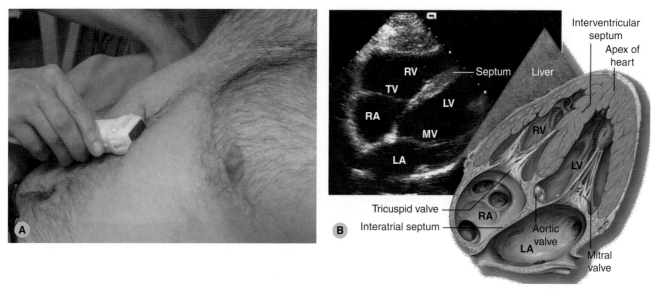

Figure 17.11. Subcostal echocardiographic view. (See color insert.) LA, left atrium; LV, left ventricle; MV, mitral valve; RA, right atrium; RV, right ventricle; TV, tricuspid valve. *(Images and illustrations reproduced from FEEL-UK with permission)*

Pulseless Electrical Activity/Cardiac Standstill (Figs. 17.13 and 17.14)

During cardiac arrest the presence or absence of coordinated cardiac motion (that which would be compatible with cardiac output) can only be inferred from palpation of the pulse or the presence of a pulse pressure waveform in the presence of invasive arterial blood pressure monitoring. Echocardiography in the pulseless patient may occasionally demonstrate coordinated cardiac activity (Figure 17.13). In other cases, despite electrical activity, there is no detectable cardiac motion

(cardiac standstill). This difference may be important, because where there is no cardiac motion, the prognosis is poor, even if a potentially treatable cause of cardiac arrest is identified. Cardiac standstill may be confirmed using an M-mode image through the heart, as shown in Figure 17.14.

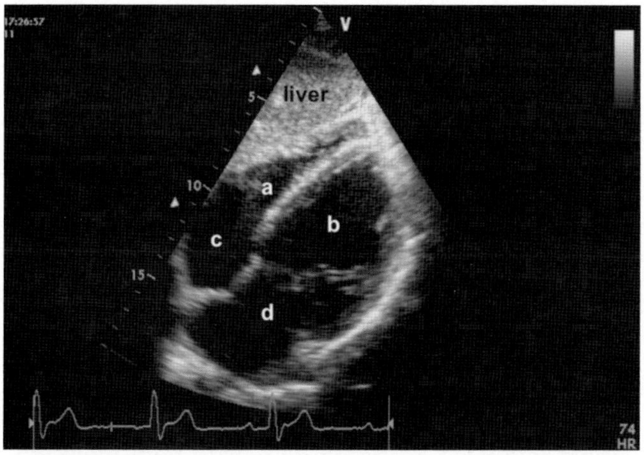

Hypovolemia

Figure 17.15 shows a subcostal four-chamber view in a septic patient with severe hypovolemia as demonstrated by the small, collapsed ventricles.

In the critical care setting, additional images may be obtained to confirm the diagnoses. By turning the probe counterclockwise, one obtains the subcostal short-axis view of the inferior vena cava. Measurement of the inferior vena cava diameter (<1.6 cm) and its collapsibility with respiration can help confirm hypovolemia, but this is not within the scope of periresuscitation echocardiography in cardiac arrest.

Pericardial and Pleural Collections

A parasternal long-axis view in a patient following cardiac surgery with both pleural and pericardial collections is shown in Figure 17.16. Differentiating between pleural and pericardial collections can be difficult. The two layers of the pericardium (parietal and visceral) need to be visualized. Since the visceral pericardium is very thin, this can be challenging. In the

Figure 17.12. Subcostal four-chamber view of a normal heart. The key structures are labeled: a, right ventricle; b, left ventricle; c, right atrium; d, left atrium.

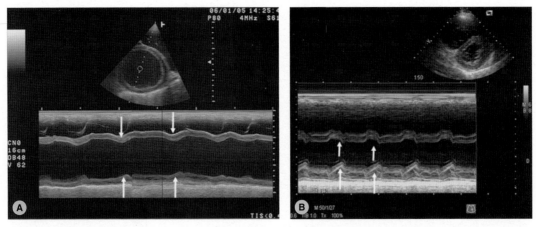

Figure 17.13. **(A)** M-mode of the patient with pulseless electrical activity due severely decreased left ventricular function. **(B)** M-mode of the patient with pulseless electrical activity due to right ventricular failure and fairly well preserved left ventricular function.

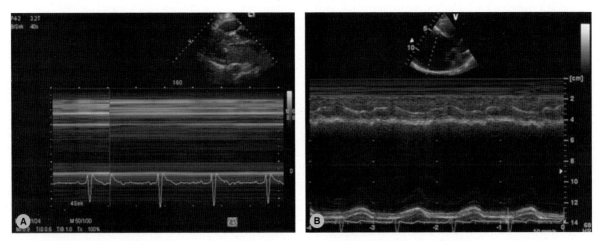

Figure 17.14. M-mode echocardiogram demonstrating **(A)** primary pulseless electrical activity (PEA) (no pulse or wall motion visible, regular rhythm) and **(B)** secondary PEA (no pulse, wall motion visible, regular rhythm) on a single image.

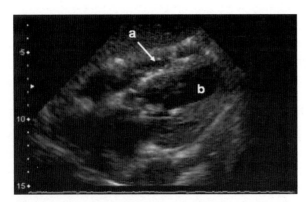

Figure 17.15. Subcostal four-chamber view in a septic patient with severe hypovolemia. This echocardiographic finding indicates an underfilled right (a, *arrow*) and left ventricular cavity (b).

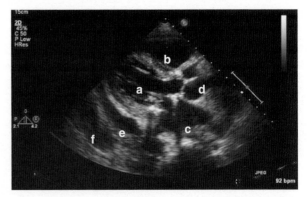

Figure 17.16. A parasternal long-axis view in a patient following cardiac surgery with both pleural and pericardial collections. The key structures are labeled: a, left ventricular cavity; b, right ventricular outflow tract; c, left atrium; d, ascending aorta; e, pericardial collection; f, pleural collection.

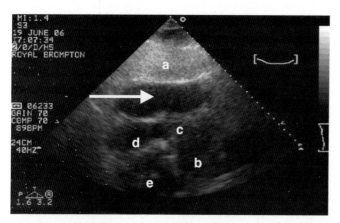

Figure 17.17. The image shows a subcostal view in a patient who experienced a cardiac arrest with pericardial tamponade. The key structures are labeled: a, liver; b, left ventricle; c, right ventricle; d, right atrium; e, left atrium. There is an echo-free space between the right ventricle and the liver (*arrow*), representing a pericardial collection.

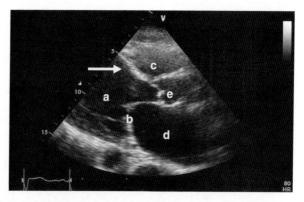

Figure 17.18. A parasternal long-axis view of a patient who had sustained a prior myocardial infarction. The arrow demonstrates the interventricular septum. The key structures are labeled: a, left ventricle; b, mitral valve; c, right ventricular outflow tract; d, left atrium; e, aortic valve and ascending aorta.

periresuscitation setting, the clinician must balance the certainty of the echocardiography diagnosis against the risk of intervention if the diagnosis is wrong, bearing in mind that cardiac tamponade is a clinical diagnosis.

Figure 17.17 shows an example of a subcostal view in a patient who experienced a cardiac arrest with pericardial tamponade. Cardiac tamponade is due to a pericardial collection causing increased intrapericardial pressure. The actual volume of the collection is not as relevant as the rate of accumulation and consequent pressure rise. Although the collection shown in Figure 17.17 is not large, it accumulated rapidly, resulting in a sharp rise in intrapericardial pressure and clinically evident tamponade (cardiovascular collapse and cardiac arrest).

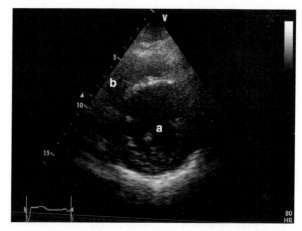

Figure 17.19. A parasternal short-axis view of the same patient with prior myocardial infarction.

Anterior Myocardial Infarction

A parasternal long-axis view of a patient who had sustained a prior myocardial infarction is shown in Figure 17.18. The interventricular septum (*arrow*) is thin and bright (echogenic), suggesting a previous myocardial infarction. A parasternal short-axis view of the same patient with a prior myocardial infarction is provided in Figure 17.19.

Massive Right Ventricular Dilatation

A parasternal short-axis view in a patient with severe pulmonary hypertension and subsequent right heart failure is shown in Figure 17.20, demonstrating that

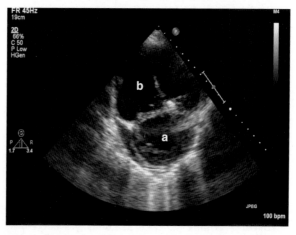

Figure 17.20. A parasternal short-axis view in a patient with severe pulmonary hypertension and subsequent right heart failure. Left ventricular cavity (b); Right ventricular cavity (b).

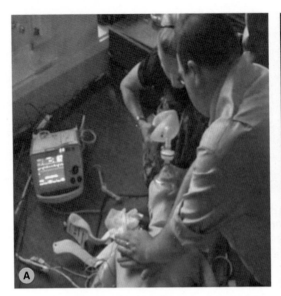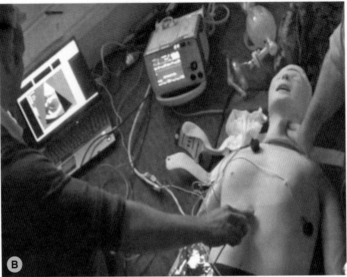

Figure 17.21. (A) A typical setting for focused echocardiography evaluation in life support (FEEL) training is shown. **(B)** An ultrasound simulator serves for real-time imaging on a manikin.

the right ventricle is significantly larger than the left, which appears small and D-shaped. This is suggestive of right ventricular pressure overload, and in the case shown, resulted from pulmonary hypertension secondary to recurrent pulmonary emboli.[11]

FUTURE DEVELOPMENTS

Echocardiography provides a diagnostic tool that allows immediate identification of the causes of cardiac arrest, and can potentially increase survival. However, literature supporting periresuscitation echocardiography is limited. Research demonstrating improved outcomes in cardiac arrest with the use of echocardiography will enhance its widespread applicability. In order to fulfill this vision, a coordinated response by relevent stakeholders that assures adequate equipment and training, even in the prehospital setting, will be necessary (Figure 17.21). Progressive miniaturization of ultrasound equipment together with the use of telemedicine is likely to drive implementation of this potentially lifesaving diagnostic test to become commonplace in resuscitation in the future.

ACKNOWLEDGEMENTS

The section on Echocardiography Anatomy contains anatomic drawings of the heart and echocardiographic images from the *Yale Atlas of Echocardiography* with kind permission; see http://www.med.yale.edu/intmed/cardio/echo_atlas/contents/index.html (access date: October 1, 2009).

References

1. A position statement: echocardiography in the critically ill. On behalf of a Collaborative Working Group of the British Society of Echocardiography (BSE). *J Intensive Care Soc.* 2008;9(2). Available at: www.journal.ics.ac.uk/pdf/0902197.pdf

2. Price S, Via G, Sloth E, et al; World Interactive Network Focused on Critical UltraSound ECHO-ICU Group. Echocardiography practice, training and accreditation in the intensive care: document for the World Interactive Network Focused on Critical Ultrasound (WINFOCUS). *Cardiovasc Ultrasound.* 2008;6:49. Available at: www.cardiovascular ultrasound.com/contents/6/1/49

3. Breitkreutz R, Walcher F, Seeger F. Focused echocardiographic evaluation in resuscitation management: concept of an advanced life support-conformed algorithm. *Crit Care Med.* 2007;35:S150–S161.

4. Cholley BP, Vieillard-Baron A, Mebazaa A. Echocardiography in the ICU: time for widespread use! *Intensive Care Med.* 2005;32:9–10.

5. Breitkreutz R, Uddin S, Steiger H, et al. Focused echocardiography entry level: new concept of a 1-day training course. *Minerva Anesthesiol.* 2009;75(5): 285–292.

6. Via G, Breitkreutz R, Price S, Daniel T; WINFOCUS ECHO-ICU Group (World Interactive Network Focused on Critical UltraSound ECHO ICU Group). Detailed echocardiography (echo) protocols for the critical patient. *J Trauma.* 2009;66(2):589–590.

7. Jones AE, Tayal VS, Sullivan DM, Kline JA. Randomized controlled trial of immediate versus delayed goal-directed ultrasound to identify the cause of nontraumatic hypotension in emergency department patients. *Crit Care Med.* 2004;32:1703–1708.

8. Jensen MB, Sloth E, Larsen KM, Schmidt MB. Transthoracic echocardiography for cardiopulmonary monitoring in intensive care. *Eur J Anaesthesiol.* 2004;21:700–707.

9. Joseph MX, Disney PJ, Da Costa R, Hutchison SJ. Transthoracic echocardiography to identify or exclude cardiac cause of shock. *Chest.* 2004;126:1592–1597.

10. Neri L, Storti E, Lichtenstein D. Toward an ultrasound curriculum for critical care medicine. *Crit Care Med.* 2007;35:S290–S304.

11. Torbicki A, Perrier A, Konstantinides S, et al. Guidelines on the diagnosis and management of acute pulmonary embolism: the Task Force for the Diagnosis and Management of Acute Pulmonary Embolism of the European Society of Cardiology (ESC). *Eur Heart J.* 2008;29:2276–2315.

Web Resources

Yale Atlas of Anatomy: www.med.yale.edu/intmed/cardio/echo_atlas/views/index.html

P. Barbier, Echo by Web: www.echobyweb.com

Eric Sloth's FATE Protocol: www.fate-protocol.com

World Interactive Network Focused on Critical Care UltraSound (WINFOCUS): www.winfocus.org

CHAPTER 18

Ultrasound Guidance for Common Procedures

Christian H. Butcher, MD, FCCP and Sameh Aziz, MD, FCCP, FACP

INTRODUCTION

The advent of high-quality, portable equipment has enabled the dissemination of ultrasound technology to the bedside physician. Led by a few pioneers, the development and application of diagnostic ultrasound are occurring in a variety of settings, including bedside medical-surgical care, ambulatory clinics, and medical education. In addition to its role in clinical medicine, ultrasound is quickly becoming recognized as an excellent tool to teach anatomy and physiology to students of medicine, and in several institutions ultrasound is seamlessly integrated into the medical curriculum (see Chapter 20).[1,2]

The safe performance of procedures is an important part of both medical education and medical practice. In recent years, ultrasound has improved the safety of key procedures including central venous catheter placement and thoracentesis.[3–5] This chapter will serve as a guide to the proper use of ultrasound for the performance of five common procedures, a how-to manual that can be taken to the bedside, opened to the relevant section, and placed in a convenient location to allow for frequent consultation during the procedure. Each procedure includes an anatomic review, a review of the pertinent physical examination findings, correlation with ultrasound findings, and the most common problems encountered. Reminiscent of anatomy texts taken into the gross anatomy laboratory, this book is meant to get dirty.

VENOUS CANNULATION

Introduction

Central venous catheterization is commonly performed, with an estimated 5 million central venous catheters (CVCs) placed annually in the United States.[6] In addition, peripherally inserted central catheters (PICCs) and peripherally inserted catheters sited in a midline position (midlines) have gained increased popularity as an alternative to CVCs in the care of selected patients because of their ease of insertion, longevity, and low rate of early complications.

Although venous cannulation is associated with a relatively low rate of serious complications,[6] complications do occur. However, an improved understanding of the cause of complications may help the provider reduce their occurrence. Interestingly, ultrasound has been used to guide vascular access and as a research tool to study the cause of certain complications of venous cannulation, such as the incidence of significant anatomic variation and the likelihood of puncturing the posterior venous wall.

Complications associated with vascular access procedures are well described[6] and can be categorized as patient or operator dependent (Table 18.1). Patient-dependent factors include body habitus, coagulopathy, and anatomic variation. Operator-dependent factors include the operator's level of experience, time allotted to perform the procedure, and human factors such as fatigue and lack of ultrasound guidance.[7–9] The most common complications of CVC placement include accidental arterial puncture, failed placement, malposition of the catheter tip, hematoma, pneumothorax, and hemothorax, the frequency of which varies depending on the site of catheter insertion. PICC and midline placement are also associated with hematomas, and these catheters are sometimes inserted into an artery. The most common complication of PICC line placement is malposition of the catheter tip into the ipsilateral internal jugular vein or coiling in the subclavian vein or a thoracic branch such as the thoracodorsal vein.

Complications of venous cannulation are not merely inconvenient; there are tangible repercussions, including increased costs derived from prolonged hospital and intensive care unit lengths of stay and additional procedures, such as chest tube insertion or hematoma evacuation, to treat the complications. For example, a single episode of iatrogenic pneumothorax has an attributable length of stay of 3 to 4 days.[10] Indirect costs such as additional provider time and patient suffering are also important issues to consider.

TABLE 18.1. Causes of Complications in Vascular Access: Patient Versus Operator Factors	
Patient Dependent	*Operator Dependent*
Body habitus	Experience
Coagulopathy	Time allotted for procedure
Vascular anatomic variation	Fatigue
Prior surgery with distortion of anatomy	Lack of ultrasound use

The rationale for ultrasound use to guide vascular access is robust. Legler and Nugent published a brief report describing the use of Doppler ultrasonography to locate the internal jugular vein for cannulation back in 1984.[11] Since then, two meta-analyses investigating the use of ultrasound for CVC placement,[12,13] several review articles, standardized procedure guidelines,[14,15] and results from the Sonography Outcomes Assessment Program (SOAP-3) trial have been published.[16] These and other studies clearly demonstrate that the use of two-dimensional (2D) ultrasound during central venous access is associated with fewer complications, fewer attempts before successful cannulation, shorter procedure times, and fewer failed procedures when compared to a landmark-based approach. As a result, the Agency for Healthcare Research and Quality and the British National Institute of Clinical Excellence (NICE) have issued statements advocating the use of ultrasound guidance in central venous access procedures.[17,18] A 2007 study by Wigmore et al confirms that implementation of the NICE guidelines has resulted in fewer complications.[19]

Some providers continue to resist the adoption of the ultrasound-guided technique and use ultrasound only in potentially "difficult to cannulate" patients such as the morbidly obese or when landmark-based cannulation has failed.[20] Unfortunately, it is difficult to predict which patients will be hard to cannulate, and the recognition of a failed attempt, as may arise from an occluded vessel, can be viewed only retrospectively after the failure has occurred and the patient has been adversely affected.[21] Therefore, the consideration of ultrasound up front to improve safety in all central venous access procedures is recommended. And, as evidenced by Lee et al, the technique is easily taught.[22]

Review of Ultrasound

Transducer Selection

Ultrasound transducers come in a variety of frequencies, each with different properties and clinical applications. Recall that the relationship between ultrasound frequency and the depth of tissue penetration is an inverse relationship. Thus, low-frequency ultrasound (1–3 MHz) penetrates more deeply than high-frequency ultrasound (7–10 MHz). The relationship between frequency and image detail, or resolution, is *proportional*. This means that low-frequency ultrasound has poorer resolution than high-frequency ultrasound. Therefore, high-frequency ultrasound provides a very detailed image of superficial structures, to a depth of approximately 5 cm, but cannot penetrate into deeper tissues. Alternatively, lower-frequency ultrasound is capable of reaching into deeper structures but provides a less-detailed image. These relationships form the basis for transducer selection. For percutaneous vascular access, which is a procedure that is superficial, higher-frequency transducers are ideal.

Modes

A-mode ultrasound has very few clinical applications and is not discussed further here. B-mode ultrasound uses an ultrasound probe with many active elements aligned in a specific orientation, or "array," to create a recognizable 2D image (Fig. 18.1, top). B mode is the most common mode currently employed in diagnostic medical ultrasound. M-mode ultrasound uses information obtained with B mode to create an image that demonstrates the movement of structures over time

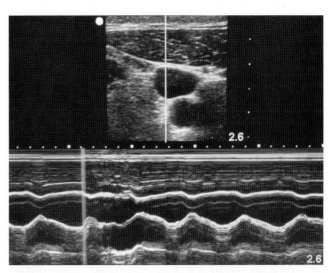

Figure 18.1. Typical B-mode (two-dimensional) image (*top*) and M-mode image (*bottom*) of the internal jugular vein.

(Fig. 18.1, bottom). The most common application of M mode is to assess valve leaflet movement and wall motion in cardiac ultrasound.

Doppler mode also has several forms. The simplest produces no image; there is only an audible signal that varies in intensity with the velocity of the structure being studied (e.g., blood). Color Doppler takes velocity information obtained by the Doppler shift and assigns color to it. Most modern ultrasound equipment uses Doppler or color Doppler in combination with B mode to both create an image and simultaneously superimpose information about blood flow velocity (Fig. 18.2 [see also color insert]). Color Doppler is very commonly used in vascular applications, such as vascular access. An important concept to understand is that the strength of the Doppler signal is related to the velocity of the target tissue (e.g., blood) and the angle of incidence, with the best estimate of velocity occurring at an angle approaching zero. If the same vessel is imaged in a plane 90° from the direction of blood flow, there is no perceived motion of blood either toward or away from the transducer, and the Doppler signal fades. Also, when the angle of incidence changes from one "side" of the 90° mark to the other side, the color of the blood within the target vessel changes (e.g., from red to blue) (Fig. 18.3). This is very important and a potential source of error when a beginner is becoming familiar with orientation and selecting a vessel for cannulation.

Techniques of Ultrasound Guidance

Ultrasound is not a substitute for a thorough knowledge of the landmark-based technique for central

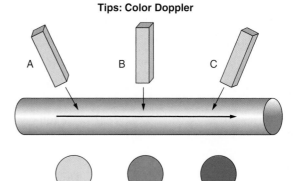

Tips: Color Doppler

Figure 18.3. The effect of varying the angle of incidence on color flow Doppler. Intensity and/or color will change depending on angle of incidence. Blood is flowing away from probe A, but if you change the angle (such as in probe C), the blood will flow toward the probe, which changes the color.

venous cannulation. Frequently, the beginner may focus on the image on the screen and be inattentive to anatomic landmarks and the position of the needle. In fact, ultrasound should be used as an educational tool to teach and confirm the landmark-based technique whenever possible. Just as computed tomography of the chest is an excellent tool to teach interpretation of the chest x-ray in a retrospective fashion, ultrasound is an excellent tool to teach landmark-based cannulation (including its limitations).

Ultrasound guidance can be categorized as static or dynamic. Dynamic guidance refers to performing the procedure in real time with ultrasound imaging viewing the needle puncturing the vessel wall. Static guidance refers to identifying the target vessel, assessing patency, and marking an appropriate insertion site with ultrasound, then cannulating blindly. For vascular access, static guidance appears to be inferior to dynamic but still better than the landmark-based technique alone.[16] Table 18.2 provides a comparison between static and dynamic guidance techniques. Dynamic guidance is more technically demanding since it requires significant eye-hand coordination.

Anatomic Review and Physical Examination Correlation with Ultrasound Anatomy and Physiology

Planes

For our purposes, there are two planes to be considered: transverse and longitudinal, which refer to the orientation of the ultrasound transducer and the image to the vessel axis. A transverse view is a cross sectional view and provides the operator with information

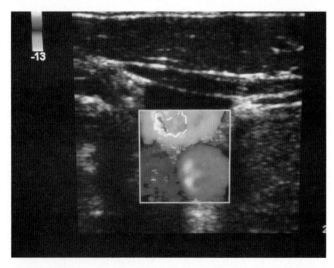

Figure 18.2. Color flow Doppler image of the internal jugular vein (*top*) and carotid artery (*bottom*). (See color insert.)

TABLE 18.2. Comparison of Static Versus Dynamic Guidance*	
Dynamic Guidance	**Static Guidance**
Ultrasonic localization and image-guided cannulation	Ultrasonic localization and marking of landmarks only
More precise and "real time"	Cannulation is not image guided
More difficult to maintain sterility	Time delay between marking and cannulation
Requires significant hand-eye coordination	Less difficult to maintain sterility
	Less technically demanding

In general, the advantages and disadvantages apply to all ultrasound-guided procedures.

about structures that lay adjacent to the vessel of interest. For example, a cross-sectional view of the internal jugular vein will enable visualization of the adjacent common carotid artery and, perhaps, the vagus nerve, thyroid gland, and trachea.

A longitudinal view will depict structures anterior and posterior to the vessel of interest and may allow for visualization of the entire needle during cannulation but does not allow simultaneous visualization of structures lateral to the vessel. All commonly utilized central veins can be visualized in either orientation. As a general rule, transverse views tend to be easier for the novice to learn ultrasound-guided cannulation, but complications such as puncturing the posterior vessel wall may be reduced by using the longitudinal view as reported by Blaivas et al[23] and commented on by Levitov et al.[24]

Recently, a study was published touting the use of a hybrid method of obliquely imaging the target vessel, the implication being that this approach may confer the benefits of both a transverse and longitudinal view.[25]

Methods of Orientation

Orientation is probably the most important step to a successful procedure. Problems with orientation can largely be prevented by ensuring proper patient, transducer, and ultrasound machine position. Most transducers have an identifiable mark, known as a *notch*, on one side. This corresponds to a mark displayed on one side of the image and allows right/left, or lateral, orientation (Fig. 18.4). Where orientation is uncertain during a procedure, a finger can be rubbed on one side of the transducer surface to produce an image and confirm the orientation. In general, the screen should be in the operator's line of sight during vessel cannulation; in practical terms, the needle should point directly at the screen during cannulation. For a subclavian line, the machine is placed on the opposite side of the patient; the machine is placed on

the ipsilateral side for an internal jugular line (Fig. 18.5). For femoral insertion, the screen can be placed on either the ipsilateral side or the contralateral side at the level of the patient's chest.

Differentiating an Artery from a Vein

Upon reviewing the vascular anatomy of the neck, recall that the common carotid and internal jugular veins travel together in the carotid sheath (along with the vagus nerve). Despite what many readers learned in anatomy, there is significant variation in the position of the vein relative to the artery. In fact, the vein is either posterior to, directly anterior to, or medial to the vein in a significant minority of patients.[15] It becomes important, therefore, to be able to differentiate artery from vein by some other means. Arteries, in general, are smaller and thicker walled than accompanying veins on ultrasound. In addition, veins are usually

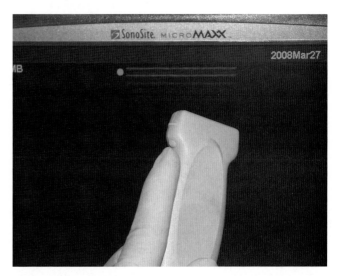

Figure 18.4. Orienting the transducer to the image. The notch on the transducer corresponds to the indicator on the screen.

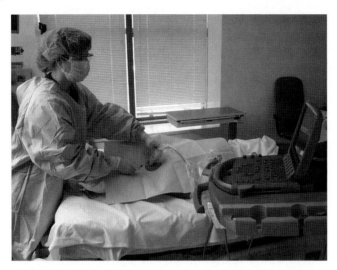

Figure 18.5. Comfort should be maximized by positioning the machine "ergonomically"; in general, the needle should be pointing toward the ultrasound image during cannulation.

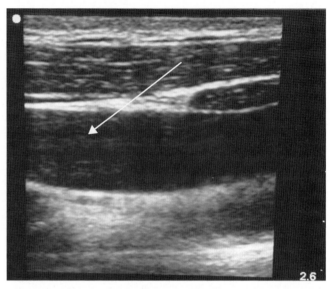

Figure 18.6. A thrombus (*arrow*), especially if chronic, can be difficult to distinguish from surrounding tissue. This is a clot in the internal jugular vein. This vessel would be impossible to compress fully, and color flow would be absent. Prior to cannulation, the entire vessel should be scanned since clot may be distal to the proposed insertion site. Both sides should be scanned, especially when placing an internal jugular line; a central line placed in a patient with a contralateral internal jugular clot greatly increases the risk of bilateral thrombus.

very easily collapsed with the application of pressure via the transducer. The character of vessel pulsation is another clue; arteries will pulsate with the cardiac cycle, and veins may pulsate with the respiratory cycle (respiratory variation in venous diameter), unless significant right-sided heart failure is present. A fourth method is to apply color Doppler to the vessel and observe the character of the color pulsation. The correct use of color flow Doppler requires that the operator know how the machine is set up and at what angle the vessel was "Dopplered." The machine can be set so that blood moving toward the transducer is either red or blue. However, if the angle of insonation of the vessel crosses a line perpendicular to the vessel, the color will change (see Fig. 18.3). It is useful to compare color Doppler signals of all vessels in the area of interest, paying close attention to the angle of the incident ultrasound beam; with a little practice arterial flow is easily differentiated from venous flow. Remember that large, rapid fluctuations in intrathoracic pressure can create very high venous blood flow velocities that can mimic arterial flow; this situation may require the use of other methods such as respiratory variation or compressibility to help differentiate the vessel type.

Occasionally, the vein cannot be visualized. The most common reason for this is hypovolemia with associated venous collapse, which can be remedied by placing the patient in the Trendelenburg position or applying a vagal maneuver or fluid administration. Other less common causes are agenesis, chronic occlusion or scarring of the vessel, and clot that is completely occluding the lumen. Clot may be difficult

to distinguish from the surrounding tissue (Fig. 18.6). In this case, a thorough examination of the proximal and distal parts of the vessel should be performed, and a formal venous Doppler procedure should be performed to evaluate for deep venous thrombosis prior to any attempted central venous cannulation. If access is critical, and vessel presence or patency cannot be assured, a different vessel should be cannulated.

Technique

Internal Jugular Vein

1. The patient is positioned appropriately. The head should be rotated slightly contralaterally, with the neck extended. Severe rotation of the neck and head should be avoided, since this may lead to significant distortion of the anatomy and may increase the amount of overlap of the carotid artery and jugular vein. The bed should be placed in Trendelenburg position, and the ultrasound machine should be placed by the ipsilateral side of the bed, at about the level of the patient's waist.

2. An initial examination of the landmarks *without ultrasound* should be performed, including selection of an insertion site. The site should then be

confirmed with ultrasound. This technique provides the operator with immediate feedback regarding landmark-based site selection and therefore facilitates teaching both the landmark-based approach and the ultrasound-guided approach. During this process, the vein should be identified and assessed for patency.

3. The patient's skin can now be prepped in sterile fashion and full barrier precautions used to maintain sterility and reduce the incidence of catheter-related infections.[26] Ultrasound use introduces another piece of equipment onto the sterile field, making the maintenance of sterility more difficult. While learning, one needs to pay special attention to this issue in order to develop good habits. A sterile ultrasound sheath should be placed on the sterile field for when an assistant hands the operator the ultrasound transducer.

4. After the patient is prepped and draped, the catheter is set up per normal routine. All ports should be flushed with bacteriostatic saline to remove air and to test for occlusion caused by manufacturing defects. The components needed for catheter insertion, including needles, wire, dilator, scalpel, catheter, and sterile transducer cover, should be arranged in an orderly fashion and within easy reach.

5. The operator acquires the transducer, places it in the sterile cover, and secures it on the sterile field. The transducer can either be "picked up" by the operator whose gloved and sterile hand is inside the transducer cover like a puppet or, alternatively, an assistant can insert the transducer in the open end of the cover. The end sheath is then extended to cover the transducer cord, and sterile rubber bands are applied to secure the sheath in place.

6. A second ultrasound examination should be performed to ensure that the original insertion site is still viable. Remember that proper orientation every time the probe is applied to the patient is essential for ensuring an appropriate procedure.

7. When cannulating the vessel, the operator uses the same insertion site and needle trajectory as he or she would when using the landmark-based approach (lateral, medial, etc.). If using the transverse plane for ultrasound guidance, which is especially good for novices, the operator must be sure to center the vessel lumen on the screen; remember that if the vessel is centered on the screen, it is directly underneath the middle of the transducer head.

8. Sometimes it is useful to perform a "mock poke" to confirm the proposed insertion site relative to the underlying vessel. This is done by laying the needle on the skin surface, then applying the transducer to it. The acoustic shadow produced by the needle should be directly over, or superimposed on, the target vessel (Fig. 18.7). The skin puncture should be approximately 1 cm proximal to the transducer, which in most cases will result in visualization of the needle tip entering the vessel without having to move the probe much. If the needle tip cannot be visualized indenting either the subcutaneous tissue overlying the vessel or the vessel itself, the operator moves the probe along the axis of the vessel while slightly "agitating" the needle; this will accentuate the image of the needle and tip. The point of the "V" caused by indenting the subcutaneous tissue above the vein with the needle tip should be directly over the vessel. The operator should be sure to visualize the tip of the needle at all times (it is very easy to misinterpret the shaft of the needle as the tip) and to move the probe axially along the vessel frequently to

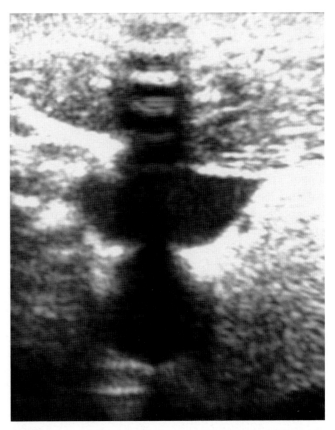

Figure 18.7. Mock poke technique. This shows a transverse view through the internal jugular vein. Note the acoustic shadow of the overlying needle.

maintain imaging of the tip. If done properly, the needle tip should be seen entering the lumen at about the same time as the flash of blood is obtained in the syringe.

9. Once the vessel has been successfully cannulated, the operator sets aside the transducer and proceeds with wire placement. Intravascular position of the wire can be confirmed with ultrasound, which can then be saved for documentation in the medical record.

10. Once the line is in place, flushed, secured, and dressed, a quick ultrasound examination of the anterior chest wall can be performed to evaluate for a pneumothorax (see Chapter 7). Pleural ultrasound specifically looking for an absence of normal "sliding pleura" is highly sensitive for identifying pneumothorax.[27]

11. The use of ultrasound should be documented in the medical record. Typically, a statement regarding the use of ultrasound to assess the location and patency of the vessel and an image of the wire or catheter in the vessel lumen is sufficient for documentation and often provides sufficient documentation for reimbursement. Additionally, a statement about the presence or absence of sliding pleura should be included.

Subclavian Vein

Typically, the subclavian vein is slightly more difficult to visualize ultrasonographically than either the internal jugular, axillary, or femoral veins. This is because of its position under the clavicle, which requires significant angulation and manipulation of the transducer to acquire a useful image. Two additional challenges are the difficulty visualizing the vein in obese patients using an infraclavicular view and the inability to adequately compress the vein to exclude the presence of clot.

In our experience, it is usually easier to visualize the subclavian with a longitudinal supraclavicular view in obese patients since an adequate transverse view or infraclavicular longitudinal view is often technically challenging. Considering the ease with which the internal jugular and axillary veins are visualized, we have largely abandoned the subclavian vein in our practice, except for specific clinical situations, such as for long-term total parenteral nutrition administration or for emergency central venous access.

Axillary Vein

Using the axillary vein for central venous access has many unique advantages over using other sites.[28–31]

Although not well-studied, since the insertion site is on the anterior chest, axillary catheterization likely shares a low incidence of catheter-related infections with the subclavian approach. Unlike the subclavian vein, using the axillary vein may be associated with fewer complications, such as pneumothorax, hemothorax, and chylothorax. The axillary vein is usually easier to compress than the subclavian vein and allows an easier recognition of clots. There is, however, the additional potential complication of causing a brachial plexus injury, particularly if a far lateral approach is used.[30] One distinct disadvantage of the axillary approach is the unique dependence on ultrasound to ensure localization and subsequent cannulation; landmark techniques are not as effective as with the other common sites used to access the central venous system. Figure 18.8 shows proper transducer placement for viewing the axillary vein transversely. As with internal jugular and subclavian access approaches, a quick postprocedure scan of the chest should be performed to ensure sliding pleura, which essentially eliminates the possibility of pneumothorax.[27]

Femoral Vein

Femoral cannulation remains a popular approach because of its relatively low incidence of life-threatening complications. However, several clinically important complications may occur that lead to significant morbidity. Accidental (or intentional for that matter) femoral arterial cannulation, especially in coagulopathic patients, may cause life-threatening retroperitoneal hemorrhage and hematoma. Inadvertent stimulation of the femoral nerve with the cannulation needle can cause intense pain. A puncture site that is

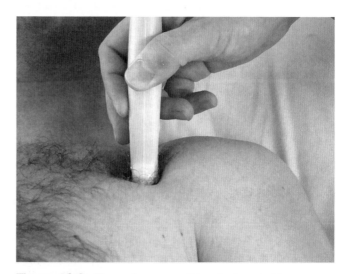

Figure 18.8. Transducer position to image the axillary vein.

too proximal can also result in inadvertent puncture of intraperitoneal structures. Ultrasound can help avoid some of these important complications.

Like internal jugular, subclavian, and axillary cannulation, the first step in successful femoral access is achieving proper orientation. The ultrasound machine should be placed in a location that encourages operator comfort. The entire area should be scanned, with identification of all vascular structures, including the femoral artery, common femoral vein, and saphenous or profunda femoris vessels if possible. Once the vein is identified, it should be evaluated for the presence of clot. Additionally, a longitudinal view of the vein should be obtained as it dives under the inguinal ligament, and the ligament itself should be marked on the skin. If a femoral hernia is not present, this step ensures that an intraperitoneal puncture will not occur (Fig. 18.9). All other steps are identical to those listed earlier for the internal jugular vein.

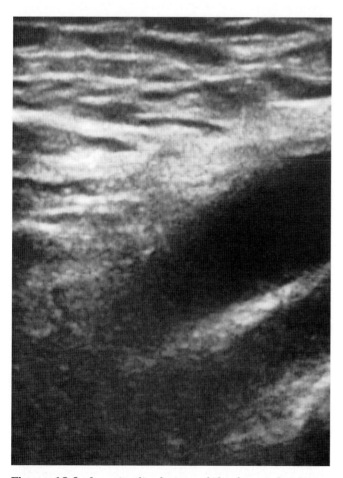

Figure 18.9. Longitudinal view of the femoral vein as it "dives" under the inguinal ligament. The inguinal ligament is the confluence of bright lines in the left upper quadrant of the image.

Common Pitfalls

The most common pitfalls encountered in ultrasound-guided vascular access are easily avoided. These include not understanding the relationship between transducer frequency and both depth of penetration and image resolution, incomplete understanding of the basics of color Doppler and how the angle of the incident ultrasound beam can alter the Doppler signal (and color), poor technique in terms of always keeping the needle tip in view during image-guided cannulation, not paying attention to equipment setup to maximize comfort and ergonomics during the procedure, and not scanning the entire vessel to exclude the presence of thrombus. These pitfalls can be avoided by proper training and subsequent practice.

LUMBAR PUNCTURE

Introduction

Lumbar puncture, first described by Heinrich Quincke, has been performed for over a century. Typically, the procedure is performed after proper positioning of the patient and careful palpation of anatomic landmarks to help locate an appropriate site for needle insertion. However, successful lumbar puncture can be difficult to achieve in certain patient populations (e.g., the morbidly obese), presumably because of obscuration of palpable anatomic landmarks such as the spinous processes. In recent years, there has been a renewed interest in augmenting the landmark-based technique with ultrasound.

The first reported use of ultrasound to help guide lumbar puncture was published in 1971 in the Russian literature.[32] Since that time, the technique remained relatively dormant until the last decade, when it was resurrected by anesthesiologists for use in guiding spinal and epidural blocks.[33–37] In fact, most of the data currently available have been reported in the anesthesia literature; incorporation of ultrasound guidance into critical care and generalist practice has been a more recent development. The main advantages of adding ultrasound guidance to the landmark-based technique are shown in Table 18.3.

Anatomic Review and Physical Examination Correlation with Ultrasound Anatomy and Physiology

Normal lumbar spinal anatomy is shown in Figure 18.10. As can be seen, the needle used for lumbar puncture must traverse the skin, subcutaneous tissues, and

> **TABLE 18.3. Advantages of Using Ultrasound Guidance for Lumbar Puncture**
>
> Allows visualization of the interspace and the exact midline as well as the target (ligamentum flavum)
>
> Allows one to easily see the required needle trajectory between the spinous processes
>
> Allows one to gauge the required needle depth prior to needle insertion
>
> Reduces failure rate
>
> Reduces procedure time

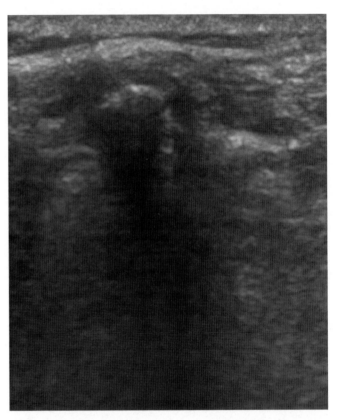

Figure 18.11. Transverse ultrasound view through the spine, clearly showing the tips of the spinous processes as well as the transverse processes.

supraspinous ligament; then it must navigate through the spinous processes and the interspinous ligament before traversing the ligamentum flavum before it enters the dural space and, finally, the subarachnoid space. Success is inherently dependent on proper needle position and angulation. Since the conus medullaris rarely extends beyond L3 in most studies, the most common site of insertion is the L3-L4 interspace. Figure 18.11 shows a transverse view through the lumbar spine at the level of L4. Note the easily distinguishable tip of the spinous process as well as the transverse processes. This transverse view facilitates identification of the midline, which can be surprisingly difficult to identify by palpation in some patients. Figure 18.12 shows a longitudinal view of the L3-L4 level. Note the appearance of the spinous processes as well as the presence of the ligamentum flavum,

which overlies the dura. In one study, the depth of the dural reflection correlated very well with needle depth during insertion.[38]

Technique

A linear array transducer works well for most patients. In our institution, we use the same 6- to 13-MHz linear array transducer used for vascular access procedures. Alternatively, a curvilinear 5-MHz transducer could be substituted. The patient is positioned appropriately, either sitting upright, leaning forward, or on the side in the lateral recumbent position (particularly if pressure measurements will be obtained). Puncture can be guided either statically or dynamically. In static guidance, an appropriate site is marked on the skin by first finding the L3-L4 level by the usual technique (palpation of the iliac crest), then marking the exact midline with a transverse ultrasound view, followed by locating and marking the appropriate interspace with a longitudinal view. Once the two marks are made, the insertion site will be the center of the "+"; it helps to make a skin indentation with a sterile instrument in case the "+" is removed during sterile preparation of

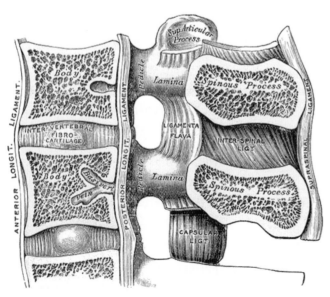

Figure 18.10. Normal spinal anatomy.

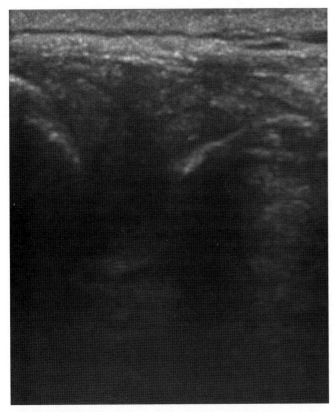

Figure 18.12. Longitudinal view through the lumbar spine. The spinous processes can be seen, as can the ligamentum flavum at the "floor" between the two vertebrae. The distance between the skin and the ligamentum flavum approximates the needle length required to enter the space and reach fluid.

the skin (see Fig 18.13). If dynamic guidance is employed, all the above steps are done, followed by needle insertion under ultrasound guidance; the needle tip can be seen to enter the area of the dural sac. As mentioned earlier, one can measure the distance from the skin to the dural reflection on the image; this has been found to correspond well to the required depth of the needle to obtain fluid. Once learned, this technique can improve success rates up to 92% as reported in one series.[38]

Common Pitfalls

This technique is relatively resistant to error. However, heavy ligamentous calcification can obscure underlying anatomy, so particular care is needed in these patients. Fortunately, calcification rarely impairs the operator's ability to identify the midline or an appropriate interspace for needle insertion. Another very common pitfall, much more difficult to overcome, is the presence of posterior spinal hardware. There are more advanced techniques to obtain

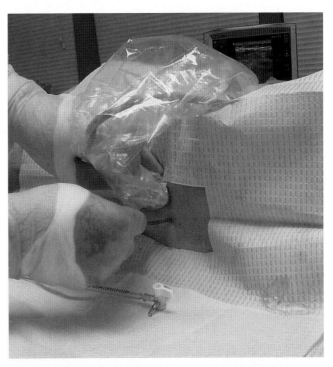

Figure 18.13. A combination of transverse and longitudinal views to mark the midline and appropriate interspace, respectively.

spinal fluid in these patients, but this is beyond the scope of this book.

THORACENTESIS

Introduction

Ultrasound-guided thoracentesis is a very useful procedure, especially in the critical care setting when visualization of pleural effusions in supine mechanically ventilated patients becomes difficult. In fact, ultrasound-guided thoracentesis was found to be a safe procedure with a lower risk of pneumothorax in comparison to blind thoracentesis in both mechanically ventilated and nonventilated patients.[4,39] Furthermore, it has been found to be a helpful adjunct when used to evaluate unsuccessful thoracentesis.[40]

Evaluation of the pleural space and pleural fluid with ultrasound is useful to help determine the nature of the effusion and help differentiate between transudative and exudative effusions. A transudative pleural effusion is usually anechoic, while an exudative effusion may have complex septation, echogenic material, or the presence of pleural thickening[41] (Figs. 18.14 and 18.15).

In addition to providing useful information about the type of fluid present, ultrasound can help with the

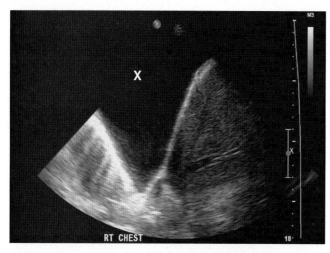

Figure 18.14. Anechoic appearance indicates an uncomplicated transudative pleural effusion. *X* marks the spot.

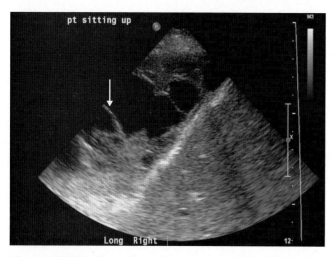

Figure 18.15. Complicated parapneumonic effusion with septation (*arrow*).

quantitative evaluation of the pleural fluid.[42] In most circumstances, this is not essential information, and, therefore, we will not discuss techniques to quantify pleural fluid any further.

Anatomic Review and Physical Examination Correlation with Ultrasound Anatomy and Physiology

The pleural space can be thought of as being roughly conical in shape, bordered by the chest wall anteriorly, laterally, and posteriorly; the mediastinum medially; and the diaphragm inferiorly. From a sonographic viewpoint, only the anterior, lateral, and posterior borders are accessible. Fluid, if it is free flowing, accumulates dependently, inferiorly and posteriorly in the upright chest and posterolaterally when the patient is supine. When fluid is present in the thorax, it is always bordered by three structures: the chest wall, the diaphragm, and the lung. Knowledge regarding the location and appearance of intra-abdominal structures, such as the spleen, liver, and kidneys, is absolutely necessary to be able to perform ultrasound-guided thoracentesis safely. The liver is shown in Figures 18.16A and 18.16B as a relatively homogenous structure bordered superiorly by the diaphragm and inferiorly by the kidneys. The kidneys are usually very easy to recognize, having an outer cortex and inner medulla. The potential space in between the liver and the right kidney (hepatorenal recess), as well as that between the spleen and the left kidney (splenorenal recess), can occasionally be confused with the pleural space (Figure 18.17), especially when large amounts of intra-abdominal fluid are present (Figure 18.18).

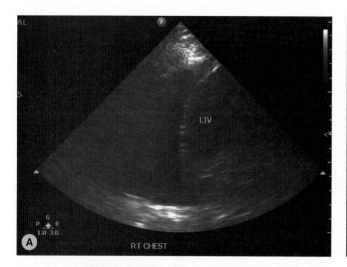

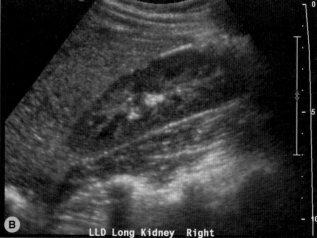

Figure 18.16. Appearance of the liver, spleen, and kidneys in relation to the diaphragm. **(A)** The different appearance of the liver from the chest ultrasound window may be confused with a pleural effusion. **(B)** Normal appearance of the liver and kidney from the chest ultrasound window.

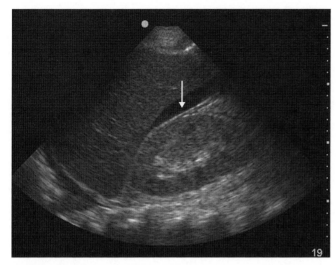

Figure 18.17. Appearance of fluid in the hepatorenal recess. This can occasionally be confused with pleural fluid (*arrow*).

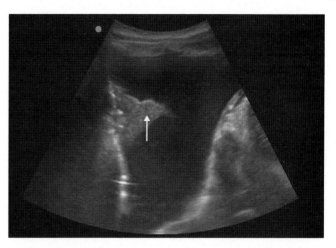

Figure 18.18. Appearance of pleural fluid confirmed by the presence of the diaphragm (hyperechoic line on the left) and the collapsed lung (compression atelectasis [*white arrow*]).

Pleural fluid usually appears homogenously black if the effusion is simple. Complex effusions may appear "speckled" or otherwise inhomogeneous. Occasionally, a spider-web appearance will be encountered, which indicates loculation. Dynamic characters are almost universally present, which include a moving diaphragm, moving lung, and movement within the effusion itself.

Technique

1. The patient is positioned appropriately. The best position for thoracentesis is with the patient sitting upright with arms elevated and extended in front, especially for nonloculated effusions. However, when ultrasound is utilized, thoracentesis becomes feasible even in the lateral and supine positions, which is helpful in assessing critically ill mechanically ventilated patients because it would be difficult to place them upright without significant ancillary support.[43,44]

2. A 3.5- to 5-MHz curvilinear ultrasound probe is used in a longitudinal orientation (perpendicular position of the ultrasound probe in relation to the underlying rib) to identify the location, quantity, and quality of the fluid, if present.[45]

3. One should scan below the effusion to identify the diaphragm, the spleen on the left side, and the liver on the right side. **Pay particular attention in order to not confuse fluid in the hepatorenal recess or the splenorenal recess with pleural fluid.**

4. The operator confirms that there is enough fluid to create a safe distance between the planned site of entry and vital organs, remembering that the diaphragm is dome shaped; if one plans to advance the needle close to it, he or she may inadvertently penetrate through it if the needle is advanced too far.

5. The operator confirms the presence of the pleural effusion by identifying at least three borders and at least two dynamic characters; usually the pleural fluid is bordered by the diaphragm inferiorly, the chest wall anteriorly, and the lung posteriorly (or medially) (Fig. 18.18).

6. M mode can be used to confirm the presence of pleural fluid using the sinusoid sign, especially with minimal pleural effusion (Fig. 18.19).[46]

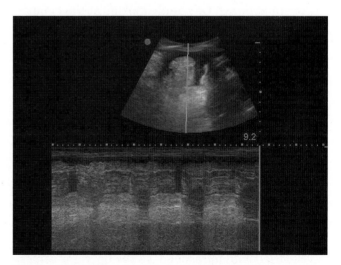

Figure 18.19. The borders of a pleural effusion are shown: diaphragm, pleura, and collapsed lung.

7. Once the position of the effusion is identified, a transverse position of the ultrasound probe is used to evaluate both the proper puncture site and the presence of any superficial vascular structures.

8. The operator plans the needle trajectory based on the location of fluid, the presence and distance of any underlying structures, and the angle of incidence of the ultrasound transducer during the examination. In general, once a good view is obtained with the transducer, the operator mentally note the position and angle of the probe; this will be the position and angle of the needle during insertion.

9. The operator cleans the site of entry with ChloraPrep and sterilely drapes it. One may use a sterile cover for the ultrasound probe to rescan the area again to confirm the optimum site of entry.

10. Using a 25- to 30-gauge needle, the operator infiltrates the skin with local anesthetic using 1% or 2% lidocaine. Using a 22-gauge, 1.5-inch needle, the operator infiltrates local anesthetic to the subcutaneous tissues and intercostal space. The catheter is inserted through the planned tract until pleural fluid is obtained and is then advanced into the pleural space while the inner needle is pulled back.

11. Once the procedure is done, the catheter is withdrawn from the pleural space.

12. Postprocedure ultrasound evaluation of the pleural space is recommended. One needs to evaluate first for the resolution of the pleural effusion and for the presence of any residual fluid, and secondly for postprocedure complications such as pneumothorax. One study looking at the comparison between chest x-ray and chest ultrasound for postinterventional pneumothorax showed that transthoracic ultrasound had a sensitivity and specificity of 100% to rule out postinterventional pneumothorax. About 16% of cases with postprocedure pneumothorax were missed with chest x-ray.[47]

A freehand technique in which real-time ultrasound guided thoracentesis is utilized (so-called dynamic guidance) is highly recommended for small pockets of pleural fluid or in patients on mechanical ventilation. This technique requires significant hand-eye coordination, however. The advantage is that needle insertion is visualized with ultrasound, so the operator can see the needle tip as it is advanced.

Pitfalls

There really are no pitfalls unique to ultrasound-guided thoracentesis. However, all the usual pitfalls of traditional thoracentesis exist, which include dry tap, re-expansion pulmonary edema, and pneumothorax. The most common causes for dry tap when ultrasound guidance is used are either poor angle selection or the presence of a complicated effusion with interpleural septation. Feller-Kopman et al found that re-expansion pulmonary edema occured more often if the patient experienced chest discomfort during the procedure, there was rapid removal of pleural fluid, or the end-expiratory pleural pressure was noted to be less than –20 cm H_2O.[48]

PARACENTESIS

Introduction

Paracentesis is a very commonly performed procedure, typically indicated as part of the initial evaluation of patients with new-onset ascites or patients with a known history of ascites who develop clinical deterioration. Using ultrasound guidance for paracentesis has been shown to decrease the duration, increase the ease, and improve the accuracy of the procedure, partly by avoiding unnecessary procedures in patients with minimal or no ascites.[49] Other advantages of ultrasound use to guide paracentesis are that it can detect as little as 10 mL of free fluid with a specificity of 100%,[50] help identify the character of the fluid, and be used to determine an appropriate point of entry[51] (Fig. 18.20). Theoretically, ultrasound

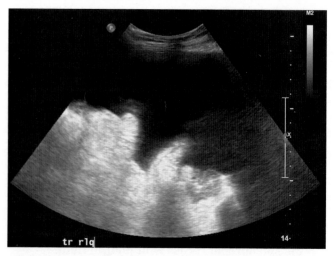

Figure 18.20. M mode of a small effusion showing the sinusoid sign (*arrow*).

guidance can help avoid puncture of vital organs, such as the liver, kidney, and spleen.

Anatomic Review and Physical Examination Correlation with Ultrasound Anatomy and Physiology

The peritoneal space is bordered by the diaphragm superiorly, the abdominal wall anteriorly and laterally, and the retroperitoneum posteriorly. Inferiorly, the peritoneal space is contiguous with the pelvis and is bordered by the pelvic floor. The abdomen presents a fairly unique challenge in that one of its resident organs, the bowel, is highly mobile. In addition, several intra-abdominal organs are highly subject to changes in intrathoracic pressure and can change position during respiration. Another challenge is that in morbidly obese patients, it is very difficult to appreciate the classic fluid wave on physical examination maneuvers. Therefore, it is quite advantageous for medical providers to know basic abdominal ultrasonographic anatomy (see Chapter 10). For our purposes, remember that the liver is separated from the right kidney by a potential space known as the hepatorenal recess. This space can fill with fluid and occasionally be mistaken for pleural fluid, with the liver being mistaken for lung. On the left side, the spleen is likewise separated from the left kidney by the splenorenal recess. The kidneys, probably the most recognizable structure on ultrasound, are located retroperitoneally and are most easily imaged from a posterolateral transducer position. Bowel, especially in patients with large fluid collections, can be seen as multiple free-floating loops. A particularly important structure to be able to recognize is the urinary bladder, which, if full, can be mistaken for ascites. The bladder typically has easily identifiable walls and may have a visible balloon if catheterized.

Technique

1. Prior to the procedure the patient is asked to empty the urinary bladder to decrease the risk of bladder perforation. Also, any coagulopathy needs to be corrected prior to commencing.[52]

2. Most of the time the procedure is performed while the patient is supine, although it can also be done with the patient in the sitting position.[44]

3. Curved array transducers are preferred for evaluation of the abdomen and to identify the quality and the quantity of ascitic fluid. Ultrasound is able to reveal as little as 100 mL of ascitic fluid[53] and can, therefore, determine a safe site of entry.

4. The left lower quadrant approach is considered to be a safe starting point. One may use color flow Doppler to evaluate for cutaneous veins at the proposed site of entry and to help avoid the inferior epigastric artery.

5. The operator performs a careful evaluation of the entire abdomen, paying particular attention to the position of the liver, spleen, bowels, and bladder; this step is key to avoiding complications.

6. The operator selects an appropriate site for needle insertion.

7. Once the site of entry is identified, the area is then cleaned and draped.

8. The transducer is sheathed in a sterile probe cover.

9. Prior to the procedure, ultrasound is used again to confirm the location of the ascitic fluid as well as the expected needle depth at which fluid should be encountered.

10. The operator introduces the needle into the peritoneal fluid using a "Z-line technique" to decrease the risk of postprocedure leak.

11. Using a free-hand technique with real-time ultrasound (dynamic guidance), the operator should try to keep the needle and the ultrasound beam in the same plane. Again, this is the key point for successful thoracentesis, paracentesis, and the longitudinal approach for central line placement (Figs. 18.21 [see also color insert] and 18.22).[54,55]

12. If dynamic guidance is used, the operator should be able to see both the needle and the catheter entering the peritoneal space in real time (Fig. 18.23).

13. Once fluid is obtained, the operator sets the transducer aside and proceeds with fluid evacuation.

Pitfalls

As with thoracentesis, the pitfalls associated with ultrasound guidance for paracentesis are the same as with the traditional technique. Large-volume paracentesis (>10 liters) is usually avoided, as it may lead to severe hypotension.[52] Damage to blood vessels can occur, with postprocedure hemorrhage that can occur from 6 to 48 hours after the procedure.[56] However, careful evaluation of superficial veins and arteries with ultrasound can help avoid bloody paracentesis and even inferior epigastric artery aneurysm. Of course, areas of previous scars and areas of intra-abdominal adhesion should be avoided.

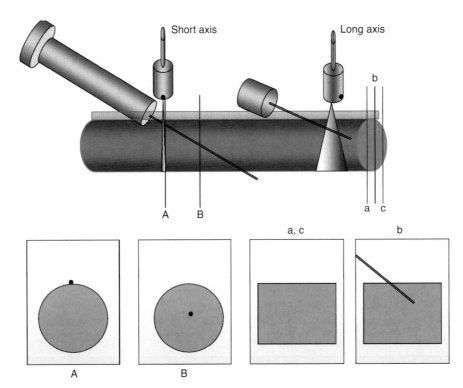

Figure 18.21. Diagram comparing transverse and longitudinal approach, illustrating the need for for the visualization of the needle tip (see color insert). In plane B needle appears in the center of the vessel while the tip has penetrated the posterior wall. (*Adapted with permission from Sameh Aziz, MD.*)

DOCUMENTATION, CODING, AND REIMBURSEMENT

It is the responsibility of the physician to select the appropriate code for the services rendered. *Current Procedural Terminology* (CPT) code 76604 can be used for diagnostic ultrasound of the chest and code 76700 for diagnostic ultrasound of the abdomen, while CPT code 76942 can be used for ultrasound-guided thoracentesis.[57]

There are two separate payment components that can be requested: the professional fee and the facility fee. The professional fee is the physician's fee for the medical services provided. The facility fee is the fee charged to offset the cost of equipment and maintenance. For most ultrasound-guided procedures, the additional professional fee attributable to ultrasound guidance is nominal. However, the facility fee can be

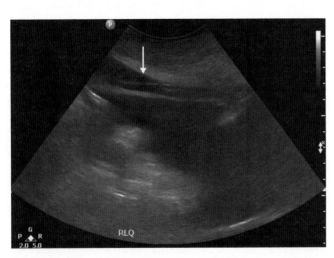

Figure 18.22. Longitudinal view of the internal jugular vein with the needle seen in the vessel lumen (*white arrow*).

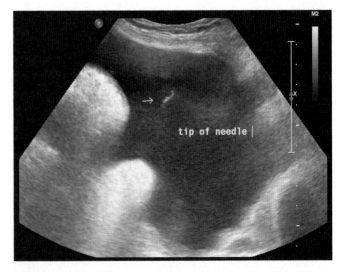

Figure 18.23. The arrow demonstrates the tip of the paracentesis needle in the peritoneal cavity during real-time guidance for paracentesis.

quite large. One caveat is that the person or group charging the facility must own the equipment. If these procedures are going to be billed to the patient, adequate documentation that ultrasound was indeed used must be permanently stored in the medical record. Adequate documentation, for example, would include a static photo of the vein before and after cannulation, showing the needle or guidewire in the vessel lumen. Video loops of the procedures may also be stored on a computer for access should an audit be performed.

FUTURE DEVELOPMENTS

Ultrasound guidance has been used for many years and with excellent success in interventional radiology suites. As these techniques become disseminated to nonradiologist practitioners, the limits of what is "standard" change. Already, nephrologists are learning to perform ultrasound-guided renal biopsy, general internists are performing ultrasound-guided liver biopsy, and critical care practitioners are aspirating abdominal abscesses. Standardized training programs will emerge, with clearly defined training requirements, to enable practitioners of varied backgrounds to acquire the skills they need to perform these procedures at the point of care, Data will very likely emerge proving that ultrasound guidance improves the outcome of the vast majority of procedures, including those discussed in this chapter, and early adapters will have a distinct advantage.

References

1. Rao S, van Holsbeek L, Musial JL, et al. A pilot study of comprehensive ultrasound education at Wayne State University School of Medicine: a pioneer year review. *J Ultrasound Med.* 2008;27(5):745–749.

2. Hoppmann R, Cook T, Hunt P, et al. Ultrasound in medical education: a vertical curriculum at the University of South Carolina School of Medicine. *J S C Med Assoc.* 2006;102(10):330–334.

3. Jones PW, Moyers JP, Rogers JT, et al. Ultrasound guided thoracentesis: is it a safer method? *Chest.* 2003;123(2): 418–423.

4. Mayo PH, Goltz HR, Tafreshi M, et al. Safety of ultrasound guided thoracentesis in patients receiving mechanical ventilation. *Chest.* 2004;125(3):1059–1062.

5. Feller-Kopman D. Ultrasound-guided thoracentesis. *Chest.* 2006;129(6):1709–1714.

6. McGee DC, Gould MK. Preventing complications of central venous catheterization. *N Engl J Med.* 2003;348: 1123–1133.

7. Polderman KH, Girbes AJ. Central venous catheter use. Part 1: mechanical complications. *Intensive Care Med.* 2002;28:1–17.

8. Merrer J, De Jonghe B, Golliot F, et al. Complications of femoral and subclavian venous catheterization in critically ill patients: a randomized controlled trial. *JAMA.* 2001;286:700–707.

9. Mansfield PF, Hohn DC, Fornage BD. Complications and failures of subclavian vein catheterization. *N Engl J Med.* 1994;331:1735–1738.

10. Light RW. *Pleural Diseases.* 5th ed. Philadelphia, PA: Lippincott Williams & Wilkins; 2007.

11. Legler D, Nugent M. Doppler localization of the internal jugular vein facilitates central venous cannulation. *Anesthesiology.* 1984;60:481–482.

12. Randolph AG, Cook DJ, Gonzales CA, et al. Ultrasound guidance for placement of central venous catheters: a meta-analysis of the literature. *Crit Care Med.* 1996;24: 2053–2058.

13. Hind D, Calvert N, McWilliams SR, et al. Ultrasonic locating devices for central venous cannulation: meta-analysis. *BMJ.* 2003;327–361.

14. Feller-Kopman D. Ultrasound-guided internal jugular access. *Chest.* 2007;132:302–309.

15. Maecken T, Grau T. Ultrasound imaging in vascular access. *Crit Care Med.* 2007;35:s178–s185.

16. Milling TJ Jr, Rose J, Briggs WM, et al. Randomized, controlled clinical trial of point-of-care limited ultrasonography assistance of central venous cannulation: the third sonography outcomes assessment program (SOAP-3) trial. *Crit Care Med.* 2005;33:1764–1769.

17. NICE guidelines. Available at: http://www.nice.org.uk/nicemedia/pdf/Ultrasound_49_GUIDANCE.pdf. Accessed December 20, 2007.

18. AHRQ evidence based practice. Available at: http://www.ahrq.gov/clinic/ptsafety/pdf/chap21.pdf. Accessed December 20, 2007.

19. Wigmore TJ, Smythe JF, Hacking MB, et al. Effect of the implementation of NICE guidelines for ultrasound guidance on the complication rates associated with central venous catheter placement in patients presenting for routine surgery in a tertiary referral centre. *Br J Anesthesiol.* 2007;99(5):662–665.

20. Muhm M. Ultrasound guided central venous access (letter). *BMJ.* 2002;325:1374–1375.

21. Forauer A, Glockner J. Importance of US findings in access planning during jugular vein hemodialysis catheter placements. *J Vasc Interv Radiol.* 2000;11:233–238.

22. Lee AC, Thompson C, Frank J, et al. Effectiveness of a novel training program for emergency medicine residents in ultrasound-guided insertion of central venous catheters. *CJEM.* 2009;11(4):343–348.

23. Blaivas M, Video analysis of accidental arterial cannulation with dynamic ultrasound guidance for central venous access *J Ultrasound Med.* 2009;28(9):1239–1244.

24. Levitov AB, Aziz S, Slonim AD. Before we go too far: ultrasound-guided central catheter placement. *Crit Care Med.* 2009;37(8):2473–2474.

25. Phelan M, Hagerty D. The oblique view: an alternative approach for ultrasound guided central line placement. *J Emerg Med.* 2008;37(4):403-8.

26. Mermel LA. Prevention of intravascular catheter-related infections. *Ann Intern Med.* 2000;132:391–402.

27. Mayo PH, Doelken P. Pleural ultrasonography. *Clin Chest Med.* 2006;27:215–227.

28. Sandhu NS. Transpectoral ultrasound-guided catheterization of the axillary vein: an alternative to standard catheterization of the subclavian vein. *Anesth Analg.* 2004;99:183–187.

29. Mackey SP, Sinha S, Pusey J. Ultrasound imaging of the axillary vein-anatomical basis for central access (letter). *Br J Anaesth.* 2003;93:598–599.

30. Galloway S, Bodenham A. Ultrasound imaging of the axillary vein-anatomical basis for central venous access. *Br J Anaesth.* 2003;90:589–595.

31. Sharma S, Bodenham AR, Mallick A. Ultrasound-guided infraclavicular axillary vein cannulation for central venous access. *Br J Anaesth.* 2004;93:188–192.

32. Bogin IN, Stulin ID. Application of the method of 2-dimensional echospondylography for determining landmarks in lumbar punctures. *Zh Nevropatol Psikhiatr Im S S Korsakova.* 1971;71(12):1810–1811.

33. Cork RC, Kryc JJ, Vaughan RW. Ultrasonic localization of the lumbar epidural space. *Anesthesiology.* 1980;52(6):513–516.

34. Currie JM. Measurement of the depth to the extradural space using ultrasound. *Br J Anaesth.* 1984;56(4):345–347.

35. Grau T, Leipold RW, Conradi R, Martin E, Motsch J. Efficacy of ultrasound imaging in obstetric epidural anesthesia. *J Clin Anesth.* 2002;14:169–175.

36. Grau T, Leipold RW, Conradi R, Martin E, Motsch J. Ultrasound imaging facilitates localization of the epidural space during combined spinal and epidural anesthesia. *Reg Anesth Pain Med.* 2001;26(1):64–67.

37. Grau T, Leipold RW, Fatehi S, Martin E, Motsch J. Real-time ultrasonic observation of combined spinal-epidural anaesthesia. *Eur J Anaesthesiol.* 2004;21(1):25–31.

38. Ferre RM, Sweeney TW, Strout TD. Ultrasound identification of landmarks preceding lumbar puncture: a pilot study. *Emerg Med J.* 2009;26(4):276–277.

39. Crogan DR, Irwin RS, Channick R. Complications associated with thoracentesis: a prospective, randomized study comparing three different methods. *Arch Intern Med.* 1990;150:873–877.

40. Weingarde JP, Guico RR, Nemcek AA Jr, Li YP, Chiu ST. Ultrasound findings following failed, clinically directed thoracentesis. *J Clin Ultrasound.* 1994;2:419–426.

41. Yang PC, Luh KT, Chang DB, et al. Value of sonography in determining the nature of pleural effusion: analysis of 320 cases. *AJR Am J Roentgenol.* 1992;159:29–33.

42. Vignon PV, Chastagner C, Berkane V, et al. Quantitative assessment of pleural effusion in critically ill patients by means of ultrasonography. *Crit Care Med.* 2005;33(8):1757–1763.

43. Nicolaou S, Talsky A, Khashoggi K, et al. Ultrasound guided interventional radiology in critical care. *Crit Care Med.* 2007;35(suppl):S186–S197.

44. Irwin RS, Rippe JM, Cerra, FB, Curley FJ, Heard, SO. *Procedures and Techniques in Intensive Care Medicine.* 3rd ed. Philadelphia, PA: Lippincott William & Wilkins;1999.

45. Feller-Kopman D. Ultrasound-guided thoracentesis. *Chest.* 2006;129:1709–1714.

46. Lichtenstein D. Ultrasound in the management of thoracic disease. *Crit Care Med.* 2007;35(5):S250–S261.

47. Reissig A, Kroegel C. Accuracy of transthoracic sonography in excluding post-interventional pneumothorax and hydropneumothorax comparison to chest radiography. *Eur J Radiol.* 2005;53(3):463–470.

48. Feller-Kopman D, Berkwitz D, Boiselle P, et al. Large-volume thoracentesis and the risk of re-expansion pulmonary edema. *Ann Thorac Surg.* 2007;84:1656–1662.

49. Nazeer SR, Dewbre H, Miller AH. Ultrasound-assisted paracentesis performed by emergency physicians vs the traditional technique: a prospective randomized study. *Am J Emerg Med.* 2005;23(30):363–367.

50. Chongtham DS, Singh MM, Kalantri SP, Pathak S, Jain AP. Accuracy of clinical maneuvers in detection of minimal ascites. *J Indian J Med Sci.* 1998;52:514–520.

51. Bard C, Lafortune M, Breton G. Ascites: ultrasound guidance or blind paracentesis? *CMAJ.* 1986;135:209–210.

52. Thomsen TW, Shaffer RW, White B, et al. Videos in clinical medicine paracentesis. *N Engl J Med.* 2006;355(19):e21.

53. Goldberg BB, Goodman GA, Clearfield HR. Evaluation of ascites assisted by ultrasound. *Radiology.* 1970;96:15–22.

54. Rumack CM, Wilson SR, Charboneau JW. *Diagnostic Ultrasound.* 3rd ed. St. Louis, MO: Elsevier Mosby;1998.

55. Levitov AB, Aziz S, Slonim AD. Before we go too far: ultrasound guided central line placement. *Crit Care Med.* 2009;37:2473–2474.

56. Webster ST, Brown KL, Lucey MR, et al. Hemorrhagic complications of large volume abdominal paracentesis. *Am J Gastroenterol.* 1996;91(2):366–368.

57. Thorwarth, Jr, WT(Editorial panel chair). Current Procedural Terminology (professional edition). Chicago: AMA press/Elsevier; 2009.

CHAPTER 19

Ultrasound Use in Pediatrics

William T. Tsai, MD and Anthony D. Slonim, MD, DrPH

INTRODUCTION

Ultrasound use is gaining popularity for bedside clinicians who wish to enhance their patients' physical examination. It is particularly useful for conditions of the head and neck, chest, abdomen, and extremities when a clinician has a specific diagnostic question or etiology that needs to be assessed. For a long time, ultrasound use has been a technology restricted to the purview of radiologists; now, it has expanded to obstetrics and gynecology, cardiology, anesthesiology, and critical care. As time progresses, it will surely establish a firm foothold in general medicine and, as described in this chapter, pediatrics.

THE DISCIPLINE OF PEDIATRICS

While there are many similarities between the disciplines of internal medicine and pediatrics, there are some important differences that have relevance to the use of ultrasound. Pediatric medicine considers both the patient and the parent or guardian as the "unit of treatment." The clinician must realize that the pediatric patient exists within a large spectrum of developmental levels. This impacts the clinician's ability to derive important historical information and his or her approach to the patient for a physical examination. Because of insufficient historical information and limitations of the clinical examination, ultrasound provides a valuable resource for pediatric patients. The consent for procedures or an examination is usually implied or granted by the guardian, but for children able to understand, appropriate assent should also be obtained from the child. Finally, one of the major benefits of ultrasound use is that it is noninvasive and painless. Nonetheless, children may be frightened by the examination itself, whether or not it engenders pain. This may be difficult for the clinician, since a child's crying may be due to many underlying causes including pain, fear, or stress.

The approach to the history and physical examination of a child requires a certain level of skill and experience to obtain a thorough assessment and interpret the information to determine if further diagnostic testing is necessary. When physical examination findings are limited because of the patient's developmental level or pain, the clinician has to determine whether the differential diagnoses are of significant enough risk to the child to warrant additional testing, recognizing that the additional testing has its own risks and benefits. Having the diagnostic equipment readily available for use by the bedside clinician provides an important method of immediately validating or refuting a diagnosis. Recently, diagnostic studies in pediatric patients that use ionizing radiation, like computerized tomography, have come under scrutiny because of their relationship to future malignancies. Ultrasound avoids this problem.

The use of ultrasonography holds great promise as an adjunct in the general physical examination of pediatric patients. Ultrasound is safe, established, and useful for the diagnosis of both simple and complex conditions. Children should very likely accept the use of the ultrasound probe and the viewing screen with relatively little distress during the examination session. Ultrasound can augment the physical examination and add to the clinician's confidence and precision when he or she is diagnosing a clinical condition or performing invasive procedures.

THE PEDIATRIC PATIENT

Disease processes in pediatrics are age specific. While it is true that a great number of disease processes, such as pneumonia, extend quite equally through the age spectrum and into adulthood, many disease processes in pediatrics, for example pyloric stenosis and congenital heart disease, are age specific.

For the bedside clinician, the age-specific nature of diseases in children requires an ability to formulate an appropriate differential diagnosis and direct the collection of ultrasonographic data. This focused physical examination applies not only to the hands-on physical examination but also to the focused ultrasonographic examination.

In addition to age-specific disease, the pediatrician must navigate age-specific development and use it to his or her advantage during the ultrasound examination. The pediatrician must be prepared to address the challenges of patient cooperation and to understand the anxiety associated with the examination based on the child's age. When using the ultrasound probe, the clinician must be prepared to use techniques for examining children and apply these to the ultrasonographic examination.

TECHNIQUES FOR FACILITATING ULTRASOUND EXAMINATION IN CHILDREN

A quiet and cooperative pediatric patient is optimal for the general ultrasonographic examination. However, this may not always be the case, and certain techniques to facilitate ultrasound examination in children may be employed.

Most children undergo sonography without difficulty. Infants and neonates should have examinations performed with a warm probe, preferably in the arms of the parent or caregiver to maintain the warm, comfortable setting of a caregiver's embrace. In infants who are crying vigorously but require a quiet examination such as in echocardiography, a sucrose solution can be used quite successfully as a calming agent. In addition, allowing the infant to breast-feed or drink from a bottle, if not contraindicated by the possible diagnoses, may enhance the sonographic examination. Toddlers and school-aged children are fascinated by the television image and usually have no problem with the ultrasound machine. All the probes employed in pediatrics are nonthreatening and can be handled by the child without a concern for damaging them.

In a relatively cooperative child, care should be given to completing the better tolerated portions of the examination prior to the more invasive portions. This may differ based on the individual personality of the child, but, in general, a cardiac ultrasound examination may need to be performed prior to speculum examination of the ears so that the patient is not agitated. In the older patient, a brief description of the ultrasound machine and examination is usually all that is necessary for the examination to be successful.

The use of moderate sedation should be reserved for the rarest of circumstances, and probably plays no role in the routine ultrasonographic examination of patients.

SPECIFIC USES OF ULTRASOUND IN CHILDREN

Head and Neck Ultrasound

Routine ultrasound of the head and neck generally is not necessary in the pediatric patient, but specific disease processes may arise in which ultrasound examination is useful (Table 19.1). The investigation of lumps and bumps of the neck may be facilitated by sonography. In a child with diffuse neck swelling, sonography may be helpful to differentiate between lymphadenitis, cervical abscess, or cystic hygroma. Midline neck lesions may reveal a fluid-filled lesion consistent with an ectopic thyroid. Ultrasound facilitates examination because gentle pressure is often all that is needed for diagnosis, while the standard physical examination may require more extensive palpation, possibly resulting in pain, a less than optimal examination, and a lack of specificity about the diagnosis. Normal ultrasound of the neck will reveal normal fat, muscle, and fascial planes, while abnormal studies may reveal fluid collections, cobblestoning, or enlarged nodes.

The endocavitary probe may be used for the intraoral ultrasound of a peritonsillar abscess. Use of the endocavitary probe requires careful topical anesthesia of the oropharynx but may assist the clinician with the diagnosis of cellulitis or abscesses and will provide guidance for the clinician prior to performing needle aspiration of a peritonsillar abscess.

Routine ultrasound of the neck is generally unnecessary but may be useful in the assessment of thyroid size, size and relationship of neck vessels, and assessment of masses for the child in whom these are a concern.

TABLE 19.1. Conditions of the Head and Neck in Children That Are Benefitted by the Use of Ultrasound
Lymphadenitis
Neck abscess
Cystic hygroma
Branchial cleft cysts
Thyroid cysts
Thyroglossal duct cysts
Torticollis
Peritonsillar abscess

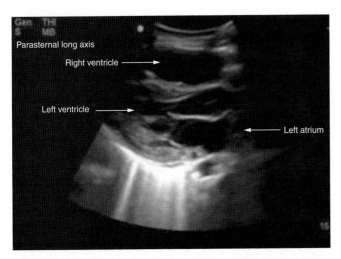

Figure 19.1. Normal parasternal long-axis view of the heart demonstrating the cardiac chambers in a child.

A high-frequency linear transducer is useful in the assessment of the soft tissues of the neck. For smaller children, transducers with smaller footprints are available that allow the clinician to insonate the small areas and crevices seen in the neck. In general, frequencies of 10 to 15 MHz are necessary depending on the depth of penetration. Color Doppler is useful in differentiating a fluid collection from the flow seen in the neck vessels.

Cardiac Ultrasound

Routine ultrasound of the heart may play a prominent role in the standard examination of the pediatric patient (Figs. 19.1 and 19.2). Its use may augment the physical examination and enhance standard cardiac

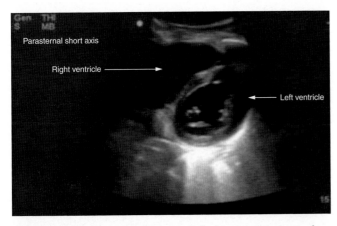

Figure 19.2. Normal parasternal short-axis view of the heart demonstrating the cardiac chambers in a child.

assessment by providing specific information on chamber number, chamber function, and the presence of pericardial effusion. More advanced assessment may take the form of identifying intra-atrial or intra-ventricular communications or using Doppler analysis in the assessment of intracardiac shunts, valve regurgitation, or vessel or outflow tract stenosis.

In the ill child, focused echocardiography is useful. The need to assess cardiac function may be underestimated in the acute care setting. Focused echocardiography, a limited echocardiogram that has as its goal the hemodynamic assessment of gross ventricular function, pericardial tamponade, ventricular dilation, and volume status, may help in guiding patient management (Table 19.2).

Spurney demonstrated that with limited training and limited echocardiographic views, noncardiologist physicians are capable of diagnosing significant pericardial effusions, decreased left ventricular systolic function, and left ventricular enlargement. Even more important is that focused bedside echocardiography offers the clinician the ability to perform repeat bedside examinations, which enables the assessment and reassessment of the adequacy and efficacy of therapy.

Thoracic Ultrasound

Routine thoracic assessment is not useful in the standard physical examination of children. However, focused thoracic ultrasound is quite helpful in identifying general pathologic conditions in pediatrics.

While initially it seems that ultrasound of the chest would be limited to the evaluation of pleural effusion, since a lung filled with air is a poor medium for ultrasound waves, lung ultrasound is quite useful in the pediatric intensive care unit for evaluating pneumothorax, effusion, and pulmonary edema.

TABLE 19.2. The Data Evaluated During a Focused Echocardiographic Examination of a Child
Chamber number
Intracardiac shunts
Cardiac function assessment
Left ventricular enlargement
Pericardial effusion
Inferior vena cava dynamics

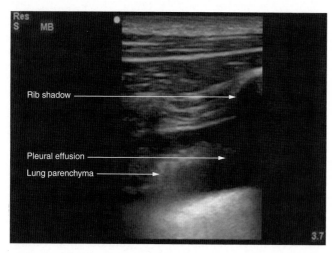

Figure 19.3. A pleural effusion can be differentiated from the lung tissue.

The assessment of pleural effusion is useful in the acute care setting because it provides timely information about the size, quality, and location of pleural effusions. In patients who are predisposed to hemodynamically significant pleural effusions, rapid assessment and procedural ultrasound-assisted drainage may be emergent and lifesaving (Fig. 19.3).

Assessments of complicated pneumonias (Fig. 19.4) can be performed quite rapidly with ultrasound and may affect the clinical management at the bedside. In distinction to standard chest x-rays, ultrasound readily identifies patients with effusion and helps to distinguish effusion from consolidation. In patients with pneumonia

with effusion, early video-assisted thoracoscopy may be necessary in the patient's management, and the use of ultrasound can help to direct this therapy. Ultrasound can also be used to characterize the quality of the fluid by distinguishing a transudate from an exudate. In children with transudative effusions, the echocardiographic picture is quite lucent with very little echogenicity within the fluid. In patients with an exudate, the echocardiographic picture is quite echogenic and may appear complex. This information can impact the management of these patients.

Pneumothorax

The assessment of pneumothorax is extremely useful and provides timely information regarding patients with thoracic air leaks. Pleural sliding or shimmering occurs on thoracic ultrasound when the visceral and parietal pleura are apposed to one another and are sliding past each other with movements of the diaphragm or mechanical ventilation (Fig. 19.5). Dynamic images of pleural sliding are quite striking, and its presence denotes the mobile apposition of the visceral pleura with the parietal pleura. The lack of sliding, however, does not prove pneumothorax, and the clinician must proceed through the differential diagnosis for the lack of lung sliding (Table 19.3).

Once it has been determined that the lack of lung sliding is due to pneumothorax, the transducer can be moved over the hemithorax to determine the extent of pneumothorax and whether the pneumothorax is loculated. Thoracic ultrasound can help determine the best and safest place to insert a chest tube or pigtail drain.

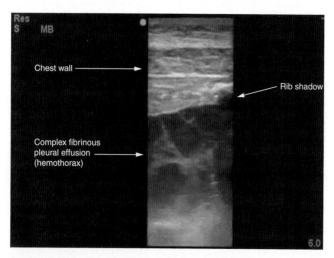

Figure 19.4. A complex pleural effusion is demonstrated.

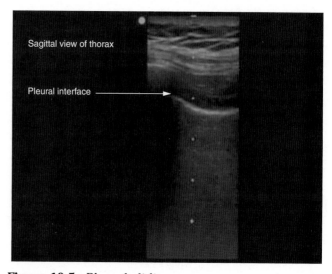

Figure 19.5. Pleural sliding.

TABLE 19.3. Differential Diagnosis for the Absence of Pleural Sliding
Pneumothorax
Pleural effusion
Pleural scarring
Poor respiratory effort
Mainstem intubation
Mainstem occlusion

TABLE 19.4. Conditions Visualized in Ultrasound of the Abdomen
Hepatomegaly
Splenomegaly
Ascites
Free intraperitoneal fluid
Kidney architecture
Bladder volume
Pyloric stenosis
Intussusception
Gallbladder disease
Abdominal masses

Abdominal Ultrasound

Much can be learned from an ultrasound of the abdominal cavity. The use of sonography may augment the routine physical examination by enabling the physician to assess liver span and spleen size in more objective ways than are currently available by the physical examination. For organs not immediately palpable, like the kidneys, ultrasound provides definitive bedside information. In pathologic conditions, ultrasound can reveal ascites, free intraperitoneal fluid (Fig. 19.6), renal pathology, liver and gallbladder pathology, uterine and ovarian pathology, intestinal pathology, and the assessment of pregnancy. With increasing experience, specific conditions such as appendicitis, pyloric stenosis, and intussusception can be identified (Table 19.4).

In the acute care setting, ultrasound is effective in determining whether free intraperitoneal fluid is present. The use of focused abdominal sonography for trauma (FAST) is quick, avoids ionizing radiation, and provides information regarding the presence of intraperitoneal blood or pericardial tamponade with four basic views of the abdomen (Chapter 10).

Musculoskeletal

Ultrasound use for the diagnosis of musculoskeletal conditions is increasing as clinicians become familiar with its use as an adjunct to the physical examination. Table 19.5 lists musculoskeletal conditions amenable to use of ultrasound. In particular, the assessment and differentiation of cellulitis and abscess are particularly valuable. With the increased incidence of methicillin-resistant *Staphylococcus aureus* infections in outpatient settings, the ability to differentiate between cellulitis and an abscess helps to determine management

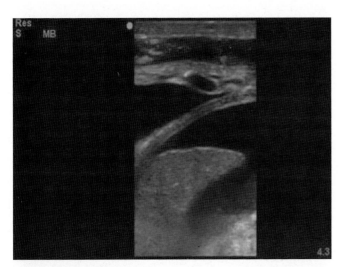

Figure 19.6. Abdominal ultrasound of left upper quadrant demonstrating significant ascites and pleural effusion. Note the clear view of the diaphragm separating fluid collections.

TABLE 19.5. Musculoskeletal Conditions Visualized on Ultrasound
Cellulitis
Abscess
Foreign body
Cysts
Fracture
Joint effusions

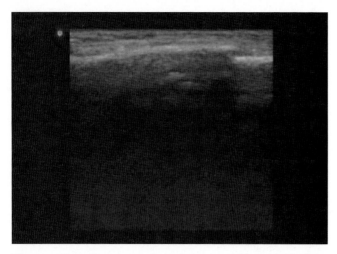

Figure 19.7. Fracture of the fifth metacarpal. The ultrasound shows a "stepoff" in the brightly echogenic cortex.

with the institution of antibiotics or whether an incision and drainage may be necessary. Ultrasound is very useful in assisting with this assessment. The depth, width, and proximity of adjacent structures can be readily assessed with ultrasonography and can be performed relatively painlessly.

The assessment of fractures from musculoskeletal injuries demonstrates some promise as an alternative to x-ray but is still being developed. The images may reveal distortions in the periosteum (Fig. 19.7) of the affected bone and may also reveal a surrounding hematoma or impingement on neurovascular structures.

The identification of radiolucent foreign bodies in the soft tissue has also become more common because of the distinct advantages over the use of static radiography and real-time fluoroscopy. Identification of organic or plastic material is quite simple with ultrasonographic guidance and assists the clinician in its localization and removal.

Procedures

While ultrasound has been extremely useful and has become a mainstream technology for procedural guidance in medical specialties such as anesthesia, critical care, and emergency medicine, it also has a role in the generalist's office. Not only can ultrasound assist in intravenous line placement by more accurately identifying the vein's location in the extremity, at the antecubital fossa, or above the antecubital fossa, but it can

also enhance vein visualization and palpation in patients with excessive adipose tissue. A bladder assessment prior to urinary catheterization may assist in eliminating unnecessary catheters due to "dry" catheterizations (Fig. 19.8). Finally, ultrasound has been used for quite some time in the placement of more invasive catheters into the deep veins, arteries, thoracic cavities, peritoneal cavities, and pericardial spaces of pediatric patients.

FUTURE

The use of ultrasound has revolutionized the practice of pediatric medicine. While its use by the generalist still remains limited in the United States, a systematic program teaching future physicians the basic principles and application of ultrasound to general pediatric patients will result in breakthroughs at every level of clinician experience. In the future, comprehensive physical examination with the aid of ultrasonography will help clinicians assess their patients and enhance their abilities to identify conditions requiring treatment. In emergency acute care settings, ultrasound use has been well-demonstrated. Its noninvasive nature, reduced side effects, lower doses of ionizing radiation, and relatively simple use will enhance the practice of future generations of physicians.

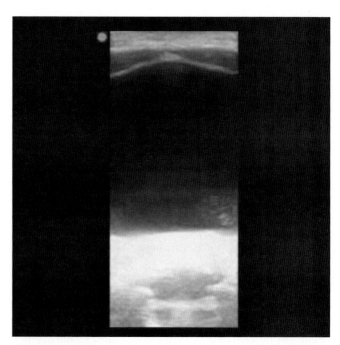

Figure 19.8. Transverse scan of the bladder demonstrating a urine-filled bladder.

Suggested Readings

Alderson PJ, Burrows FA, Stemp LI, Holtby HM. Use of ultrasound to evaluate internal jugular vein anatomy and to facilitate central venous cannulation in paediatric patients. *Brit J Anaesth.* 1993;70:145.

Ballard RB, Rozycki GS, Knudson MM, Pennington SD. The surgeon's use of ultrasound in the acute setting. *Surg Clin North Am.* 1998;78(2):337–364.

Baumann BM, McCans K, Stahmer SA, Leonard MB, Shults J, Holmes WC. Caregiver and health care provider satisfaction with volumetric bladder ultrasound. *Acad Emerg Med.* 2007;14(10):903–907.

Ceneviva G, Paschall JA, Maffei F, et al. Hemodynamic support in fluid-refractory pediatric septic shock. *Pediatrics.* 1998;102:e19.

Cervellione RM, Corroppolo M, Bianchi A. Subclinical varicocele in the pediatric age group. *J Urol.* 2008;179(2):717–719; discussion 719.

Chen L, Kim Y, Santucci KA. Use of ultrasound measurement of the inferior vena cava diameter as an objective tool in the assessment of children with clinical dehydration. *Acad Emerg Med.* 2007;14(10):841–845.

Galicinao J, Bush AJ, Godambe SA. Use of bedside ultrasonography for endotracheal tube placement in pediatric patients: a feasibility study. *Pediatrics.* 2007;120:1297.

Ganesh A, Kaye R, Cahill AM, et al. Evaluation of ultrasound-guided radial artery cannulation in children. *Pediatr Crit Care Med.* 2009;10(1):45–48.

Giss SR, Dobrilovic N, Brown RL, Garcia VF. Complications of nonoperative management of pediatric blunt hepatic injury: diagnosis, management, and outcomes. *J Trauma.* 2006;61(2):334–339.

Gudinchet F. Multimodality imaging evaluation of the pediatric neck: techniques and spectrum of findings. *Radiographics.* 2005;25(4):931–948.

Hartas GA, Tsounias E, Gupta-Malhotra M. Approach to diagnosing congenital cardiac disorders. *Crit Care Nurs Clin North Am.* 2009;21(1):27–36.

Hoppe B, Kemper MJ. Diagnostic examination of the child with urolithiasis or nephrocalcinosis. *Pediatr Nephrol.* 2008;25:403–413.

Klein MD. Clinical approach to a child with abdominal pain who might have appendicitis. *Pediatr Radiol.* 2007;37(1):11–14.

Lugo-Vicente H, Ortíz VN, Irizarry H, Camps JI, Pagán V. Pediatric thyroid nodules: management in the era of fine needle aspiration. *J Pediatr Surg.* 1998;33(8):1302–1305.

Maecken T, Grau T. Ultrasound imaging in vascular access. *Crit Care Med.* 2007;35:S17.

Menon SC, Ackerman MJ, Cetta F, O'Leary PW, Eidem BW. Significance of left atrial volume in patients < 20 years of age with hypertrophic cardiomyopathy. *Am J Cardiol.* 2008;102(10):1390–1393.

Merx MW, Weber C. Sepsis and the heart. *Circulation.* 2007;116:793.

Meuwly JY, Lepori D, Theumann N, et al. Sonographic assessment of the normal limits and percentile curves of liver, spleen, and kidney dimensions in healthy school-aged children. *J Ultrasound Med.* 2005;24(10):1359–1364.

Rudinger A, Singer M. Mechanisms of sepsis-induced cardiac dysfunction. *Crit Care Med.* 2007;35:1599.

Scaife ER, Fenton SJ, Hansen KW, Metzger RR. Use of focused abdominal sonography for trauma at pediatric and adult trauma centers: a survey. *J Pediatr Surg.* 2009;44(9):1746–1749.

Schiller NB, Shah PM, Crawford M, et al. Recommendations for quantitation of the left ventricle by two-dimensional echocardiography. American Society of Echocardiography Committee on Standards, Subcommittee on Quantitation of Two-Dimensional Echocardiograms. *J Am Soc Echocardiogr.* 1989;2:358.

Sivitz AB, Lam SH, Ramirez-Schrempp D, Valente JH, Nagdev AD. Effect of bedside ultrasound on management of pediatric soft-tissue infection. *J Emerg Med.* 2009 (in press).

Spurney CF, Sable CA, Berger JT, et al. Use of hand-carried ultrasound device by critical care physicians for the diagnosis of pericardial effusions, decreased cardiac function, and left ventricular enlargement in pediatric patients. *J Am Soc Echocardiogr.* 2005;18:313.

Steinberger J, Moller JH, Berry JM, Sinaiko AR. Echocardiographic diagnosis of heart disease in apparently healthy adolescents. *Pediatrics.* 2000;105(4 Pt 1):815–818.

Swischuk LE. Emergency pediatric imaging: changes over the years. Part II. *Emerg Radiol.* 2005;11(5):253–261.

Tatli B, Aydinli N, Caliskan M, Ozmen M, Bilir F, Acar G. Congenital muscular torticollis: evaluation and classification. *Pediatr Neurol.* 2006;34(1):41–44.

Thiru Y, Pathan N, Bignall S, et al. A myocardial cytotoxic process is involved in the cardiac dysfunction of meningococcal septic shock. *Crit Care Med.* 2000;28:2979.

Tsung JW, Blaivas M. Feasibility of correlating the pulse check with focused point-of-care echocardiography during pediatric cardiac arrest: a case series. *Resuscitation.* 2008;77(2):264–269.

Verghese ST, McGill WA, Patel RI, Sell JE, Midgley FM, Ruttimann UE. Ultrasound-guided internal jugular venous cannulation in infants: a prospective comparison with the traditional palpation method. *Anesthesiology.* 1999;91:71.

Verghese ST, McGill WA, Patel RI, Sell JE, Midgley FM, Ruttimann UE. Comparison of three techniques for internal jugular vein cannulation in infants. *Paediatr Anaesth.* 2000;10:505.

Yoo JH, Kwak HJ, Lee MJ, Suh JS, Rhee CS. Sonographic measurements of normal gallbladder sizes in children. *J Clin Ultrasound.* 2003;31(2):80–84.

BEDSIDE ULTRASONO-GRAPHY IN CLINICAL MEDICINE: PREPARING FOR AND ACHIEVING THE FUTURE STATE

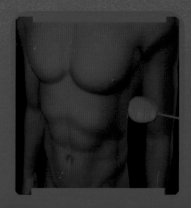

Education and Training in Portable Bedside Ultrasound: The Life Cycle of the Clinician

Richard C. Vari, PhD; Tarin A. Schmidt-Dalton, MD; Timothy A. Johnson, PhD; Apostolos P. Dallas, MD, FACP; Alexander B. Levitov, MD, FCCM, RDCS; and Anthony D. Slonim, MD, DrPH

PART 1: PORTABLE ULTRASOUND INTEGRATION INTO THE MEDICAL SCHOOL CURRICULUM

Richard C. Vari, PhD; Tarin A. Schmidt-Dalton, MD; and Timothy A. Johnson, PhD

The current utilization of ultrasound in medical education has primarily been directed at the residency level[1] or elective experiences offered to junior and senior medical students.[2–5] These experiences typically consist of didactic sessions that are designed to explain the principles of ultrasound, the advantages and disadvantages of ultrasound use in clinical medicine, and a description of how to operate the ultrasound devices. These sessions are followed by hands-on experiences with preceptors obtaining ultrasound images from various organ systems. In addition, opportunities for students to gain experience in ultrasound-guided vascular access and pelvic ultrasound have been offered. The technological progression to smaller, portable ultrasound devices has facilitated the development of experiences, courses, and integrated modules of clinical and basic science application in the earlier stages of undergraduate medical education.[5–7] Medical students, even during the first year of medical school, can demonstrate a high degree of technical competence with ultrasound and regard this training as a highly favorable experience.[4–10] Two medical schools have integrated portable ultrasound in a longitudinal fashion across the 4 years of their programs: Wayne State University School of Medicine[7] and the University of South Carolina.[11]

Some have referred to the portable ultrasound as the "stethoscope of the future"[3] because this device is being used for more and more procedures in medicine.

It is imperative, then, that medical students be trained in the appropriate use of these devices for their future careers. Application of portable ultrasound technology to instruction of the basic sciences, including anatomy, physiology, pathology, and physical examination of patients,[10] will enhance the education of students. The Virginia Tech Carilion School of Medicine (VTC), is the latest in a small group of medical schools to fully integrate a longitudinal ultrasound curriculum from the beginning of medical school.

PATIENT-CENTERED LEARNING AT THE VIRGINIA TECH CARILION SCHOOL OF MEDICINE

The patient-centered curriculum at VTC, when fully implemented, will be integrated across all 4 years of medical school. Knowledge and experience in four major educational "value domains" of professional development are provided using a variety of sound educational strategies to maximize student learning. These domains include Basic Sciences, Clinical Sciences and Skills, Research, and Interprofessionalism. Portable ultrasound education, training, and experience are integrated longitudinally over the 4 years and vertically across the four value domains and are delivered utilizing a variety of approaches including didactic presentations, small-group case learning objectives, hands-on demonstrations, cadaveric application in the anatomy laboratory, clinical skills sessions with standardized patients, interprofessional team exercises, and research projects. The portable ultrasound curriculum is based on formalized goals, objectives, and outcomes (Table 20.1) that are linked to the VTC Goals and Objectives document and the Accreditation Council for Graduate Medical Education core

TABLE 20.1. Virginia Tech Carilion School of Medicine (VTC) Portable Ultrasound Goals, Objectives, and Outcomes

These goals and objectives pertain to ultrasound and were taken from the VTC Goals and Objectives document that has all six Accreditation Council for Graduate Medical Education (ACGME) core competencies and the core areas identified by the Institute of Medicine (IOM) in their report on Health Professional Education (2003).

ACGME Core Competency: Patient Care
IOM Core Area: Patient-centered Care and Quality Improvement

Goal: Graduates will be physicians who are skilled in providing care to individual patients.

Objective 5: Students will acquire basic procedural clinical skills.

Outcomes: Graduates will be able to perform the following basic clinical skills including but not limited to:

Administering injections	Inserting and removing Foley catheters
Performing phlebotomy	Inserting, suctioning, and removing nasogastric tubes
Suturing	Starting intravenous and central venous lines
Performing lumbar punctures	Performing cardiopulmonary resuscitation
Applying casts	Scrubbing for surgery
Performing intubations	

Portable Ultrasound Goals and Objectives

Goal: Graduates will be equipped with:

- Understanding of the fundamental principles of medical ultrasound and image formation
- Basic knowledge of appropriate transducer manipulations
- Ability to incorporate ultrasound information into the examination and evaluation of patients
- Ability to communicate results to others and provide documentation for medical records

Objective: Graduates will acquire basic point-of-care ultrasound skills, incorporate ultrasound information in patient evaluation and procedural skills (ultrasound guidance), and use this information to improve care with emphasis on patient safety.

Outcomes: Graduates will be able to perform:
- Focused assessment of transthoracic echocardiography
- Vascular ultrasound and ultrasound-guided central and peripheral venous and arterial catheterizations
- General ultrasonography of the upper airway, chest, abdomen, retroperitoneal space, and small parts
- Ultrasound-guided thoracentesis, paracentesis, arthrocentesis, and lumbar puncture

competencies. Portable ultrasound competencies, appropriate to the level of student learning, are a part of the formal student assessment program.

The VTC patient-centered curriculum is divided into two main phases with multiple blocks varying in duration and content. Phase 1 begins with a 1-week orientation period, continues for nine consecutive blocks, and is chronologically similar to the first 2 years of medical school. The focus of the Basic Sciences curriculum during the first four blocks (Year 1) is on learning the normal structure and function of the human body. This is accomplished using an organ systems approach and a mixture of problem-based learning cases, lectures, discussion sessions, and laboratories. A typical weekly schedule for phase 1 is presented in Figure 20.1. Students meet in small groups (seven students) three times per week with a faculty facilitator and process written "paper" patient cases in a problem-based learning format. Lectures and laboratories, while reduced in number compared to more traditional medical curricula, support the learning objectives of these cases and overall block objectives. A major highlight of this curriculum occurs at the end of each week, when all of the students are assembled

	Monday	Tuesday	Wednesday	Thursday	Friday
8–9	Lecture	Lecture	Lecture	Lecture	Patient case work
9–10	Lecture	Lecture	Patient case work	Lecture	
10–11	Patient case work	Laboratory		Laboratory	Patient wrap-up
11–12					
12–1	Lunch	Lunch	Lunch	Lunch	Lunch
1–2	Research	Unscheduled	Research	Unscheduled	Research
2–3	Interprofessionalism		Clinical sciences		Clinical sciences
3–4					
4–5					

Figure 20.1. A typical weekly schedule during phase 1 at the Virginia Tech Carilion School of Medicine.

together at the "case wrap-up" session with an actual patient who has the disease that was studied in the patient case work that week and a physician. This experience provides an opportunity for the students to place their learning in the context of a real patient, to interact with the patient on a personal level, to extend their learning utilizing up-to-date best practices highlighted by the physician, and to observe positive physician role modeling. The second four blocks (Year 2) are focused on pathobiology and also use an organ systems approach. By using this approach in conjunction with patient cases in a problem-based learning format, an introduction to pathobiology becomes an added learning benefit while students are focused on normal structure and function in Year 1; and a review of normal structure and function while the students are focused on pathobiology in year 2 promotes student learning in a cumulative reinforcement educational model. This process of learning basic sciences is similar to other curricula currently in operation.[12,13]

Clinical Sciences and Skills is taught in phase 1 using multiple and varied approaches including lectures, panel discussions, movies and reflection, simulation models, standardized and real patients, and objectives in patient case-work cases. Students learn history taking and fundamental physical examination skills in Year 1 and then focus these skills on the pathologic symptoms of the various systems in Year 2. Also beginning in Year 1, each student is assigned to an ambulatory clinic and preceptor and attends this clinic for 2 half days every block: Longitudinal Ambulatory Care Experience. This experience continues throughout phase 1 and provides an immediate introduction to the clinical practice of medicine and a longitudinal opportunity for patient continuity, progressive assessment of clinical skills, and professional mentorship.

The fundamental principles and application of research are taught in Phase 1 using multiple and varied approaches including lectures, problems, experiential learning activities, and objectives in patient case-work cases. Students are exposed to researchers from various disciplines in a longitudinal seminar series entitled "Research Live." Students learn the basics of various techniques in structured research rotations. Students are guided in their self-selected project by a research mentor and small committee of basic and clinical scientists who will provide regular feedback to the students on their progress. Each student is required to complete a scholarly project that is hypothesis driven, provide a written document suitable for publication, and present his or her work in an appropriate venue.

Beginning in Phase 1 and continuing throughout the curriculum at VTC, the foundational principles and theoretical and practical application of interprofessionalism are intimately woven into the program. This value domain emphasizes activities that are focused on the development of professionalism in medical students, roles of the health profession, public health, acute and chronic disease, systems change, and patient safety.

Block IX of Phase 1 is a 14-week period during which students continue their research project S, enroll in selected transitional clinical experiences, participate in structured interprofessionalism activities that may include community-based service learning or global health programs, or take classes needed for the master of science degree.

Phase 2 begins in July of a typical Year-3 schedule and has students completing a series of rotations in the traditional clinical disciplines. Following block X, students are assessed on clinical and communication skills in a multistation objective structured clinical examination. This information is formative and used to help structure the student's experience in subsequent blocks of required clinical experiences and electives. Following the objective structured clinical examination, students will have 4 weeks to continue their research

projects and/or participate in interprofessionalism activities. Specific attention is devoted to ensuring that basic science concepts are revisited in phase 2 in an integrated problem-solving manner involving patient cases and interactive sessions with basic science and clinical faculty. Beginning in July of the fourth year, students will complete a series of required and elective clinical experiences (block XI).

ULTRASOUND INTEGRATION INTO THE CURRICULUM

The integration of portable ultrasound objectives into Phase 1 is presented in Figure 20.2. In terms of basic sciences, the sessions in the first four blocks are devoted to understanding the fundamental concepts of ultrasound physics, familiarizing oneself with operational

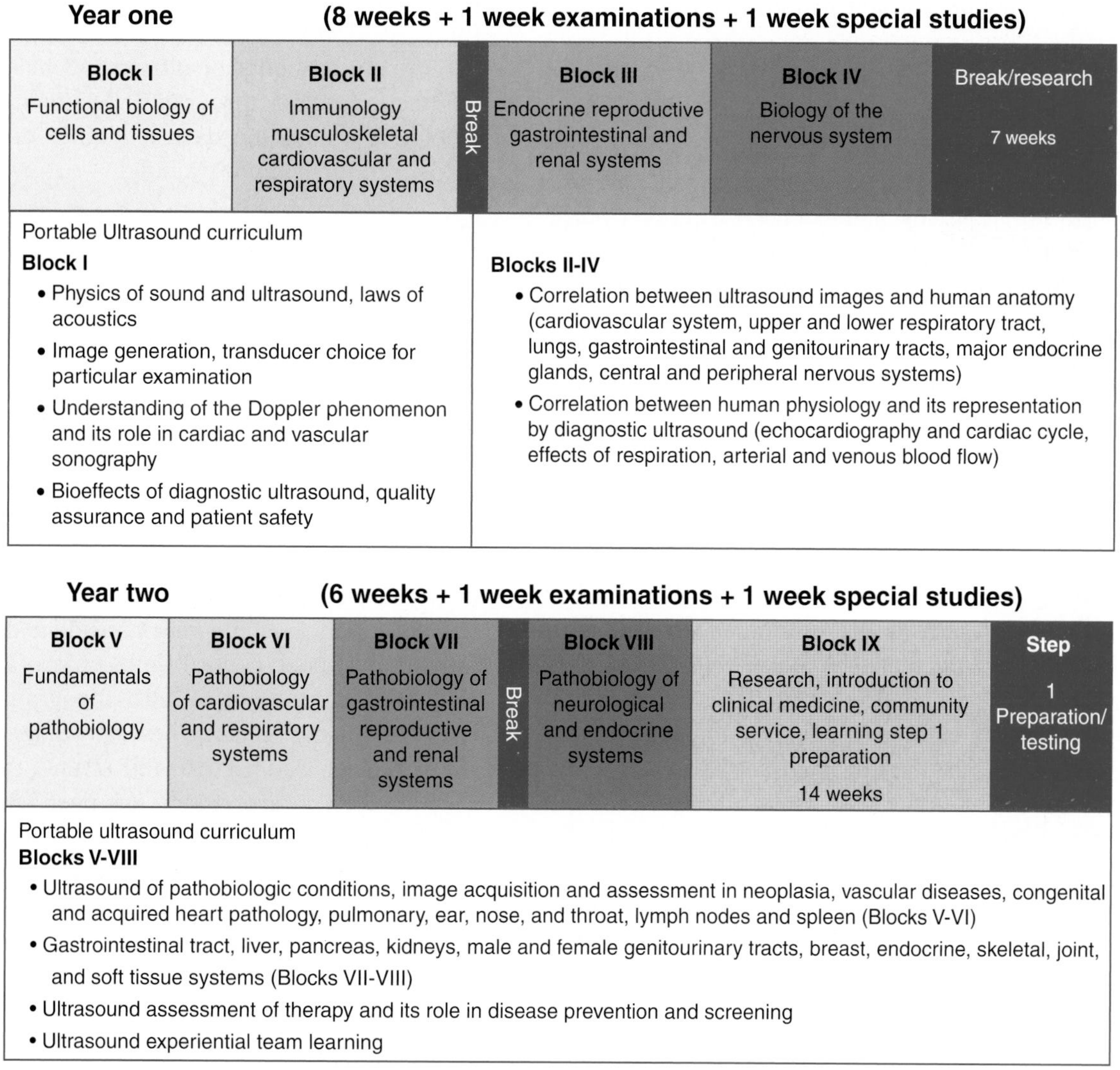

Year one   **(8 weeks + 1 week examinations + 1 week special studies)**

Block I	Block II	Break	Block III	Block IV	Break/research
Functional biology of cells and tissues	Immunology musculoskeletal cardiovascular and respiratory systems		Endocrine reproductive gastrointestinal and renal systems	Biology of the nervous system	7 weeks

Portable Ultrasound curriculum

Block I
- Physics of sound and ultrasound, laws of acoustics
- Image generation, transducer choice for particular examination
- Understanding of the Doppler phenomenon and its role in cardiac and vascular sonography
- Bioeffects of diagnostic ultrasound, quality assurance and patient safety

Blocks II-IV
- Correlation between ultrasound images and human anatomy (cardiovascular system, upper and lower respiratory tract, lungs, gastrointestinal and genitourinary tracts, major endocrine glands, central and peripheral nervous systems)
- Correlation between human physiology and its representation by diagnostic ultrasound (echocardiography and cardiac cycle, effects of respiration, arterial and venous blood flow)

Year two   **(6 weeks + 1 week examinations + 1 week special studies)**

Block V	Block VI	Block VII	Break	Block VIII	Block IX	Step
Fundamentals of pathobiology	Pathobiology of cardiovascular and respiratory systems	Pathobiology of gastrointestinal reproductive and renal systems		Pathobiology of neurological and endocrine systems	Research, introduction to clinical medicine, community service, learning step 1 preparation 14 weeks	1 Preparation/ testing

Portable ultrasound curriculum
Blocks V-VIII
- Ultrasound of pathobiologic conditions, image acquisition and assessment in neoplasia, vascular diseases, congenital and acquired heart pathology, pulmonary, ear, nose, and throat, lymph nodes and spleen (Blocks V-VI)
- Gastrointestinal tract, liver, pancreas, kidneys, male and female genitourinary tracts, breast, endocrine, skeletal, joint, and soft tissue systems (Blocks VII-VIII)
- Ultrasound assessment of therapy and its role in disease prevention and screening
- Ultrasound experiential team learning

Figure 20.2. Integration of portable ultrasound experiences into Phase 1 at the Virginia Tech Carilion School of Medicine.

aspects of the devices, and applying the technology to learning gross anatomy. Since the blocks are designed by organ systems, application of portable ultrasound technology will provide appropriate breadth of human anatomy and added depth of learning. The second year of Phase 1 is devoted to pathobiology, and the portable ultrasound integration is focused more on the abnormal structural findings associated with the various disease processes in a given organ system.

Portable ultrasound is not just restricted to learning anatomic structures and pathologic defects in the basic sciences. Application of portable ultrasound technology is a key element in teaching clinical skills. For example, a greater understanding of normal cardiac valve function, blood flow, and other cardiovascular physiologic processes can be gained through the visualization of ultrasound images. All of the organ systems in year 1 have particular structures that lend themselves to ultrasound applications. The use of ultrasound imaging to confirm abnormal physical findings (murmurs, consolidated lung, arterial bruits, etc.) will further enhance the understanding of pathology. These early experiences with ultrasound technology will lay the groundwork for expanded clinical skills applications of portable ultrasound in clinical rotations, required courses, and electives wherever possible in Phase 2. Certainly, the use of portable ultrasound will be an essential component in the critical care and radiology experiences.

As noted, ultrasound is a thread that runs through the full length of the curriculum at VTC. Initially, students are taught the basics of ultrasound including the theory of operation, clinical and research applications, unique capabilities, and application to instruction of basic sciences and clinical skills. Those curricular components are reinforced with hands-on experiences, first as a tool to better "see" and later as a tool to "probe." Along the way, students are instructed on new techniques provided by this technology and afforded an opportunity to develop appropriate skills using simulation manikins, standardized patients, and, indeed, themselves. As their skills mature and as their educational program advances, students will expand their use of this technology. For some, their research will utilize the most significant capabilities of ultrasound, either as an imaging tool or as a sophisticated measurement tool (cardiology, obstetrics/gynecology, surgery, etc.). Regardless of how advanced any student's course of study becomes, because of the integrated and longitudinal nature of the ultrasound curriculum at VTC, each graduate will view ultrasound as part of the physician's tool chest and an integral part of the medical landscape.

PART 2: GRADUATE MEDICAL EDUCATION AND BEYOND

Apostolos P. Dallas, MD, FACP; Alexander B. Levitov, MD, FCCM, RDCS; and Anthony D. Slonim, MD, DrPH

Graduate Medical Education

While medical student training in portable ultrasound is in its nascent stages with only a few medical schools offering any training and a scant few offering well-thought-out curricula, resident and fellow ultrasound education is more significantly advanced. In 1999, the American Medical Association affirmed that ultrasound imaging was within the scope of practice of appropriately trained physicians. The real question is the extent to which training programs are producing appropriately trained physicians. Certain specialties have embraced this training, even mandating it for their residents, while others have just begun to explore the benefits of ultrasound in their graduate medical education programs. Residency programs in emergency medicine have led other disciplines with respect to ultrasound training.

Emergency Medicine

The literature for ultrasound techniques and assistance in emergency medicine dates back over 15 years. The first emergency medicine ultrasound curriculum was published in 1994.[14] Since then, multiple studies have demonstrated the efficacy of ultrasound use in the emergency department. For instance, while no clear consensus exists for ultrasound-guided central venous catheter placement for emergency medicine residents, a novel training program composed of a brief Web-based instructional module and a practical session was effective in enhancing emergency resident competency in ultrasound-guided central venous catheter placement.[15] The focused assessment with sonography for trauma (FAST) examination is the best known technique for the evaluation of trauma with ultrasound. Although accuracy for FAST interpretation has been widely reported, the learning curve for emergency medicine residents had not been well described. Ma et al reported that over 18 months, the accuracy of FAST interpretation among emergency medicine residents increased steadily so that by 12 months (or 35 examinations), their accuracy approached previously reported accuracy rates.[16] A focused 6-hour echocardiography training course significantly improved emergency medicine residents' scores on written and practical examinations that tested essential components of goal-directed transthoracic echocardiography performance and interpretation,[17] and emergency medicine residents with appropriate training can accurately determine aortic diameter and the presence of abdominal aortic aneurysms.[18] Less-well-recognized or practiced techniques can be taught easily in emergency medicine residency programs. Ocular sonography, for instance, is highly accurate for diagnosing and ruling out ocular pathology such as penetrating globe injuries, foreign objects, retinal detachments, central retinal artery occlusions, lens dislocations, and increased intracranial pressure.[19,20]

Emergency medicine residents with structured ultrasound rotations, didactics, and mentors demonstrated improved performance on written examinations.[21] The more scans the residents performed, the better were their test scores; however, didactic training in excess of 15 hours produced no further improvement in resident test scores. The American College of Emergency Physicians published guidelines for ultrasonography in 2001.[22] Additionally, the Clinical Practice of Emergency Medicine (EM model) defines the scope and body of knowledge of the specialty.[23] This document, a collaborative effort of the American Board of Emergency Medicine, the Society for Academic Emergency Medicine, the American College of Emergency Physicians, the Council of Emergency Medicine Residency Directors, the Emergency Medicine Residents' Association, and the Residency Review Committee for Emergency Medicine, specifically states that bedside ultrasound is a necessary skill and is within the scope of practice of emergency medicine physicians. Despite this, a 2001 survey of 122 emergency programs found that while most residencies offer ultrasound training, it is variable and not uniform.[24] Because of this variability and because the EM model listed ultrasound but not the manner of teaching it, the same institutions developed the Scope of Training Task Force. Its goal was to define emerging areas of clinical importance including emergency medicine ultrasound and to address the issue of emergency medicine ultrasound training.[25] Besides teaching the technique itself, other concerns include quality assurance, performance, and reimbursement of emergency physician-performed ultrasonography.[26] Minimum training requirements exist and are being evaluated for their effectiveness.[27]

Obstetrics and Gynecology

Current practices in obstetrics and gynecology require the use of ultrasound. Residency programs do offer required training in obstetric ultrasound imaging, but education in gynecologic imaging is limited. Guidelines for obstetric/gynecology resident ultrasound training have been developed by the American College of Obstetrics and Gynecology, the International Society of Ultrasound in Obstetrics and Gynecology, the Association of Program Directors in Radiology, the American Institute of Ultrasound in Medicine (AIUM), and the Council on Resident Education in Obstetrics and Gynecology. These organizations suggest knowledge domains, but specific components of a structured curriculum are not defined. Comprehensive curricula have been developed to meet the AIUM accreditation standards such as that described by the University of New Mexico.[28]

Internal Medicine

The use of ultrasound in internal medicine training programs demonstrates significant variability. The use of ultrasound guidance for central venous catheter placement has been associated with fewer complications and improved success rates. A cross-sectional survey evaluating the frequency of ultrasound guidance for central venous catheter placement found than over 90% of residents at a teaching hospital used ultrasound for placement with a greater than 80% success rate.[29] Ultrasound training for central venous catheter placement has become a standard in some training programs. Internal medicine residents can be trained to image the abdominal aorta for aneurysms using portable ultrasound devices. After only three to four one-on-one sessions with an instructor, residents were able to measure abdominal aortic diameter within 5 mm of the instructor's measurements.[30] In the intensive care unit, after only a 3-hour didactic course and 5 hours of hands-on training, residents were able to adequately appraise left ventricular systolic dysfunction, left ventricular dilatation, right ventricular dilatation, pericardial effusion, and pleural effusion. The only case of tamponade was diagnosed by a resident.[31] In another study, residents' positive predictive values and sensitivities for echocardiography were slightly less than for echocardiographer-performed scans.[32] These authors concluded that training guidelines and competency evaluations were needed if these devices were to be used by nonechocardiographers for clinical decision making. Certainly, not all training is created equal. Limited training (4 hours didactic and 20 studies) made internal medicine residents more accurate predictors of elevated right atrial pressures with ultrasound than with physical examination alone.[33] Pilot studies have also shown the clinical impact of ultrasound in the ambulatory setting, where medical decisions were reinforced in 76% and changed in 40% of patients based on the use of ultrasound devices.[34]

While much evidence supports ultrasound use in internal medicine resident training, internal medicine residency programs and internal medicine organizations have not produced widespread, published curricula or national guidelines. Such guidelines would expand the use of a significant tool in the internist's diagnostic and therapeutic armamentarium.

Anesthesia

Portable ultrasound use in anesthesia has centered mostly on its use in nerve blocks. During resident teaching, ultrasound-aided peripheral nerve–stimulated blocks required less time for completion than did nerve stimulator–guided blocks.[35] Ultrasound use resulted in fewer needle insertions and vessel punctures. Anesthesia residents were able to independently identify a series of anatomic structures in a live model using ultrasound after a 4-week regional anesthesia rotation that incorporated a standardized ultrasound curriculum for peripheral nerve blockade.[36] Recently, the American Society of Regional Anesthesia and Pain Medicine and the European Society of Regional Anaesthesia and Pain Therapy Joint Committee published recommendations for education and training in ultrasound-guided regional anesthesia.[37] Recommendations included residency-based pathways for obtaining training to gain the knowledge and skills necessary for clinical competence in ultrasound-guided regional anesthesia. Didactic and experiential components were seen as necessary, and mechanisms to oversee training and to ensure quality through peer review were also highlighted.

Surgery

Ultrasound has many uses in surgery. To facilitate its application in surgical practice, the American College of Surgeons developed an ultrasound educational program. These courses, geared toward practicing surgeons, have been both popular and effective.[38] A handful of residency training programs have also incorporated this educational tool. The FAST examination has standardized ultrasound use in trauma. Surgical residents have also proven to be as accurate (94%) as radiologists in recognizing echogenicity, diameter, and margin criteria of patients' breast lesions and in differentiating between benign and malignant

lesions.[39] Ultrasound has become indispensable not only for breast lesions but also for a variety of breast problems.[40] After only 1 hour of introduction to abdominal ultrasound, surgeons in training performed valid and reliable ultrasound examinations of the gallbladder in patients admitted with acute abdominal pain.[41]

Clearly, ultrasound training in graduate medical education represents a wide continuum from mandated to helpful to hardly explored. With the advent of smaller, more portable machines, a more knowledgeable faculty, the continued development of curricula, and additional support from national organizations through guidelines, portable ultrasound teaching will continue to expand in graduate medical education.

BEYOND GRADUATE MEDICAL EDUCATION

While undergraduate and graduate medical education programs provide structures to achieve the educational objectives associated with bedside ultrasound use for medical students, residents, and fellows, the structures for postgraduate training and education are not so neatly defined, nor are the specific objectives, knowledge base, skills, and aptitudes for using ultrasound in patient care. The result is that individual institutions determine their own guidelines for credentialing and privileging providers in these techniques and considerable variability at the bedside results.

A few important concepts are germane to any discussion of new techniques that physicians are interested in adding to their repertoire of privileges. Competence is the knowledge, skill, and ability to use ultrasound for patient benefit. It is usually defined by major professional societies as the standards that will be upheld. Unfortunately, many professional societies have not provided specific guidance, and because ultrasound can be used across multiple medical specialties, there are no overriding standards across specialties. Certification is the process by which competence is recognized. In the United States, there is no certifying body for bedside ultrasound use; hence, a process for certification detailing the criteria and standards does not exist. Credentialing is a process whereby a hospital or specific entity validates the training, certifications, and licenses to perform work. Privileging is a more specific aspect of the medical staff function that highlights the specific activities that the provider can perform. This is usually displayed in a list, and hospitals will usually require some information as to the provider's competence and credentials to perform those procedures. Usually, this is satisfied by successful completion of appropriately credentialed undergraduate and graduate medical education programs. However, when the provider obtains skills after formal training, and there are no nationally accepted standards, variability in the process emerges. Training is the method of obtaining the necessary knowledge and skills to be able to perform ultrasound. There are a of very well done and independent courses that provide physicians with the knowledge and skills for performing bedside ultrasound. Without certification of these training programs, however, inconsistency in the knowledge and skills of providers will remain, and local hospitals will be left to their own methods in determining competence. A more deliberate approach is needed for ensuring that patients are cared for by providers who know how to use these techniques safely and effectively for patient care and have demonstrated those abilities.

Any effort at defining training for attending physicians must acknowledge the time, cost, and opportunity costs of taking time away from practice to obtain the necessary skills. Ultrasound training requires both cognitive and practical components, and not everyone needs to know how to use ultrasound for diagnosis across all body regions. A simple approach might be to identify what areas of a physician's practice can be enhanced with the use of ultrasound and for the physician to learn, practice, and become proficient in those areas with the most value. For example, intensive care practitioners can benefit from ultrasound use for guiding invasive procedures. Rheumatologists may benefit from musculoskeletal ultrasound, and pediatricians may want to focus on cardiac imaging. Reading about these techniques, learning about them in "mini-fellowship programs," and practicing them under supervision are all useful methods for achieving competence. Without standardized programs for certification, learners must maintain careful records of what they learned and how many procedures they performed so that they can provide this documentation to their local institution during the credentialing and privileging process.

Training

Ultrasound training requires that the learner get experience in the basics of ultrasound physics, using the equipment, troubleshooting its problems, and ensuring the necessary skills for the adequate acquisition of images. One of the major benefits of bedside ultrasound is that the physician performing the procedure is the same person obtaining the images; however, this is also one of the major limitations of bedside ultrasound. Hands-on training is essential in achieving familiarity with these devices and being successful in acquiring images. Physicians inexperienced in image acquisition have a duty to ensure that the image is of sufficient quality to make a diagnosis or to appropriately refer the patient for better images or diagnostic testing so that diagnostic errors are not made. In addition, the physician needs to be cognizant of the biases inherent with having performed other elements of the assessment himself or herself. Taking a history and performing a physical examination provide important information related to the differential diagnosis. They can also bias the physician's interpretation of the ultrasound images.

While obtaining good-quality images is critical for diagnosis, it is insufficient. The bedside sonographer also needs to be proficient in image interpretation. A working knowledge of the regional anatomy is critical as a foundational element. Understanding the three-dimensional anatomic relationships and their ultrasonographic representation is also essential and takes practice. The ultrasonographer-clinician must be able to identify artifacts and recognize his or her own limitations in terms of image interpretation, referring to an expert or consulting with a radiologist when there is doubt.

Training Programs

This book was organized as a guide for the novice physician-ultrasonographer. It was intended as a "how to" manual that would allow physicians, at different points in their lives, either as medical students, residents, fellows, or postgraduate attending physicians, to have the essential knowledge elements in one place while they gain proficiency with bedside ultrasound. Importantly, the book does not need to be read from "front to back." After mastering the basic principles in Section 1, readers can skip to other sections, depending on the relevance to their practice. This book also provides only one aspect of training. Mastery of ultrasound use at the bedside can be accomplished only with practice. Holding the probe, maneuvering the dials, and manipulating the images are all important parts of training and developing confidence and competence in ultrasound use. Readers are encouraged to incorporate this book with practical experiences, either in a formalized course or under supervision in their own institutions that provide them with the practical tools for performing these procedures.

Level 1

Cognitive skills should include:

• A basic knowledge of ultrasound physics

• Understanding of the indications for the examination

• A basic knowledge of appropriate transducer choices and manipulations

• Basic spatial orientation and anatomic relationships

• Basic ability to distinguish adequate and inadequate images

• Ability to distinguish between anatomic structures, positions, and pathology

• Ability to communicate results to others and provide documentation for medical records

Training requirements should include but not be limited to:

• For physicians already in practice, 32 hours of formal ultrasound education

• For physicians in training, a 1-month rotation in point-of-care ultrasound

• Perform and interpret 25 supervised ultrasounds per body region or procedure

• Progress to level 2 within 1 year

Skills necessary to demonstrate level 1 competence:

• Ability to independently choose proper transducer and ultrasound system settings to perform an ultrasound on that body region

• Performance of an adequate bedside two-dimensional examination

• Ability to independently obtain adequate two-dimensional images

• Demonstration of competence to distinguish between normal and abnormal structures

• Ability to incorporate knowledge obtained from bedside study into the care of patients

• Letter from supervising physician attesting to level 1 competence

Level 2

Cognitive skills should include:

• All requirements for level 1 competence

• Detailed knowledge of ultrasound physics, including Doppler (continuous wave, pulsed, and color)

• Detailed knowledge of appropriate transducer choice and manipulations

• An advanced ability to distinguish adequate and inadequate images

• An ability to assess normal and abnormal arterial and venous flow patterns

• An advanced ability to recognize pathologic correlates of disease

Training requirements should include but not be limited to:

• For physicians already in practice, an additional 32 hours of formal ultrasound education

• For physicians in training, an additional 1-month rotation in point-of-care ultrasound

• Perform and interpret an additional 25 supervised and 25 unsupervised ultrasounds including continuous wave, pulsed, and color flow Doppler studies

• All unsupervised procedures are subject to random review by a level 3 mentor or supervisor

• Procedures resulting in an inability to reach diagnosis, misreads, or complications are subject to mandatory review by a level 3 mentor or supervisor

Skills necessary to demonstrate level 2 competence:

• Ability to independently choose proper transducer and ultrasound system settings to perform an ultrasound on the specified body region

• Performance of adequate bedside two-dimensional and Doppler examinations

• Ability to independently obtain adequate two-dimensional images and Doppler flow velocity measurements for specified examinations

Figure 20.3. A model training program describing the knowledge, training, and skills needed for three levels of competence in bedside ultrasound. This approach provides a template that can be applied to each body region.

- Competence to distinguish between normal and abnormal structures and blood flow patterns
- Ability to diagnose common pathologic conditions relevant to that body region
- Ability to incorporate knowledge from the bedside study into the care of patients
- Letter from supervising physician attesting to level 2 competence

Level 3

Cognitive skills should include:
- Detailed knowledge of concepts described in level 2
- Additional 16 hours of ultrasound education annually

Training requirements should include but not be limited to:
- Yearly performance and interpretation of at least 50 ultrasounds excluding ultrasound-guided arterial and venous cannulations
- Active participation in vascular laboratory case reviews with other level 3 operators
- Serving as a mentor or supervisor to level 1 and 2 operators
- Assuming responsibility for quality control and participating in ultrasound education
- Reaccreditation every 3 years for all level 3 operators is highly advisable

Figure 20.3. *(Continued)*

Model Training Program

A model training program highlighting the knowledge, training, and skills at three levels of competence is provided as an example (Fig. 20.3). Level 1 competence is the entry level for the novice ultrasonographer. Level 2 competence is a level that demonstrates a moderate level of experience, and Level 3 competence demonstrates significant experience and some levels of expertise related to bedside ultrasound (see Fig. 20.3).

One can achieve different levels of training in different ultrasound techniques or advance simultaneously in all body regions. This template merely provides an attempt at describing the cognitive, procedural, and skill-based objectives and criteria that can be applied to different ultrasound examinations.

Ultrasound-friendly simulation platforms and specially adapted cadavers provide additional opportunities for advancing invasive skills and sparing patients the "see one, do one, teach one" approach previously popular in the field of procedural education. Professional societies in concert with the AIUM and the American Board of Medical Specialties will need to respond to the pressing needs of the medical community by developing the necessary sets of guidelines for training and credentialing physician-sonographers across the various medical specialties.

References

1. American College of Radiology. ACR standards for performing and interpreting diagnostic ultrasound examinations. In: *Standards.* Reston, VA: American College of Radiology; 1996:235–236.
2. Robert Wood Johnson Medical School, Department of Emergency Medicine. Available at: http://rwjms.umdnj.edu/education/current_students/academics/fourth_year_electives/fourthyearelectives_PNB/EMED9010_EmergencyUltrasoundElective.pdf. Accessed February 28, 2010.
3. SUNY Downstate to institute ultrasound training for all medical students. http://www.newswise.com/articles/view/549835/. Accessed February 18, 2010.
4. Fernandez-Frackelton M, Peterson M, Lewis RJ, Pwerez JE, Coates WC. A bedside ultrasound curriculum for medical students: prospective evaluation of skill acquisition. *Teach Learn Med.* 2007;19(1):14–19.
5. Arger PH, Schultz SM, Sehgal CM, Cary TW, Aronchick J. Teaching medical students diagnostic sonography. *J Ultrasound Med.* 2005;24:1365–1369.

6. Wittich CM, Montgomery SC, Neben MA, et al. Teaching cardiovascular anatomy to medical students by using a handheld ultrasound device. *JAMA.* 2009;288:1062–1063.

7. Rao S, van Holsbeeck L, Musial JL, et al. A pilot study of comprehensive ultrasound education at the Wayne State University School of Medicine. *J Ultrasound Med.* 2008;27:745–749.

8. Kobal SL, Trento L, Baharami S, et al. Comparison of effectiveness of hand-carried ultrasound to bedside cardiovascular physical examination. *Am J Cardiol.* 2005;96:1002–1006.

9. Yoo MC, Villegas L, Jones DB. Basic ultrasound curriculum for medical students: validation of content and phantom. *J Laparoendosc Adv Surg Tech.* 2004;14(6):374–379.

10. Shapiro RS, Ko PP, Jacobson S. A pilot project to study the use of ultrasonography for teaching physical examination to medical students. *Comput Biol Med.* 2002;32:403–409.

11. Hoppmann R, Cook T, Hunt P, et al. Ultrasound in medical education: a vertical curriculum at the University of South Carolina School of Medicine. *J S C Med Assoc.* 2006;102:330–334.

12. Hoffmann K, Hosokawa M, Blake R, Headrick L, Johnson G. Problem-based learning outcomes: ten years of experience at the University of Missouri-Columbia School of Medicine. *Acad Med.* 2006;81(7):617–625.

13. Christianson CE, McBride RB, Vari RC, Olson L, Wilson HD. From traditional to patient-centered learning: curriculum change as an intervention for changing institutional culture and promoting professionalism in undergraduate medical education. *Acad Med.* 2007;82:1079–1088.

14. Mateer J, Plummer D, Heller M, et al. Model curriculum for physician training in emergency ultrasonography. *Ann Emerg Med.* 1994;23:95–102.

15. Lee AC, Thompson C, et al. Effectiveness of a novel training program for emergency medicine residents in ultrasound-guided insertion of central venous catheters. *Can J Emerg Med Care.* 2009;11:343–348.

16. Ma OJ, Gaddis G, et al. How fast is the focused assessment with sonography for trauma examination learning curve? *Emerg Med Australas.* 2008;20(1):32–37.

17. Jones AE, Tayal VS, Kline JA. Focused training of emergency medicine residents in goal-directed echocardiography: a prospective study. *Acad Emerg Med.* 2003;10(10):1054–1058.

18. Costantino TG, Bruno EC, Handly N, Dean AJ. Accuracy of emergency medicine ultrasound in the evaluation of abdominal aortic aneurysm. *J Emerg Med.* 2005;29(4):455–460.

19. Blavais M, Theodoro D, Sierzenski PR. A study of bedside ocular ultrasonography in the emergency department. *Acad Emerg Med.* 2002;9(8):791–799.

20. Blavais M, Theodoro D, Sierzenski PR. Elevated intracranial pressure detected by bedside emergency ultrasonography of the optic nerve sheath. *Acad Emerg Med.* 2003;10(4):376–381.

21. Costantino TG, et al. Predictors of success in emergency medicine ultrasound education. *Acad Emerg Med.* 2003;10(2):180–183.

22. American College of Emergency Physicians. Emergency ultrasound guidelines 2001. Available at: www.acep.org. Accessed February 28, 2010.

23. Hockeberger RS, Binder LS, Graber MA, et al. Model of the clinical practice of emergency medicine. *Ann Emerg Med.* 2001;37(6):745–770.

24. Counselman FL, Sanders A, Slovis CM, et al. The status of bedside ultrasonography training in emergency medicine residency programs. *Acad Emerg Med.* 2003;10(1):37–42.

25. Heller MB, Mandavia D, Tagal VS, et al. Residency training in emergency ultrasound: fulfilling the mandate. *Acad Emerg Med.* 2002;9(8):835–839.

26. Moor CL, Gregg S, Lambert M. Performance, training, quality assurance, and reimbursement of emergency physician-performed ultrasonography at academic medical centers. *J Ultrasound Med.* 2004;223(4):459–466.

27. Jang T, Aubin C, Nunheim R. Minimum training for right upper quadrant ultrasonography. *Am J Emerg Med.* 2004;20(6):439–443.

28. Hall R, Ogburn T, Rogers RG. Teaching and evaluating ultrasound skill attainment: competency-based resident ultrasound training for AIUM accreditation. *Obstet Gynecol Clin North Am.* 2006;33(2):305–323.

29. Nomua ST, Sierzenski PR, Nare JE, et al. Cross-sectional survey of ultrasound use for central line catheter insertion among resident physicians. *Del Med J.* 2008;80(7):255–259.

30. Riegert-Johnson DL, Bruce CJ, Montori VM, et al. Residents can be trained to detect abdominal aortic aneurysms using personal ultrasound imagers: a pilot study. *J Am Soc Echocardiogr.* 2005;18(5):394–397.

31. Vignon P, Dugard A, Abraham J, et al. Focused training for goal-oriented hand-held echocardiography performed by non-cardiologist residents in the intensive care unit. *Intensive Care Med.* 2007;33(10):1795–1799.

32. DeCara JM, Lang RM, Koch R, et al. The use of small personal ultrasound devices by internists without formal training in echocardiography. *Eur J Echocardiogr.* 2003;4(2):141–147.

33. Brennan JM, Blair JE, Goonewordena S, et al. A comparison by medicine residents physical examination versus hand-carried ultrasound for estimation of right atrial pressure. *Am J Cardiol.* 2007;99(11):1614–1616.

34. Croft LB, Duvall WL, Goldman ME. A pilot study of the clinical impact of hand-carried cardiac ultrasound in the medical clinic. *Echocardiography.* 2006;23(6):439–446.

35. Tracy TA, Edlow JA. Ultrasound guidance with nerve stimulation reduces the time necessary for resident peripheral nerve blockade. *Emerg Med Clin North Am.* 2004;22(3):775–796.

36. Orebaugh SL, Bigeleisen PE, Kento ML, et al. Impact of a regional anesthesia rotation on ultrasonographic identification of anatomic structures by anesthesiology residents. *Acta Anaesthesiol Scand.* 2009;53(3):364–368.

37. Sites B, Chan V, Knudson MM, Rozycki GS, et al. The American Society of Regional Anesthesia and Pain Medicine and the European Society of Regional Anaesthesia and Pain Therapy Joint Committee recommendations for education and training in ultrasound-guided regional anesthesia. *Reg Anesth Pain Med.* 2009;34(1):40–46.

38. Staren ED, Knudson MM, Rozycki GS, et al. An evaluation of the American College of Surgeons' ultrasound education program. *Am J Surg.* 2006;191(4):489–496.

39. Raghavan K, Shah AK, Cosgrove JM. Intraoperative breast problem-focused sonography, a valuable tool in the training of surgical residents. *J Surg Educ.* 2008; 65(5):350–353.

40. Fine RE, Staren ED. Updates in breast ultrasound. *Surg Clin North Am.* 2004;84(4):1001–1034.

41. Eiberg JP, Grantcharov TP, Eriksen JR, et al. Ultrasound of the acute abdomen performed by surgeons in training. *Minerva Chir.* 2008;63(1):17–22.

CHAPTER 21

The Future of Bedside Ultrasound

Ashot E. Sargsyan, MD

INTRODUCTION

Ultrasound is unique in terms of its universality and variation in operator expertise. In the traditional imaging paradigm, the operator's abilities and many other factors shape the clinical impact of a particular study, placing it anywhere from nondiagnostic or belated to highly specific and rich in essential anatomic detail. Its "free-hand" nature with commensurate dependence on the operator's performance has earned it a stigmatic label of "operator dependent," commonly perceived as undependability. This feature of ultrasound imaging, combined with typically still-image-based, delayed interpretation, has led to undeservedly modest expectations as compared to its true potential, especially in emergency medicine.

At the same time, we are witnessing rapid growth and recognition of ultrasound performed by nonradiologist physicians, which, in some medical specialties, is becoming a part of discipline-wide standards of care. Success in "nontraditional" ultrasound applications is reported in numerous publications, most of which have relevance to emergency medicine settings or resource-poor environments. The modality works near flawlessly when used to answer specific clinical questions at the time of real-time examination, and many of its success stories are born and evolve when the physician takes the probe into his or her hands to find the answer to one important clinical question: Intra-abdominal bleeding? Testicular torsion? Esophageal intubation? Abdominal aortic aneurysm? Biliary obstruction? Globe rupture? Many such questions are asked every day in various health care settings, but without ultrasound only a fraction get answered instantaneously. Whether the physician is reimbursed for the added procedure or ultrasound is used as a "visualizing stethoscope," an immediate answer to the critical question saves time and resources and, quite often, improves the outcome of illness or trauma.

As a generous source of real-time anatomic and functional information, ultrasound imaging shares the pedestal only with physical examination itself, and naturally fits in the process and logic of patient examination by a physician; its results are complementary or confirmatory to other physical examination techniques. Previous chapters of this remarkable volume offer ample evidence and specific directions for physicians as they add bedside ultrasound to their patient examination routines.

For the examining physician, working with a live ultrasound image is an advantage that was largely unclaimed for decades. As late as in 2001, the Emergency Ultrasound Guidelines of the American College of Emergency Physicians (ACEP), while calling for ultrasound training of emergency physicians, stated: "Not only must EPs know how to interpret ultrasound images; they need to know how to obtain them too." While technically correct, the phrase in its context fails to recognize that image acquisition and interpretation are inseparable, and in fact, it is their concurrence and unity that ensure the success of bedside ultrasound. Real-time search of target views through probe manipulation allows the physician to observe anatomic structures in their natural motion; over a short time the process becomes intuitive and natural. This training effect of real-time scanning explains the steep learning curve reported in bedside ultrasound trials, as it compensates quickly for the lack of comprehensive training in radiology. Physicians develop the skills to translate patterns on the live screen into anatomic and pathologic concepts very quickly, since by virtue of our education and practice we are well-prepared to perceive such information correctly. The main teaching goal in the author's experience is assisting the physician in training to identify and describe the patient's organs and tissues, rather than signs and patterns on the screen. Real-time ultrasound video must not be "read" like an electrocardiogram strip or a computed tomography scan, because it is a live anatomic view of the patient being scanned. Once one begins seeing and describing live anatomy instead of the image on the screen, the risk of diagnostic errors drops dramatically, and medical knowledge becomes an internal filter that rejects erroneous conclusions, serving as a primary quality assurance mechanism. Fortunately, the 2008 update of the earlier-mentioned guidelines no longer separates image acquisition as an added nuisance or challenge and seems to respect appropriate scanning experience without separating it from "image interpretation."

This chapter offers a high-level review of factors that will likely determine further evolution of bedside ultrasound, with limited analysis of their effect and significance. With minimal, if any, controversy, most thoughts herein will point to the obvious—bedside ultrasound is here to stay and will hold a major role in shaping the practice of medicine in the 21st century. Whether you are a medical student or a fully accomplished specialist, this text is yet another assurance of the essential benefits that your practice and your future patients are receiving with the help of this outstanding manual. In order to highlight the versatility of bedside ultrasound, provoke new ideas, and, certainly, reward you with some leisure reading, its use in human space flight is described in a separate section.

HISTORY, TRENDS, AND A GLIMPSE INTO THE FUTURE

The notion of bedside sonography (variably called point-of-care, focused, physician-performed, or hand-carried) dates back to the advent of real-time gray-scale scanners in the 1980s. Technical limitations and poor mobility of early devices, lack of appropriate evidence, and regulatory constraints prevented its rapid spread at that time. Because of differences in tradition, bedside ultrasound initially gained more acceptance in countries where it had evolved as a prerogative of physicians, and at the same time, more expensive tomographic modalities were in extremely short supply. While very few instruments were of truly "hand-carried" size, relatively lightweight cart-based mobile systems were already available for quick in-hospital response or transporting in a passenger-size car. Smaller units of the 1980s and 1990s with basic image-only capability were often used in lieu of stationary devices wherever affordability considerations overweighed the need for advanced features. Early uses of focused ultrasound included support of triage and rapid follow-up, diagnosis of early and late postoperative complications, and trauma; merits of rapid ultrasound techniques were also demonstrated in mass casualty situations. Unfortunately, the early experience of physician-performed bedside ultrasound was sporadic and remained largely unreported.

Toward the end of the 20th century, the amount of quality evidence on ultrasound imaging and its ever-broadening scope reached a critical level, eliciting a new wave of interest among nonradiologist physicians, in addition to the comprehensive ultrasound services offered by imaging facilities. This new notion coincided with further miniaturization of microelectronic technology in general and of transducer technology and commensurate digital data processing in particular. It was only a matter of time now for the United States and Western European companies to respond to the rising demand by offering, in a rapid sequence, several lines of hand-held, battery-powered devices with reasonable image quality. In a number of areas, including prehospital diagnosis and telemedicine, improvement of patient outcomes was clearly shown, fueling further growth of interest worldwide. The reemergence and rapid growth of bedside emergency ultrasound did not take place on account of routine radiologic ultrasound services, but rather as a response to a new, unmet demand and an opportunity to improve patient care—a demand revealed by high-level clinical and experimental evidence. To an extent, bedside ultrasound tended to replace some other diagnostic modalities, which were losing the competition in direct comparison of accuracy, invasiveness, speed, cost, required personnel, repeatability, and overall perception of adequacy. Such was the case with the focused assessment with sonography for trauma (FAST) examination that largely replaced diagnostic peritoneal lavage and partly abdominal computerized tomography in blunt abdominal trauma, playing a championing role in the current unstoppable expansion of bedside ultrasound.

Market analysts report a steady growth in sales of ultrasound equipment worldwide, with a stronger rise in the portable sector. Based on the current trends in both sales and utilization, experts predict further major rises in the medical industry's investments in ultrasound equipment, with the share of hand-carried devices doubling in the next several years. These forecasts are widely available and remarkably consistent. However, seemingly straightforward implementation of bedside ultrasound in medical practice at large is still in the early stages. Further growth is assured by the numerous factors that operate in a complex interplay; the most significant ones are listed in Table 21.1 and discussed in the following sections.

Evidence

Evidence published in peer-reviewed literature will continue to drive further expansion and broader recognition of bedside ultrasound. In some applications, such as the FAST examination and diagnosis of pneumothorax, the amount of high-level evidence is overwhelming; in others, only anecdotal reports have been published. The latter will be gradually supplanted by solid high-level evidence, including results of prospective clinical trials that will address not only the accuracy of specific

TABLE 21.1. Factors That Determine Further Evolution of Bedside Ultrasound

Evidence	Accumulation of published evidence that upholds the accuracy of focused ultrasound techniques in a growing number of clinical scenarios in prehospital, hospital, and ambulatory settings and supports their integration in the routine practice of physicians and facilities
Acceptance	Broadening acceptance, advocacy, and endorsement by professional organizations, with commensurate improvement of the regulatory climate. Issuance of policies that require ultrasound training as part of specialty residency programs, define pathways to proficiency and quality management requirements, and provide implementation guidelines to enable credentialing by medical systems and facilities and appropriate reimbursement
Education	Emergence and evolution of learning and teaching opportunities for physicians, including fellowships, e-learning tools, textbooks, dedicated courses, lectures, and journal articles
Equipment	Continued improvement of imaging instruments in terms of image quality, user-friendliness, versatility, compliance with industry standards, mobility, and affordability
Telemedicine	Evolution and cost-effective operation of teleultrasound arrangements, whereas ultrasound is performed by a nonphysician in a prehospital or limited-resource setting, with real-time or deferred image transmission for review and decision making by a centrally located physician
Maturation	Secondary effects of the growing number of ultrasound-proficient physicians and facilities, cross-training, and full integration of ultrasound in daily practice

ultrasound techniques in reference to "gold standard" imaging alternatives or objective clinical results, but also the technical, logistical, quality assurance, training and proficiency, and other aspects that work together to determine acceptance of any new technique in medical care. Since bedside ultrasound is performed by nonradiologist physicians, specific evidence is important in ensuring the accuracy of ultrasound when performed by "inexperienced" or "minimally trained" individuals in comparison with colleagues having considerable experience (e.g., emergency physicians after ultrasound fellowship). Typically, the published data are favorable and acceptable in terms of sensitivity and specificity of the results as well as time to acquisition of target views. What we know today allows us to expect that further evidence will uphold the accuracy of rapid, focused ultrasound techniques in a growing number of clinical scenarios and conditions. Articles of interest are published predominantly in journals dedicated to emergency medicine, trauma, critical care, and limited resource medicine (space, military, wilderness, etc.). In response to the obvious demand, a number of textbooks already have been published, and even a dedicated peer-reviewed journal was founded in 2009 by the World Interactive Network Focused on Critical UltraSound (WINFOCUS)—the *Critical Ultrasound Journal* (Springer).

Let us note, however, that in the absence of alternative imaging capability, objective information from bedside ultrasound can be extremely helpful in many more conditions than currently recognized. Physicians practicing in limited-resource settings may be compelled to consider ultrasound applications without strong evidence to their accuracy, realizing that images obtained from a particular patient may be anywhere in the continuum of diagnostic confidence, from nondiagnostic to highly specific. As mentioned earlier, a physician's medical knowledge is a potent quality assurance mechanism, which allows using applications of ultrasound imaging with less than ideal specificity and sensitivity—as long as expectations from the study are appropriate and the level of general ultrasound expertise is sufficient for real-time anatomic correlation and for adequate perception of diagnostic confidence.

Acceptance

In 1998, the American College of Surgeons published an official statement called "Ultrasound Examinations by Surgeons." In 1999, the American Medical Association House of Delegates through its Resolution 802 affirmed that ultrasound was within the scope of practice of all appropriately trained physicians. The 2008 Policy Statement of the ACEP pronounced emergency ultrasound performed and interpreted by emergency physicians "a fundamental skill in the practice of emergency medicine" and defined the availability of ultrasound equipment in emergency departments as a "requisite to the optimal care of critically ill and injured patients." The document listed "core" and "emerging" applications, stressed the importance of a continuous quality management process, and suggested a training curriculum for emergency physicians. For each recommended application, this document listed sources of evidence that had led to its inclusion in the document. Other national medical organizations that have moved to integrate ultrasound in practice of nonradiologist physicians include the Society of Academic Emergency Medicine, the American Association of Clinical Endocrinologists, and the American Society of Breast Surgeons. Decisive steps taken by these highly influential organizations enable medical systems and facilities to establish their credentialing, training, and quality assurance mechanisms in order to integrate bedside ultrasound into routine practice and optimize patient care, upholding its major role outside of radiology services. As of today, the 2008 ACEP Policy Statement stands out as the most comprehensive document that is used by other professional organizations to facilitate integration of bedside ultrasound and could be easily adapted to cover every important aspect of its implementation and integration.

During the last two decades, the attitude of the radiologic community toward bedside ultrasound has gradually shifted from opposition to reluctant tolerance and, more recently, to acceptance and support. The initial opposition was directed mainly at ultrasound use by nonradiologists in lieu of comprehensive ultrasound studies, rather than at the emergency focused ultrasound and was based on quality, patient safety, and reimbursement considerations. However, our subject is primarily the area of focused emergency ultrasound, where radiology department routines could not adapt to take advantage of the real-time nature of newly emerging rapid techniques in acute conditions such as blunt abdominal trauma. These techniques promised better outcomes only if used within the very limited time frame in parallel with and as part (but not on account) of rapid patient assessment and resuscitation. Recognition of bedside ultrasound by the American Institute of Ultrasound in Medicine (AIUM) was issued as an official statement "Training Guidelines for Physicians Who Evaluate and Interpret Diagnostic Ultrasound Examinations," approved on March 16, 2008. These guidelines defined training and proficiency levels that would render a physician qualified to independently perform ultrasound examinations. Also important is the content of the AIUM "Practice Guideline for the Performance of the FAST Examination" (2007) and other guidelines on the use of focused ultrasound.

Growing acceptance, advocacy, and endorsement by professional organizations will facilitate further implementation of ultrasound, improvement of the regulatory climate, adoption of policies that require ultrasound training as part of specialty residency programs, definition of pathways to proficiency, and quality management requirements, and will provide implementation guidelines to enable credentialing by medical systems and facilities. A major step in the acceptance of bedside ultrasound will be the integration of ultrasound in the training curricula of medical students in two ways—as an emergency imaging technique and as a teaching tool in clinical anatomy and physiology, clinical pathology, and in a number of clinical disciplines.

Education

Guidelines and position statements of the professional organizations mentioned earlier specify the minimum amount and type of training or exposure/experience in the given specialty area that would qualify a physician for conducting focused emergency ultrasound procedures. These concrete "catch-up" requirements are very important at this stage of bedside ultrasound implementation, with expertise, not equipment, being in short supply. Along the same lines, paramount also is the current trend of year-long "ultrasound fellowships" for emergency physicians that aim to create a cohort of ultrasound mentors that will qualify facilities for bedside ultrasound and spread the culture of bedside ultrasound nationwide. In a 2009 survey, Stein et al found that most (66%) California emergency departments do not use bedside ultrasound; of those that do, the majority do not have any quality assurance programs as recommended by 2008 ACEP guidelines. Compared with community emergency departments, academic emergency departments are more likely to use bedside ultrasound, to have physicians credentialed in ultrasound use, and to have quality assurance programs. These data constitute the best evidence in support of the earlier-mentioned "catch-up" measures, such as ultrasound fellowships. For 2009, there were over 40 fellowship positions advertised in the United States.

As the acute demand for basic ultrasound expertise is gradually satisfied in the next 3 to 5 years, the medical community will fully embrace the notion of bedside ultrasound and will eventually recognize that basic ultrasound knowledge and skills can and should be taught to medical students as a primary skill of a physician, with further natural enhancement and specialization during residency and subsequent practice.

Indeed, early introduction of ultrasound in medical schools and its broad use is warranted by the very nature of this imaging modality and by virtually every factor listed in Table 21.1. Besides better emphasizing ultrasound in the limited radiology course or elective rotation and in clinical specialty rotations, very attractive opportunities are in store to use ultrasound as a teaching tool, from basic disciplines like human anatomy and physiology to pathology and clinical specialties. With a token of imagination, it is easy to appreciate the potential of ultrasound to reinforce the student's knowledge of normal anatomy. In fact, ultrasound is the only modality in existence that can show live anatomy, in motion, to a class of first-year students: the anatomy professor equipped with an ultrasound machine wearing a headset with a microphone, scanning a healthy volunteer and displaying the live ultrasound image and the probe position side by side on a big screen, describing viscera and their relationships, tracking vessels as they branch and pulsate, identifying muscles in their fascial compartments with their insertion points, pointing out potential spaces such as the costophrenic angle or the rectouterine pouch—the list is endless. It will not be long before this vision becomes a reality, making physicians jealous and wishing they could go back to school. After taking such an ultrasound-enriched anatomy course, students not only will know anatomy and physiology better but also will be ready to see and understand ultrasound images with pathologic contents. They will then hold the ultrasound probe in a steady hand naturally and confidently while still in clinical rotations. Ultrasound will be part of their essential patient examination skills when they graduate. Needless to say, many of them will use an ultrasound machine on their very first day of residency, and will have an ultrasound device on their shopping list as they begin to practice. There is not much fantasy in this description, as it is a very realistic prospect; some medical schools are already implementing some of its elements (Fig. 21.1 [see also color insert]). Conceivably, there is no better place for this vision than this book and this particular chapter.

In our experiments for the U.S. space program, we have used not only healthy volunteers but also commercially available ultrasound phantoms and specialized simulated structures "home-made" at our facility to teach basic ultrasound concepts and use of equipment, with remarkable success. The concept of real-time planar representation of a three-dimensional structure is easily understood. In our experience with the International Space Station (ISS) crews, the skill of ultrasound probe manipulation to visualize and describe the contents of a "black box," once acquired, appears to become a permanent ability that does not noticeably fade over time. Embedding a human scanning practice session in the preflight training of

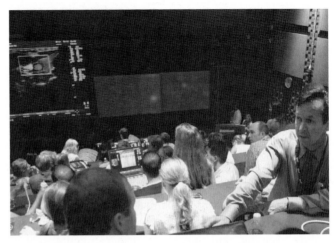

Figure 21.1. Demonstration of bedside ultrasound techniques to a group of medical students at Wayne State University School of Medicine in Detroit, Michigan (2006). (See color insert.)

astronauts introduces essential confidence to perform both limited ultrasound procedures independently and full-fledged protocols when guided by experts from Mission Control in real time.

Returning to today's reality, we can conclude that all the educational opportunities for physicians, largely influenced by the other factors outlined earlier, will facilitate broad implementation of bedside ultrasound in medical practice in the United States and worldwide. Fellowships, dedicated courses, continuous medical education lectures, e-learning tools, textbooks, and journal articles will all be variably used by physicians as appropriate for a given specialty, phase of their careers, places of practice, and many other circumstances. As with other clinical skills, peer mentoring and cross-training will continue to play a huge role in the emergence of the first ultrasound-savvy generation of modern physicians.

Equipment

In some countries, ultrasound utilization already exceeded x-ray modalities as far back as in the late 1990s, and the trend of both net and relative growth in ultrasound use shows no signs of weakening. Some industry analysts predict that sales of portable ultrasound devices will be increasing at a faster pace than those of ultrasound equipment in general, at a compound annual growth rate of over 15% from 2007–2008 to 2012–2015, largely on account of the uses for emergency medicine, surgery, critical care, and regional anesthesia. Continued improvement of imaging instruments in terms of image quality, user-friendliness and versatility, compliance with industry standards, mobility, and affordability will all contribute to the progress of bedside ultrasound.

For each user community and health care setting, equipment priorities are somewhat different. For example, portability and mobility are a primary consideration for military, prehospital, and wilderness applications, while user friendliness, versatility, and digital data handling features rank higher in the hospital emergency department and intensive care unit settings. The complex interplay and mutual dependency among the demands of the clinical world, research and development, manufacturing technology, and market factors are thoroughly studied and analyzed by market research firms and widely publicized by the press, trade journals, and specialized literature. We will refrain from turning this chapter into an "ultrasound buying guide," and stop at stating that for each health care setting or medical specialty, the industry and the secondary market offer a wide choice of equipment at unprecedented value.

Telemedicine

Evolution and operation of teleultrasound arrangements have played a substantial role in the development and popularization of focused ultrasound techniques. Teleultrasound will likely play a modest but substantial part of non–radiologist-performed ultrasound in the future, whereas the operator in a prehospital or limited-resource setting is a nonphysician or a physician not qualified to interpret ultrasound data, and ultrasound images are streamed or transmitted for review and consultation by a centrally located qualified physician. Many of the indications for ultrasound, such as assessment of abdominal trauma or fractures, are highly relevant to limited-resource environments, such as remote, sparsely populated and hence underserved locations; military operations; disaster sites; industrial facilities; and various ships and expeditions.

The inability to obtain objective diagnostic information complicates treatment and triage decisions. This disadvantage for patients located outside of major metropolitan areas often results in delayed or inappropriate treatment or unnecessary evacuation. Such evacuation could be prevented if a reliable diagnosis of a benign, nonthreatening condition is made onsite and/or timely and appropriate treatment is available, advantageous, and associated with higher probability of anatomic and functional recovery. The cost of medical evacuation may be orders of magnitude higher than that of the hardware, communications, and associated attributes of operational readiness.

Indeed, no expertise is often available at a medically underserved site to adequately perform and interpret imaging data, even if ultrasound equipment is available. The lacking image acquisition and interpretation expertise must therefore be provided by means of remote guidance using communications networks of various transmission capacities. For example, NASA researchers have systematically developed and tested a real-time remote guidance methodology to augment the medical support of space crews—an example of a setting where ultrasound is the only available imaging modality, no qualified physicians are available onsite, and timely diagnostic decisions have major health, safety, mission success, and financial implications.

Many real-time telemedicine and teleultrasound arrangements of the past did not survive as "standby" capability because of lack of funding, maintenance, and other requisites of operational readiness; besides, their cost-effectiveness was not always assessed with correct metrics and methodology. Facts of preventing unnecessary evacuation or surgery, early diagnosis, shortened disability, or improved outcome were not translated into figures that accountants and administrators could operate with. As the cost of portable imaging devices and communication links further declines, the initial investment to create teleultrasound capability will become affordable at many more locations. Future teleultrasound systems will be established primarily to satisfy the demand for focused bedside ultrasound techniques (as opposed to traditional ultrasound imaging protocols), with emergency physicians and other nonradiology specialists performing guidance and interpretation as part of emergency patient consultation; radiologists could be consulted only in cases where comprehensive or highly specialized imaging becomes necessary.

Internet access rapidly becomes ubiquitous; besides ensuring the essential teleultrasound links (two-way audio, one-way video streaming), today's data links allow the remote operator to access digital resources for just-in-time training, reference tools, and instruction. Another benefit of universal digital connections is the possibility to control and adjust the ultrasound device remotely from the central location, thereby allowing the operator to focus on probe manipulations only. Remotely controllable ultrasound devices have already been tested and have shown promise for use in rural clinics that are part of distributed medical networks.

Maturation

The last but not the least important group of factors includes all the secondary effects of the growing number of ultrasound-proficient physicians and facilities, the rapid integration of ultrasound into their daily practices, and, over time, the full absorption of bedside ultrasound into the routine of patient care. Cross-training of physicians and the visibility of positive impacts will, as a chain reaction, catalyze further interest toward bedside ultrasound in each facility, medical system, and area. Cross-pollination will also result in some spread of bedside ultrasound to most disciplines, including general and family practice, and will become a means of maintaining a competitive edge and a higher quality and efficiency of patient care.

Another advantage of physician-performed ultrasound is its real-time flexibility. Unlike referral-based examinations by a standard scanning and image acquisition protocol, bedside ultrasound follows the thinking process of the physician-operator, seeking the answer to the primary question and moving, as time and experience permit, on to secondary questions and broader organ/system assessment. While in emergency trauma time is the most precious resource, other disciplines will more easily take advantage of the growing multiplicity of bedside ultrasound techniques and possibilities. Naturally, accrual of imaging experience will lead to broadening of the scope of bedside ultrasound in the practice of particular physicians, facilities, and disciplines.

ULTRASOUND IN THE LIMITED-RESOURCE ENVIRONMENT OF HUMAN SPACE FLIGHT

Management of health problems in limited-resource environments, including space flight, faces challenges in both available equipment and expertise onsite. The medical support for future ventures outside low Earth orbit is still being defined; ultrasound imaging is a strong candidate since its feasibility and potential in human space flight have been well demonstrated by American, European, and Russian scientists. Recent trials on the ISS prove that ultrasound can be used not only to study space physiology but also operationally for focused diagnostic evaluation in many foreseeable medical problems. Notwithstanding the inherent complexity of space operations, weightlessness, and lack of expertise onboard, ultrasound is seen as a powerful resource to mitigate risks and protect the mission. Since 1999, NASA researchers have tested and validated the clinical utility of abdominal, retroperitoneal, and thoracic ultrasound in preliminary animal experiments and human observations in parabolic flight, in order to study the "microgravity normal" ultrasound data, human factors, and

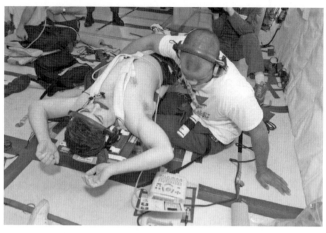

Figure 21.2. NASA astronaut Robert L. Curbeam conducting a focused ultrasound examination of the urinary system in parabolic flight using a Sonosite-180 hand-held ultrasound system. The volunteer is on a Crew Medical Restraint System with straps to ensure stability during gravity transitions and scanning; the operator is also restrained. Note another researcher in the background using a self-scanning technique. *(Image courtesy of NASA)*

microgravity-specific aspects of data collection and interpretation (Fig. 21.2). The behavior of liquids, gases, organs with alterable positions, and their interfaces were given special attention. These investigations suggested that accuracy of ultrasound in hemothorax, pneumothorax, and hemoperitoneum are not degraded during microgravity conditions and may even be enhanced because of the different distribution of blood or air in the absence of gravitational effects (Fig. 21.3).

This section summarizes the NASA experience in the use of ultrasound to augment the medical support of space crews. Just-in-time training and real-time expert guidance have allowed nonphysician astronauts to perform over 150 hours of ultrasound examinations on the ISS, including abdominal, cardiovascular, facial and ocular, musculoskeletal, and thoracic examinations. Some of the trials supported by NASA have influenced acceptance and implementation of focused ultrasound methodologies in medicine at large. The training and guidance methods used on the ISS were also adapted for terrestrial use in professional sporting venues, the Olympic Games, austere locations including Mt. Everest, and some emergency medical systems. Many present and future solutions developed by space medicine are adaptable to terrestrial medicine including emergency, rural, and military settings that share features of limited resources, lack of adequate alternative imaging, operational complexity and urgency,

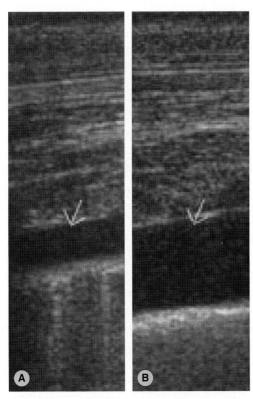

Figure 21.3. An anterior ultrasound view in a hemothorax model in normal gravity **(A)** and microgravity **(B).** The layer of pleural blood in massive hemothorax is thicker in B because of more uniform distribution in the absence of gravity. Because of this redistribution, the focused technique to rule out small hemothorax includes multiple windows and is not limited to the costophrenic angle. (Advanced Diagnostic Ultrasound in Microgravity Investigation.)

and separation from major medical facilities. First and foremost, however, these efforts benefit the space program itself as the agency plans to develop future exploration programs requiring robust medical risk mitigation capability and increased medical self-sufficiency.

INTERNATIONAL SPACE STATION

The ISS Human Research Facility Ultrasound System was flown in the spring of 2002 as a multipurpose research tool. Later in the same year, the NASA operational medical organization and NASA researchers demonstrated the possibility to rely on crewmembers of nonmedical backgrounds to obtain clinical ultrasound data with only minimal training, if supported through real-time remote guidance. During development of the methodology, e-learning software, and reference tools, multiple trials were conducted in laboratory conditions and parabolic flight. On September 13, 2002, ISS Expedition 5 NASA Science Officer Peggy A.

Whitson, PhD, having trained only in basic equipment operation, performed diagnostic-quality ultrasound examinations of the abdomen, chest, superficial tissues, and vascular system under remote guidance from Mission Control (Fig. 21.4). Focused procedure segments included a FAST examination, a pneumothorax protocol, and ureteral patency demonstration, among others. The live image from the ultrasound device, besides the monitor in the space vehicle, was streamed to the guiding ultrasound expert in Mission Control. Optimal probe position was guided by voice commands to achieve target views; equipment settings were also adjusted through voice commands to optimize image quality. A language free from medical terms and jargon was used, and basic rules of operational radio communication were observed. Notably, Dr. Whitson acquired a full set of required images in the first autonomous ultrasound of a thyroid gland in space flight after only a brief verbal instruction.

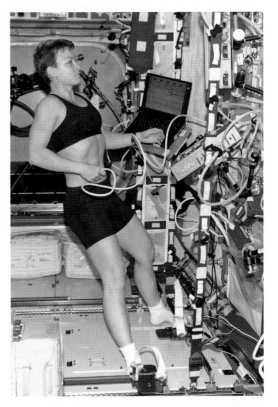

Figure 21.4. Astronaut Peggy A. Whitson, PhD, Expedition 5 NASA International Space Station (ISS) science officer, participates in a test to validate the use of the Human Research Facility (HRF) Ultrasound for potential medical contingencies (September 13, 2002). In this image Whitson was scanning herself with the guidance from the ultrasound expert on the ground. The HRF was located in the Destiny laboratory on the ISS. In 2008 it was moved to the European Columbus module. *(Image courtesy of NASA)*

The remote guidance protocols were expanded in scope during Expedition 7 to instruct and guide astronaut Edward Lu, PhD, to perform the first successful simulation of stress echocardiography in space using a cycle ergometer. During the same expedition, the crew conducted musculoskeletal, vascular, and peripheral nerve imaging of upper extremities in space. Thorough image quality assessments were made for the first time in space-based ultrasound to understand the effects of image degradation during transmission of the signal by data relay satellites and electronic systems onboard and on the ground. These highly successful sessions provided the bulk of background data for subsequent trials on the ISS, highlighting numerous possibilities for further improvements.

In 2003, NASA funded the Advanced Diagnostic Ultrasound in Microgravity (ADUM) flight investigation (principal investigator, S.A. Dulchavsky, Henry Ford Hospital, Detroit, MI). U.S. and Russian crewmembers received a 1-hour didactic and a 1- to 2-hour "hands-on" practice session in the Payload Development Laboratory of the NASA Johnson Space Center (Houston, TX) prior to their flight, using a flight-modified ultrasound system identical to the one on the ISS (HDI-5000, Philips Healthcare, Seattle, WA). Remote guidance in these practice sessions was done with a 2-second delay to simulate space-to-ground communications, included extensive use of equipment-specific and application-specific reference tools ("cue cards"), and followed special linguistic rules and modes of verbal discourse. The cue cards visualized locations of specific equipment controls, basic probe manipulation techniques, and anatomic sites for initial probe placement for various examinations. A comprehensive instructional e-learning program (On-Orbit Proficiency Enhancement, or OPE) was also developed for just-in-time refresher training of crewmembers prior to each on-orbit session, in order to maximize their performance. OPE consists of modules for familiarization with the ultrasound equipment and its setup, general principles, anatomy, and limited individualized techniques for various organ systems. The adaptive menu of the system allows the user to "drill down" to the learning area of interest, greatly simplifying the just-in-time learning process for medical emergencies. Animation, easily replayed and reviewed, allows the main story threads to be quickly absorbed, including a host of auxiliary information such as positioning of the subject. Anatomy, cue cards, helpful hints, and target images are also included. The original ISS version (2004) was developed with bilingual (English-Russian) capabilities to facilitate completion in the operator's native language.

The program records operator-specific performance metrics in an Excel database after each use; this information was downlinked to the experiment team prior to each actual imaging session to highlight areas where additional coaching or attention might be required and also served as a component of the quality management system. A sample page of the OPE e-learning tool is shown in Figure 21.5 (see also color insert).

NASA astronaut C. Michael Foale, PhD (Expedition 8), performed cardiac, vascular, and thoracic examinations, which could have been used to exclude a significant number of disease conditions in these areas. Expedition 9 crewmembers Col. E. Michael Fincke and Col. Gennady I. Padalka were rapidly trained (approximately 2 hours) to expand the list of validated ultrasound capabilities on the ISS by adding musculoskeletal ultrasound examinations to the list, resulting in the first-ever peer-reviewed publication submitted to a journal directly from a space vehicle. This crew also performed the first autonomous ultrasound examination to record some vascular effects of fluid redistribution in prolonged microgravity. In Commander Fincke's words, "the training and OPE refresher course is excellent and should be expanded on future flights. This method could be used in medical emergencies on the ISS to guide crewmembers." The research team worked with Expedition 10 crewmembers Leroy Chiao, PhD, and Col. Salizhan S. Sharipov to demonstrate ultrasound techniques applicable to dental and sinus infections and eye trauma during spaceflight (Fig. 21.6) and tested a new ultrasound pupillometry technique with a multipurpose system to measure and record the pupillary light reflex. Their findings were received by the *Journal of Trauma* directly from orbit and were featured as the lead article in the May 2005 issue. In the concluding sessions of the ADUM experiment, Expedition 11 crewmember John L. Phillips, PhD, performed a full echocardiographic examination with an unprecedented degree of autonomy (minimal guidance because of technical interruptions in video transmission). Dr. Phillips, after using the OPE program to refresh his ultrasound proficiency, was able to autonomously attain quality diagnostic visualization of the heart with voice guidance alone, heavily relying on recognition of memorized patterns and on-orbit reference tools.

Convincing evidence was thus accumulated to realize the promise of the combined application of brief familiarization training, real-time telementoring, and computer technology to allow diagnosis, staging, and monitoring of a wide variety of serious medical conditions in resource-poor environments. With this capability, the outcome of a medical contingency could be changed drastically, and

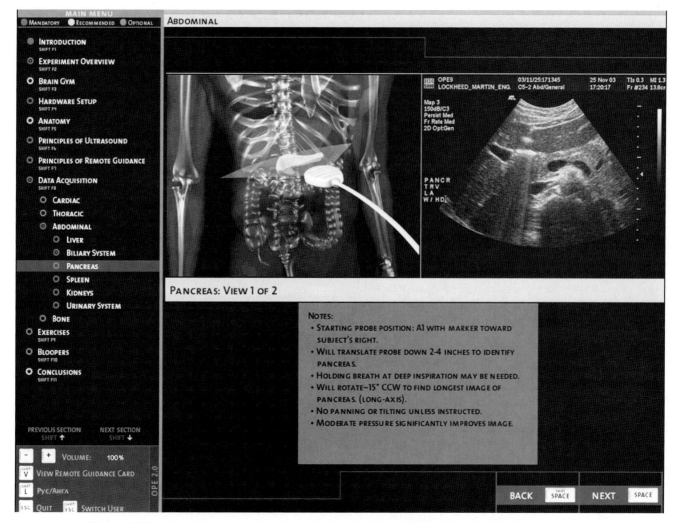

Figure 21.5. Sample page of the On-Orbit Proficiency Enhancement (OPE) e-learning tool (see color insert). Note the menu prescription with mandatory, recommended, and optional items to best prepare the operator for a specific imaging session. (Advanced Diagnostic Ultrasound in Microgravity Investigation.)

an unnecessary evacuation could be prevented. Based on new terrestrial and space-based evidence, ultrasound imaging was included in the medical requirements for the ISS; its current use hinges on real-time remote guidance of the operator from the Mission Control Center to conduct focused ultrasound examinations, a bridge that connects the modestly trained remote nonexpert ultrasound operator with an advanced expert in a single virtual working environment.

NASA METHODOLOGY IN PROFESSIONAL SPORTS, THE OLYMPICS, AND AUSTERE ENVIRONMENTS

The OPE program was later modified for use in sporting venues for diagnosis of musculoskeletal trauma.

A sports-specific introductory segment was constructed, and ultrasound setup instructions were modified from the high-end ISS equipment to the portable ultrasound systems selected for the sporting events (GE Logiqbook, GE Healthcare, Milwaukee, WI). Additional reference cue cards were created to focus on potential musculoskeletal injuries to the shoulder, knee, and ankle. Full musculoskeletal ultrasound examinations were initially obtained on over 30 professional athletes (professional hockey players and others). Examination quality and completeness were assessed by remote ultrasound experts viewing the real-time ultrasound video stream. All examinations were initiated with the probe topographically positioned at anatomic reference points as depicted on the cue card. The athletic trainers were instructed to manipulate the ultrasound probe by an experienced

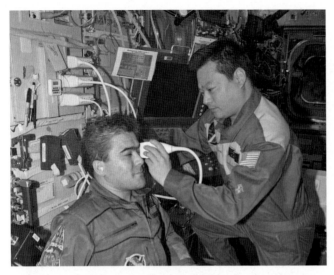

Figure 21.6. International Space Station Expedition 10 NASA science officer Leroy Chiao, PhD, and Col. Salizhan S. Sharipov during a demonstration of ultrasound techniques applicable in eye trauma evaluation in spaceflight. The ultrasound image on the screen is removed. *(Image courtesy of NASA)*

sonologist through voice commands to achieve the desired images. The remote-guided musculoskeletal ultrasound examinations were completed by the non-physician operators in less than 15 minutes at each site (groin, knee, ankle, elbow, or shoulder). Operator and subject positioning and setup of portable battery-powered equipment were accomplished in less than 2 minutes in most cases. There was a usual 0.5- to 1-second transmission delay for video, which did not impact the conduct or quality of ultrasound examinations. Full-resolution imagery conforming to the Digital Imaging and Communications in Medicine (DICOM) standard was saved at intervals during the examination and then downloaded after completion of the experiment. All downloaded DICOM data packages and video streams were subsequently deemed adequate for professional interpretation by musculoskeletal ultrasound radiologists.

Recently, athletic trainers at the Olympic Training Facility in Colorado Springs used the same techniques to rapidly diagnose a knee injury in an Olympic wrestler, to diagnose a shoulder injury in a speed skater, and to exclude a shoulder injury in a weight lifter. These techniques were expanded during the Winter Olympic Games in Torino, Italy, and the Summer Olympic Games in China. A modified version of the training program used on the ISS was utilized to familiarize U.S. Olympic Committee athletic trainers with musculoskeletal ultrasound. Portable ultrasound devices were placed in a variety of athletic venues in Torino and Beijing and

provided onsite diagnostic capabilities for a wide variety of injuries sustained during the Olympic Games.

The OPE e-learning program was modified for use on Mt. Everest to include a pulmonary section to facilitate pulmonary ultrasound examination for signs of high-altitude pulmonary edema (HAPE). Two comprehensive pulmonary ultrasound examinations were performed at high altitude by minimally trained ultrasound operators with remote guidance in order to assess the subjects for HAPE. This newly emerging technique consisted of quantifying the amount of comet tail artifacts in approximately 15 anatomic points of each lung of the subject. The examinations were completed in less than 15 minutes each and were of adequate diagnostic quality to identify pulmonary edema via comet tail artifact development. Both climber-subjects were asymptomatic; however, both demonstrated evidence of moderate pulmonary edema, since a growing number of comet tail artifacts is known as an indicator of increased lung water content. This was a very specific experiment; however, it proved that, should there be a traumatic injury in either of the climbers, the same setup would have allowed performing musculoskeletal ultrasound immediately. Further miniaturization of equipment and ubiquity of digital communications will certainly facilitate inclusion of a ultrasound capability in the medical support of expeditions, remote industrial facilities, and other isolated, resource-poor locations.

CURRENT NASA RESEARCH IN ULTRASOUND FOR INTERNATIONAL SPACE STATION AND FUTURE PROGRAMS

In the absence of radiographic or other imaging capability, ultrasound is the only objective information source that can be extremely helpful in the diagnosis, assessment, and appropriate management of a known or suspected illness or injury in a space flight. While the published accuracy data for ultrasound in a given condition may be low or even nonexistent, a particular imaging study in the hands of an advanced medical team may be of high diagnostic confidence. Therefore, in the limited-resource environment of space flight, even less specific and sensitive applications of ultrasound are not discounted. NASA researchers collaborate with major clinical and academic centers to assess new methodologies, and these efforts result in substantial new evidence.

For example, NASA researchers were involved in efforts to prove the high sensitivity and specificity of ultrasound in even limited pneumothorax; recent

NASA-funded investigations in terrestrial and microgravity conditions have confirmed the previously reported correlation between intracranial pressure and optic nerve sheath diameter measured by ocular ultrasound. The aerospace and Earth applications of these noninvasive techniques are immediate. Similarly, NASA is exploring the capability of multipurpose ultrasound systems to evaluate the ocular fundus, including the condition of the optic nerve disc and presence of its edema. These methodologies assume special importance in conditions when "gold standard" methods such as optical coherence tomography or retinal photography are not immediately available or practical; besides, they allow studying long-term effects of microgravity on some aspects of physiology that did not receive deserved attention because of lack of appropriate technology during past space missions.

In a number of ISS ultrasound sessions, opportunities arose to attempt partial and complete autonomy in data acquisition (no communication with the operator). The success of these attempts in relatively simple (complete thyroid ultrasound by terrestrial standards) and complex (echocardiography) protocols support the notion of the current NASA-funded effort—to create an effective digital information resource to support diagnostic ultrasound by inexperienced operators in conditions of complete autonomy. Many, and perhaps the majority, of the elements of remote expert guidance can be placed in a multimedia computer-based structure, and the real-time interaction with an expert can be replicated in an interaction with an adaptive knowledge databank. Reassured by our previous successes and, in particular, autonomous data acquisition segments of our experiments, we undertook to develop a comprehensive image catalog, which will allow nonexperts to perform and interpret focused ultrasound examinations for space-relevant medical conditions with a higher degree of autonomy. The intuitive ultrasound catalog builds on the previous experience of the ADUM research program on the one hand and published medical evidence on the other. The catalog includes specific ultrasound images that can be rendered to the operator in organ- or system-specific categories (such as musculoskeletal, urinary, or renal) and, in topographical organization (thoracic, anterior neck, etc.), as well as in syndrome- or condition-specific classification (blunt abdominal trauma, jaundice, dysuria, etc.). A rich, multimedia educational platform with topographic cue cards, reference images, animations, and short video segments will be provided to the user in optimized and validated sequence to quickly prepare and perform a focused ultrasound examination. Crewmembers' own preflight images will be included if desired for automatic or visual comparisons and trend detection; space-relevant pathologic images will also be included (such as images representing a urinary obstruction, a fracture, or synovial fluid collection) to allow preliminary differential diagnosis onsite. The catalog also will provide a searchable archive of images for research or medical purposes. The first-generation catalog architecture and functionality have been developed with significant input from operational space medical personnel. Reference-normal and pathologic imagery are currently being populated to allow functional testing of the autonomous functionality of the program in appropriate cohorts. Crewmember-performed ultrasound with increased autonomy will provide additional medical capability for the current space program, and may be essential for future, exploration-class space flights lacking real-time guidance capability. The intuitive ultrasound catalog appears to provide a scalable, interactive diagnostic platform for current and future space missions, and can be operated on any computer. The terrestrial applications of the product appear to be abundant, and will be investigated and pursued when feasible. This is the next logical phase of NASA's sustained effort to make ultrasound available to sites lacking proper expertise. In the development of the future systems, NASA researchers will carefully monitor and rely on the progress in terrestrial bedside ultrasound applications; at the same time, "spinoffs" from ultrasound methodologies developed for the space program, along with the experience in teleultrasound and training/expertise delivery systems, will continue to contribute to the area of bedside ultrasound at large.

CONCLUSIONS

Although most medical imaging procedures employed by the radiologic community are appropriate and readily transferable to emergency medicine, the very logic of bedside ultrasound departs from standardized comprehensive protocols toward limited, focused data acquisition driven by clear priorities of the moment. Ultrasound is of proven accuracy in focused examinations that answer a specific diagnostic question for immediate treatment decisions, such as the FAST examination.

It is no surprise that the array of recognized bedside applications of ultrasound will grow in the next several years to include traumatic injuries and other macroscopic pathology of parenchymal, musculoskeletal, and vascular structures in most anatomic regions of the body. In numerous clinical investigations, a wider range of conditions is being defined in which rapid examinations performed by nonradiologist physicians can influence treatment decisions and optimize care. These innovations will be embraced by clinicians with increasing willingness, since the way is already paved, and the notion of imaging by nonradiologist physicians is no longer perceived as unconventional. In our radiation-conscious society, bedside ultrasound probably will become the alternative first-line modality in a number of conditions where radiographic methods such as computed tomography hold the "gold standard" position, especially in younger individuals. Pneumothorax, uncomplicated fractures, urolithiasis, and biliary disease are among excellent candidates for such a shift in diagnostic approach to emergency patient evaluation. Even at lower sensitivity, acute appendicitis could be another high-prevalence condition where bedside ultrasound can assist in preoperative diagnosis in appropriate clinical situations and especially in younger age groups.

The potential of bedside ultrasound will be gradually realized in settings with limited resources. Examples of such settings include rural and remotely located medical clinics, scientific outposts, ocean-going vessels, and prisons. In these and similar settings, bedside ultrasound improves the quality of care and outcomes and often reduces overall medical care costs. Distinct focused ultrasound techniques, as a natural part of the patient evaluation sequence, will assist in triage decisions when medical evacuation or invasive last-resort interventions can be lifesaving in some cases and unnecessary or even detrimental in others. Trauma is the number one cause of morbidity among personnel in deployments to remote areas and is the primary cause of evacuations to definitive care facilities from remote sites. Traditional diagnostic imaging capabilities are limited or nonexistent in these settings; excessive size and weight prevent inclusion of x-ray capability in the battlefield, smaller seafaring vessels, or spacecraft. However, today's small, portable ultrasound systems provide an alternative diagnostic imaging capability applicable to medical care in such environments.

The U.S. space program is an extreme but excellent user, testbed, and example for the development and popularization of bedside ultrasound techniques because ultrasound is the only imaging option available to the space crews. In a number of trials and experiments, NASA researchers have demonstrated that ultrasound can be used by a general surgeon to reliably detect pneumothorax and have investigated its accuracy in fracture detection with extremity trauma, patient assessment in ocular and craniofacial trauma, and other conditions; our works have facilitated inclusion of ultrasound training in certain medical school, residency, and professional society curricula and requirements. The current NASA experience in bedside ultrasound by nonradiologist operators supports the hypothesis that modest training in ultrasound can result in diagnostic-quality examinations when directed by an expert with remote guidance experience. This expert must possess extensive knowledge of all aspects of the specific ultrasound application and advanced hands-on imaging experience to ensure consistent, composed, and efficient conduct of the focused examination. Many radiologists, emergency physicians, surgeons, and other specialists will soon possess such expertise to further contribute to the growing development and implementation of technology and methodology of bedside ultrasound that holds a great promise for the medicine of the 21st century.

Ending this text on a very optimistic note, the author wishes to express measureless gratitude to colleagues at NASA Johnson Space Center and Wyle Integrated Science and Engineering in Houston, TX; the Henry Ford Hospital in Detroit, MI; and the Foothills Medical Center in Calgary, Canada, for their essential contributions to the area of focused ultrasound, including the work described in this chapter.

Suggested Reading

American College of Surgeons. Ultrasound examinations by surgeons. *Bull Am Coll Surg.* 1998;83(6):37–40.

Blaivas M. A new point of care ultrasound journal. *Crit Ultrasound J.* 2009;1(1):1–2.

Chiao L, Sharipov S, Sargsyan AE, et al. Ocular examination for trauma; clinical ultrasound aboard the International Space Station. *J Trauma.* 2005;58(5):885–889.

Dulchavsky SA, Schwarz KL, Kirkpatrick AW, et al. Prospective evaluation of thoracic ultrasound in the detection of pneumothorax. *J Trauma.* 2001;50:201–205.

Dyer D, Cusden J, Turner C, et al. The clinical and technical evaluation of a remote telementored telesonography system during the acute resuscitation and transfer of the injured patient. *J Trauma.* 2008;65(6):1209–1216.

Foale CM, Kaleri AY, Sargsyan AE, et al. Diagnostic instrumentation aboard ISS: just-in-time training for nonphysician crew members. *Aviat Space Environ Med.* 2005;76(6):594–598.

Hussain P, Deshpande A, Shridhar P, et al. The feasibility of telemedicine for the training and supervision of general practitioners performing ultrasound examinations of patients with urinary tract symptoms. *J Telemed Telecare.* 2004;10(3):180–182.

Kwon D, Bouffard JA, van Holsbeeck M, et al. Battling fire and ice: remote guidance ultrasound to diagnose injury on the International Space Station and the ice rink. *Am J Surg.* 2007;193(3):417–420.

Levitov AB, Mayo PH, Slonim A. *Critical Care Ultrasonography.* New York, NY: McGraw-Hill Professional; 2009.

Lichtenstein DA, Pinsky MR, Jardin F. *General ultrasound in the critically ill.* Berlin, Heidelberg: Springer; 2004.

Sarkisian AE, Khondkarian RA, Amirbekian NM, Bagdasarian NB, Khojayan RL, Oganesian YT. Sonographic screening of mass casualties for abdominal and renal injuries following the 1988 Armenian earthquake. *J Trauma.* 1991;31(2):247–250.

Staren ED, Knudson MM, Rozycki GS, et al. An evaluation of the American College of Surgeons' ultrasound education program. *Am J Surg.* 2006;191(4):489–496. (ACS Ultrasound Educational Program "Bluebook": http://www.facs.org/education/ultrasoundbluebook.pdf.)

Stein JC, River G, Kalika I, et al. A survey of bedside ultrasound use by emergency physicians in California. *J Ultrasound Med.* 2009;28:757–763.

Su MJ, Ma HM, Ko CI, et al. Application of teleultrasound in emergency medical services. *Telemed J E Health.* 2008; 14(8):816–824.

Glossary of Terms

Absorption: Conversion of ultrasound energy into heat.

Acoustic variables: Parameters that define a sound wave, such as pressure and density, that change rhythmically.

Active element: Integral part of all ultrasound transducers. Also called a crystal, it is made of piezoelectric material (lead zirconate titanate or PZT) that converts electrical energy into ultrasound and vice versa.

AIUM: American Institute of Ultrasound in Medicine.

AIUM 100-mm test object: Standard phantom used for quality assurance.

Akinetic: Organ or its part that should be moving, but is not.

ALARA: **A**s **L**ow **A**s **R**easonably **A**chievable. American Institute of Ultrasound in Medicine principle limiting possible bioeffects of acoustic radiation.

Aliasing: Sampling error characteristic of the inability of pulsed wave Doppler to accurately measure high flow velocities.

A-mode ultrasound: Antiquated mode of ultrasound used to depict the position of a reflector as well as the strength of the returning echo by its amplitude. Seldom used in modern practice.

Ambiguity (range): Characteristic of continuous wave Doppler describing its inability to define the position of the sample. Caused by an overlap between transmitting and receiving beams.

Amplification (receiver gain): Increases the signal strength in the receiver of the ultrasound system and therefore the overall brightness of the image.

Amplitude: The difference between the average value of the acoustic variable and its maximum value through the duration of the sound wave; the "loudness" of the ultrasound.

Analog image: Image on the screen of the cathode-ray tube (TV screen) prior to any computer processing.

Anechoic: Area producing no echo reflections and appearing black on the ultrasound image.

Archiving: Storage of images.

ARDMS: American Registry for Diagnostic Medical Sonography. The registry institutes certifying examinations and upholds competency standards for diagnostic sonographers (medical, cardiac, and vascular).

Array transducer: Transducer with multiple active elements, arranged in a certain order.

Artifact: Image errors or any image that differs from true anatomy of the reflector. Can be caused by malfunction of the ultrasound system, physical limitations of ultrasound, or operator error.

ASE: American Society of Echocardiography. Institutes certifying examinations and upholds competency standards for interpretation of echocardiograms.

Attenuation: Reduction of amplitude of an ultrasound wave as it propagates through the medium.

Attenuation coefficient: Attenuation in negative decibels per 1 cm travel. In soft tissues **0.5 dB/cm/MHz.**

Augmentation: Increase in venous flow with distal compression; a sign of venous patency.

Axial resolution: The minimal distance between two objects that are positioned along a line parallel to the ultrasound beam where both can be distinguished as separate objects. Defines longitudinal or depth resolution or the distance between two reflectors, measured in millimeters, at which the reflectors are still imaged as separate. It is measured as a half of the ultrasound pulse length with typical values in diagnostic ultrasound of **0.05 to 0.5 mm.**

Backing material: Damping material consisting of a layer of epoxy resin impregnated with tungsten placed behind the active element of the ultrasound transducer. It improves axial resolution by decreasing pulse duration (after-ringing), much like a hand placed on a guitar string.

Banding: Hyperechoic artifact within the focal zone. Appears as a bright horizontal stripe.

Beam (ultrasound beam): Bundle of acoustic radiation transmitted by the transducer, caused by wavelet interactions and shaped like an hourglass.

Bernoulli equation (simplified): Converts maximal flow velocity into a pressure gradient. Used to assess the severity of either valvular or vascular stenosis. **Pressure gradient (mm Hg) = 4 × [Max flow velocity (m/sec)]^2**

Bioeffects: All patient-related effects of acoustic radiation.

Bistable image: Black-and-white image characterized by excessively high contrast and a narrow dynamic range (see *dynamic range*).

B-mode ultrasound: Imaging mode where echoes are represented by dots, with the brightness corresponding to the strength of the signal. Though two-dimensional ultrasound is often called B mode, this use of the terminology is technically incorrect.

Case: The outer shell of the transducer that prevents electrical injury to the patient and the operator.

Cavitation (stable and unstable): Biologic effect of the ultrasound on the tissues caused by expansion and bursting of air microbubbles in tissue.

Color Doppler: Pulsed Doppler technique that converts flow velocity information into color. Colored Doppler measures the "mean" velocity of the moving reflector.

Color map: Depicts the direction and velocity (sometimes also variance) of the flow with relationship to the transducer. It is presented as a colored stripe in the corner of the image. The upper color represents maximal flow velocity toward the transducer; the lower color represents maximal flow velocity away from the transducer.

Compensation (also known as TGC or DGC [time or distance gain compensation]): Image processing technique that is used to selectively amplify distant (deeper) and therefore weaker echoes, making all similar reflectors look the same, irrespective of the depth.

Compression: Image processing technique that diminishes the difference between the strongest and the weakest echo signal (the brightest and the darkest parts of the image) by reducing the dynamic range.

Constructive interference: Summation of two in-phase sound waves to form a wave with greater amplitude.

Continuous wave Doppler (CW): Nonimaging ultrasound modality measuring flow velocity by Doppler shift. One active element continuously emits and the other receives ultrasound signals. CW measures maximal (peak) flow velocity but cannot measure velocity at a selected point of flow because of signal overlap (range ambiguity).

Convex (curved) array transducer: Transducer with active elements arranged in an arc and activated in the same manner, as in a linear array transducer. Curved array transducers tend to be lower-frequency abdominal transducers characterized by a large image both in the near and far field with a blunted or trapezoid sector image.

Crosstalk: Doppler mirror-image artifact.

Crystal: Active element of the ultrasound transducer.

Curie point (temperature): The temperature (360°C) at which the active element irreversibly loses its piezoelectric properties. As a result, the transducer should never be exposed to heat sterilization.

Decibel (dB; 0.1 Bell): Unit of amplitude or intensity. In audible sound, it is perceived as loudness. The decibel scale is logarithmic and relative, such that a 3-dB difference indicates a twofold change in the intensity or loudness of a sound, while a 10-dB difference indicates a 10-fold change in the intensity or loudness of a sound.

Demodulation: Image processing technique that makes echo signals suitable for screen display.

"Diagnosis of existence": Checking for the presence of a lesion or structure. This approach defines the present state of the art in diagnostic ultrasound.

"Diagnosis of identification": Using ultrasound for identification of the nature of a lesion or structure (i.e., malignant vs. benign). Major direction of the development in future ultrasound applications.

Diffraction: The ability of sound to spread in more or less concentric circles in all directions. Higher-frequency sounds (ultrasound) diverge less than lower-frequency sounds. Diffraction allows a listener to hear sound around corners.

Digital converter: Converts images into a digital format for archiving and display.

Display (screen, glass): That part of the ultrasound system where the image is observed.

Divergence: Spreading out of the ultrasound beam beyond the focal point. Higher-frequency transducers produce less divergence.

Doppler effect: Change in frequency of the emitted or reflected sound produced by the moving object. If the object is moving toward the receiver, the frequency increases (positive Doppler shift); if it is moving away, the frequency decreases (negative Doppler shift).

Doppler packets (ensembles): Series of multiple pulses in colored Doppler.

Doppler transducer: Utilizes Doppler effect (frequency difference between emitted and reflected ultrasound) to measure the velocity of the moving reflector.

Dosimetry: Study of the biologic effects of acoustic radiation.

DSP: Digital signal processor. Improves ultrasound image quality.

Dyskinetic: Organ or its part moving in the direction opposite to what is expected (e.g., aneurysmal dilatation during systole).

dV/dP: Compliance.

Duplex imaging: Modality providing an anatomic image and Doppler flow information simultaneously.

Duty factor (DF): Percentage of time when the transducer emits sound (usually **0.1% to 1%** in imaging and pulsed Doppler transducers). If DF is 0%, the system is off; if it is 100%, continuous wave Doppler is on.

Dynamic frequency tuning: An imaging technique utilizing higher-frequency signals to visualize superficial structures and lower-frequency signals to image deeper structures.

Dynamic range: The ratio of the strongest to the weakest signal in the ultrasound system (image gray scale). The narrower the dynamic range, the higher is the image contrast.

Echo: Any reflected sound.

Echocardiography (echo): Ultrasound study of the heart, so named by cardiologists to differentiate the cardiac examination from other applications of ultrasonography.

Echoencephalography: Archaic A-mode technique used to detect the position of midline brain structures in head trauma.

EMBUS: Endobronchial ultrasound is a form of endoscopic ultrasound. Combination of optical bronchoscope and ultrasound system (used in diagnosis of lung lesions).

Endoscopic ultrasound: Combination of an optical endoscope and ultrasound system within one instrument.

Energy (acoustic): Amount of energy (acoustic radiation) delivered by the sound beam into the tissue, proportional to the bioeffects of the ultrasound radiation.

Enhancement: Low attenuation artifact resulting in a hyperechoic (bright) image distal to a hypoechoic structure.

Five-chamber view: Apical echocardiographic view that visualizes the atria, ventricles, and aorta. Useful for measurement of stroke volume and aortic flow velocity.

Focus or focal zone: Narrowest area (waist) of the hourglass-shaped ultrasound beam. Technically, the focus is a single point in the middle of the focal zone. The narrower the focus, the better is the lateral resolution of the image.

Focusing: Techniques diminishing the size of the focus (acoustic lenses in single-crystal transducers [fixed focus] or electronic focusing in phased array probes [adjustable focus]). Focusing improves lateral resolution.

Fraunhofer or far zone: The area of the ultrasound beam distal to the focus where there is beam divergence.

Frequency: The number of sound oscillations (periods) occurring per unit of time (1 second). It is measured in hertz (one period per second). This parameter is reciprocal to the period. (Frequency × Period = 1) Any sound with a frequency >20,000 Hz is an ultrasound; diagnostic ultrasound frequency is between 2,000,000 and 20,000,000 Hz (2 to 20 MHz). Sound with a frequency <20 Hz is an infrasound. Neither ultrasound nor infrasound is audible.

Fresnel or near zone: The area of the beam between the transducer and the focus (where the beam is converging).

Footprint (acoustic footprint): Area of the direct contact between the transducer and the surface of the skin. Curved array probes, used in the abdominal ultrasound, have the largest footprint.

Fourier transform: Form of spectral analysis of Doppler signal.

Frame: One complete sweep of the mechanical or the phased array two-dimensional transducer. The frame is a basic element of the movie of the mobile reflector.

Frame rate: Number of frames produced by the ultrasound system per unit of time. Measured in hertz, it should not be confused with the frequency of the ultrasound wave. The higher the frame rate, the more fluid is the motion and the more "real time" is the two-dimensional image. Higher frame rates result in better temporal resolution.

Gain (receiver gain): A knob controlling amplification. Higher gain increases screen brightness (see amplification).

Ghosting: Doppler artifact caused by registering the movements of adjacent structures rather than the flow of blood.

Harmonic imaging (tissue harmonics, THI): Technique utilizing echoes with frequencies that are multiples of that of the emitted signal for image formation. The frequency of the emitted sound is known as fundamental (Ff); therefore, harmonic frequency will be the fundamental frequency × 2, × 4 etc. (i.e., if Ff = 2 MHz, then with THI the image will be formed from the echoes with the frequency of 4 MHz). THI signals are generated in the tissues, eliminating some artifacts and very often (but not always) improving the overall quality of the image.

Heterogeneous: Displaying multiple echo characteristics throughout the image or area of an image.

Homogeneous: Displaying the same echo characteristics throughout the image or area of an image.

Huygen principle: Explains the formation of the hourglass shape of the ultrasound beam by the algebraic sum of the constructive and destructive interference of the individual wavelets within the beam.

Hyperechoic: Containing more echoes than usual or expected, resulting in a brighter image.

Hyperkinetic: Moving more than expected.

Hypoechoic: Containing fewer echoes than usual or expected, resulting in a darker image.

Hypokinetic: Moving less than expected.

Impedance: Calculated by multiplying density and propagation speed and measured in rayls. Impedance describes the sound transmitting and reflecting properties of the medium. The boundary between two mediums with different impedance will produce reflection, but the boundary between two mediums with identical impedance will produce no reflection. The greater the difference in impedance, the greater is the reflective property of the boundary. Impedances of 1,200,000 to 1,800,000 rayls are usual at human tissue boundaries.

Intensity: Power over area (measured in watts/cm^2). Power correlates with bioeffects. Multiple ways of measuring intensity exist, but SPTA (spatial peak, temporal average) best predicts thermal energy transfer and therefore thermal bioeffects.

Jellyfish sign: Chest ultrasound term that describes compressed lung visualized floating in pleural fluid undulating with the respiratory cycle.

Jet: High-velocity Doppler flow signal (high pitch and amplitude) due to valvular or vascular (arterial) stenosis.

Knobology: Knowledge of the particular controls of the ultrasound. Controls differ greatly from one ultrasound system to another and require specific training that is unique to each device.

Laminar (parabolic) flow: Bullet-shaped, orderly flow of blood through a vessel, where the blood at the center of the vessel moves faster than that at the periphery, but the movement is in parallel lines. Associated with a spectral Doppler envelope with a thin outer line that delineates a clear space or spectral window. Distinguished from disturbed or turbulent flow associated with an obstructive lesion.

Lateral resolution (angular or transverse resolution): The minimal distance between two objects that are positioned along a line perpendicular to the ultrasound beam where both can be distinguished as separate objects.

Line density: The number of ultrasound beams (lines) per unit of surface forming two-dimensional images. Increased line density improves spatial but reduces temporal resolution.

Linear array: Common transducer design that uses a series of piezoelectric elements arrayed in a straight line. Neighboring elements are excited simultaneously resulting in individual scan lines that are parallel to one another. Often used in vascular transducers, linear arrays are usually high-frequency probes designed to visualize relatively shallow structures. They are characterized by a square image.

Lobes (side and grating): Artifacts caused by the echoes of ultrasound beams transmitted in a secondary direction (other than that of the main axis).

Long-axis plane: In echocardiography, the ultrasound plane that is parallel to the long axis of the left ventricle (LV). This is defined by a line that goes through the LV apex and the center of the base of the LV intersecting with the center of the aortic valve. In vascular and general ultrasound, the plane that parallels the longest dimension of the anatomic structure.

Lung flapping: Chest ultrasound term that describes compressed lung visualized floating in pleural fluid undulating with the respiratory cycle.

McConnell sign: Diffuse hypokinesis of the right ventricular free wall sparing the apex. It is an echocardiographic finding suggestive of pulmonary embolism.

Mirror-image artifact: In two-dimensional imaging, where an object adjacent to a curved tissue plane is duplicated on the other side of the curved surface in mirror orientation; most commonly seen adjacent to the diaphragm or other highly reflective boundary (mirror). In Doppler imaging, a symmetric spectral image on the opposite side of the baseline from the true signal (cross-talk).

M-mode ultrasound: An early application of diagnostic ultrasound that utilizes a single line of ultrasound interrogation with the signal plotting reflector position against the time. Useful for high temporal resolution of rapidly moving cardiac structures (i.e., valves).

Moderator band: A normal right ventricular (RV) structure housing the right bundle that can be confused with a mural RV thrombus.

Nyquist frequency limit: Pulsed wave Doppler frequency at which aliasing occurs. Nyquist frequency limit (kHz) = Pulse repetition frequency (PRF)/2.

Ocular (ophthalmic) ultrasound: Ultrasound examination of the eye. Requires lower output power (ocular or ophthalmic settings) on the ultrasound system because of biologic effects.

Oscillation: A rhythmic change in a parameter that may produce a wave.

PACS: **P**icture **A**rchiving and **C**ommunication **S**ystem. Digital archiving.

Period: Time needed to complete one wave cycle. This parameter is reciprocal to frequency (Frequency × Period = 1); a typical value in diagnostic ultrasound is $1 - 5 \times 10^{-7}$ sec.

Phased array transducers: Transducer design where the image sector is triangular, and both focusing and steering are achieved electronically. A relatively high-frequency phased array transducer offers good real-time images of moving structures. This transducer type has a small acoustic footprint, so that it is useful for imaging through the intercostal spaces as in echocardiography.

Piezoelectricity: The property of some natural and man-made materials to generate an electrical impulse in response to mechanical stress or to deform when the electrical impulse is applied (**reverse piezoelectric effect**).

Pixel: The smallest distinct element of the digital picture or movie. Increased pixel density of the image improves image quality (spatial resolution).

Power Doppler: Colored Doppler modality detecting presence of flow regardless of direction or velocity (used to detect presence or absence of flow in ischemic organs). The only colored Doppler modality not susceptible to aliasing.

Processing (signal processing): Conversion of the ultrasound signal into the image.

Pulse repetition frequency (PRF): The number of pulses emitted by imaging or pulsed wave transducer per unit of time (usually 1 second); measured in hertz. Not to be confused with the frequency of the ultrasound waves.

Pulsed wave Doppler (PW): Single-crystal Doppler modality offering range resolution but subject to aliasing.

Range equation: Distance to the boundary (mm) = time of flight (μsec) × 0.77 (mm/μsec); used by the ultrasound system to position the object on the screen (13 μsec flight = 1 cm depth).

Range resolution: Ability to identify the location of the pulsed wave Doppler sample.

Rayleigh scattering: Equal reflection in all directions occurring when the reflector is significantly smaller then the wavelength of the ultrasound.

Reflection: Return of ultrasound beam (energy) from the reflective boundary to the source in a form of an echo.

Refraction: Change in the direction of the ultrasound beam when it encounters a boundary with different propagation speed at an angle. Governed by Snell's law.

Refraction artifact: Side-by-side copy of the anatomic structure.

Regional wall motion abnormalities (RWMAs): Echocardiographic term indicating segmental ventricular wall contractile dysfunction; often associated with coronary artery disease.

Reverberation artifact: Multiple, equally spaced, hyperechoic horizontal lines ("venetian blinds") perpendicular to the direction of the ultrasound beam. Caused by the presence of two strong adjacent reflectors (i.e., parietal and visceral pleura).

Ring-down (comet tail) artifact: Solid hyperechoic vertical line (form of reverberations).

Ringing: Internal vibrations of the active element that continue after the echo signal has been received. Ringing deteriorates the image quality. Ringing is reduced by backing of "damping" material in the transducer.

Sagittal view: Long-axis view.

SAM: Systolic anterior motion of the mitral leaflet (sign of hypertrophic cardiomyopathy).

Scattering: Reflection of sound in all directions.

Sector: Imaging area in two-dimensional studies. Limiting sector size improves temporal resolution.

Segmental Doppler, Doppler segmental pressure (DSP) analysis: Flow velocity detection in specific places usually utilized in arterial studies to detect the location of a stenotic area.

Shadowing: Hypoechoic vertical linear artifact caused by the ultrasound beam encountering a high attenuation reflector (i.e., gallstone).

Short-axis plane: Plane perpendicular to the long axis; also referred to as the transverse or cross-section plane. In echocardiography and vascular ultrasound, the imaged organ appears round.

Snell's law: Governs refraction (see refraction). Sine (transmission angle): Sine (incident angle) = Propagation speed A: propagation speed B where A and B are two layers at the boundary.

Spatial resolution: Ability to show image in more detail (see pixel).

Spectral waveform analysis: Graphic display of flow velocity against time.

Speed of sound: Propagation speed (in soft tissue = 1,540 m/sec).

TEE: Transesophageal echocardiogram.

Tissue elastic imaging (elastometry): Developing technology that uses ultrasound to detect physical properties (hardness) of the tissues (i.e., breast). May become useful in early breast cancer detection.

Transcranial Doppler (TCD): Doppler study designed to detect the flow velocity of intracranial arteries (can be used to diagnose vasospasm after intracranial trauma or to document brain death).

Transmission: Onward propagation of the unreflected portion of the ultrasound beam at the reflective boundary.

Transverse view: Short-axis plane.

TTE: Transthoracic echocardiogram (ultrasound of the heart).

Turbulent flow: Chaotic disorganized flow pattern indicative of vascular stenosis or valvular heart disease. In colored Doppler echocardiography, turbulent flow is also called **mosaic** flow pattern.

Two-dimensional imaging (2-D): Two-dimensional images offering gray-scale "slices" of anatomic structures in the plane of the steered or serially activated ultrasound beam. Sometimes also called B-mode imaging, which is technically incorrect.

Two-dimensional phased array transducers: Used to form three-dimensional and three-dimensional real-time (four-dimensional) images.

Velocity: Directional speed.

Vortex shed: Area distal to the jet where laminar flow becomes disturbed.

VTI: Velocity time integral. Used in calculation of the stroke volume and cardiac output.

Wave: Rhythmic transmission of energy (measured as an oscillating parameter) through the medium.

Wavelength: Length of the single cycle within the wave measured in the units of distance (mm). Wavelength (mm) = 1.54 mm/frequency (MHz) in human tissues (0.1 – 1 mm is typical).

Window (acoustic window): The part of the body surface through which the ultrasound image is obtained.

Z transform: Algorithm for spectral analysis.

Zone: Ultrasound image for fixed focus transducers (**near** = from the transducer to the focus, **far** = beneath or deeper than the focus). For multifocus transducers, the zone division is not as well defined. In most portable intensive care unit systems, there are two separate knobs that control near and far field gain. These gain areas correspond to the near and far zone.

Zoom: The ability to enlarge the image of the structure for close-up view. Preprocessing zoom increases the number of pixels per squared centimeter and does not deteriorate the spatial resolution; postprocessing zoom increases the size of the individual pixels and worsens the resolution.

Algorithms

GUIDANCE FOR ULTRASOUND PROBE SELECTION (SEE ALSO CHAPTER 3)

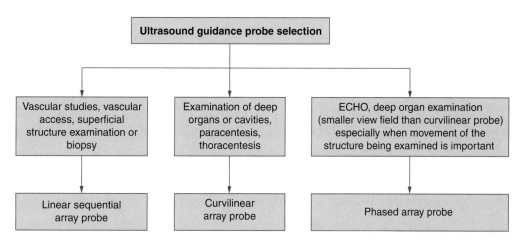

DIAGNOSTIC ALGORITHM FOR EYE COMPLAINTS AND VISUAL LOSS

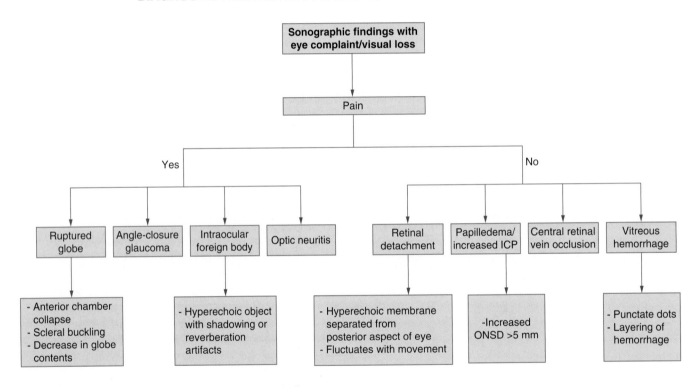

Note: ICP, intracranial pressure; ONSD, optic nerve sheath diameter

DIAGNOSTIC ALGORITHM FOR OCULAR ULTRASOUND

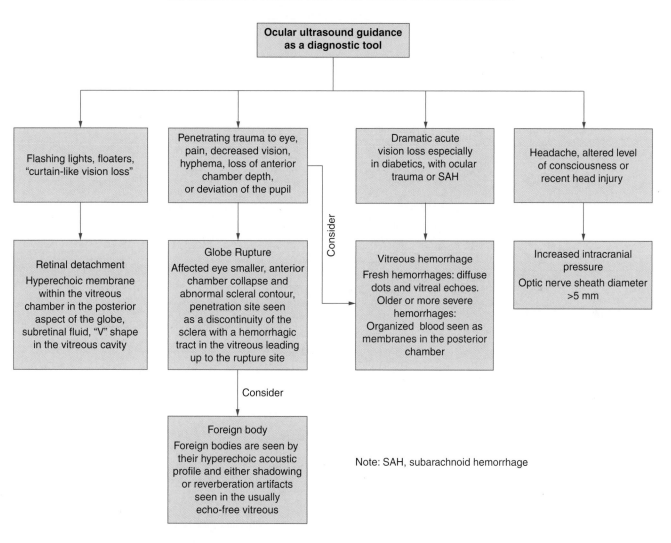

Note: SAH, subarachnoid hemorrhage

DIAGNOSTIC ALGORITHM FOR CHECKING ENDOTRACHEAL TUBE (ET) PLACEMENT

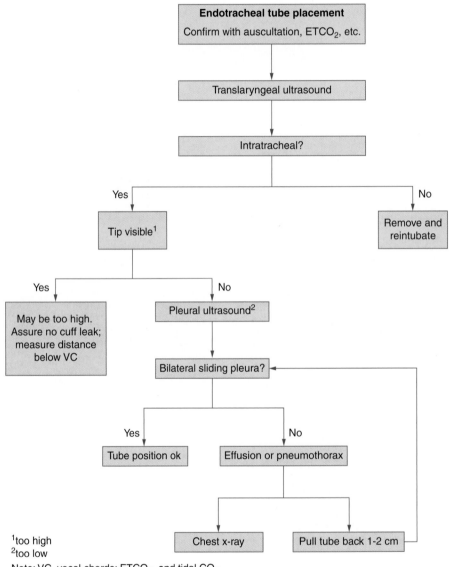

Endotracheal tube placement
Confirm with auscultation, $ETCO_2$, etc.

Translaryngeal ultrasound

Intratracheal?

Yes — Tip visible[1]

No — Remove and reintubate

Yes — May be too high. Assure no cuff leak; measure distance below VC

No — Pleural ultrasound[2]

Bilateral sliding pleura?

Yes — Tube position ok

No — Effusion or pneumothorax

Chest x-ray

Pull tube back 1-2 cm

[1]too high
[2]too low
Note: VC, vocal chords; $ETCO_2$, end tidal CO_2

DIAGNOSTIC ALGORITHM FOR DYSPNEA

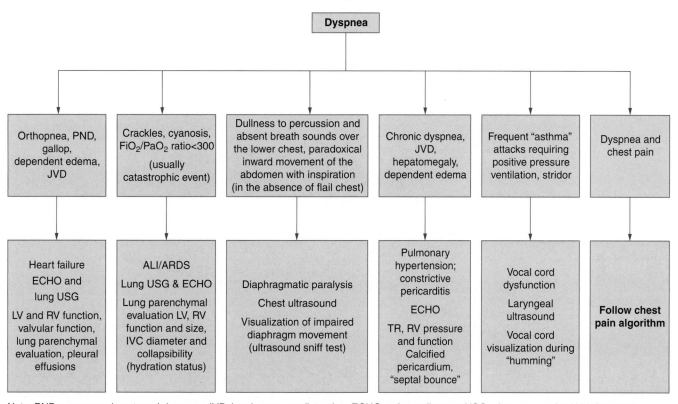

Note: PND, paroxysmal nocturnal dyspnea; JVD, jugular venous distention; ECHO, echocardiogram; USG, ultrasonography; LV, left ventricle; RV, right ventricle; IVC, inferior vena cava; TR, tricuspid regurgitation

DIAGNOSTIC ALGORITHM FOR CHEST PAIN

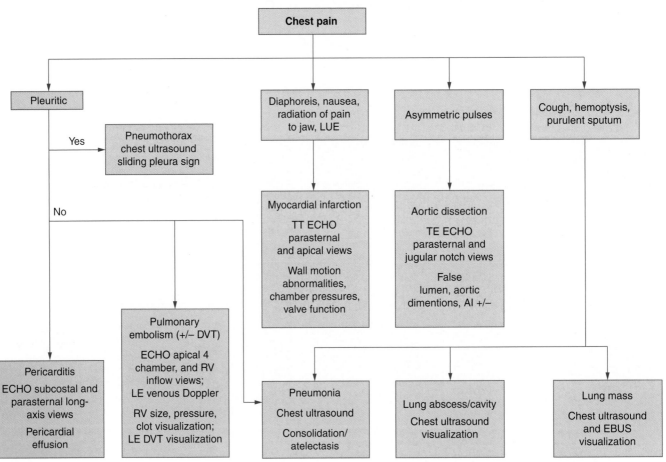

Note: LE, lower extremity; ECHO, echocardiography; RV, right ventricle; DVT, deep vein thrombosis; EBUS, endobronchial ultrasound; TT, transthoracic; TE, transesophageal

DIAGNOSTIC ALGORITHM FOR ACUTE CORONARY SYNDROME (ACS)

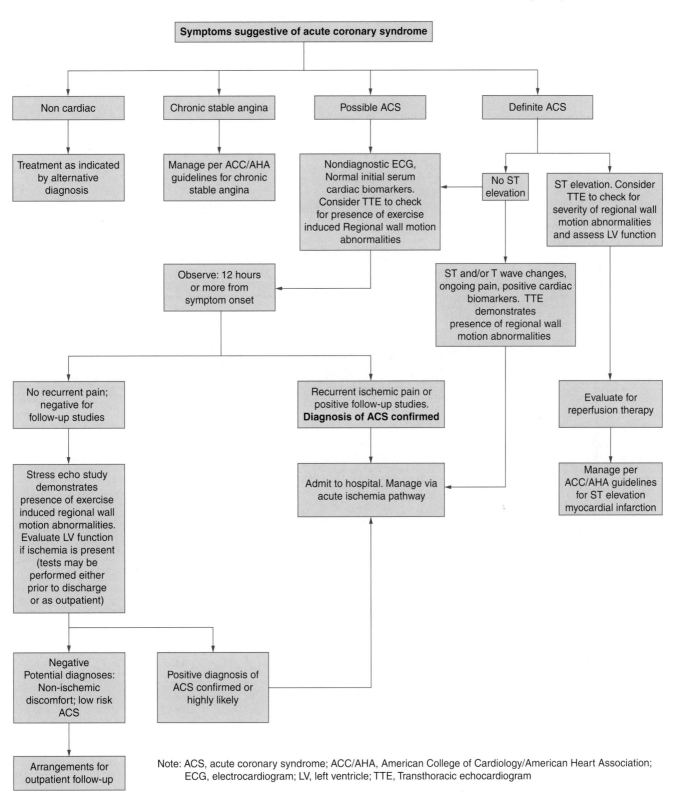

Note: ACS, acute coronary syndrome; ACC/AHA, American College of Cardiology/American Heart Association; ECG, electrocardiogram; LV, left ventricle; TTE, Transthoracic echocardiogram

DIAGNOSTIC ALGORITHM FOR SYNCOPE

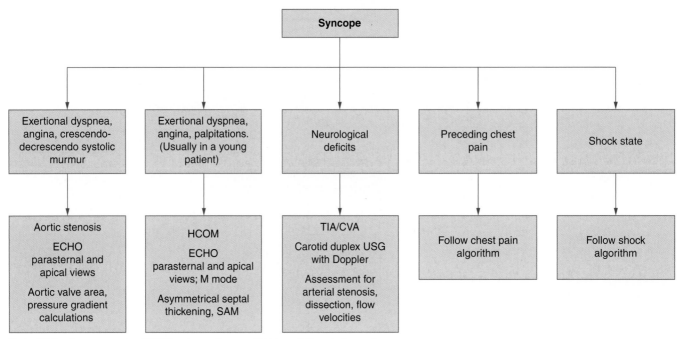

Note: USG, ultrasonography; ECHO, echocardiogram; SAM, systolic anterior motion

DIAGNOSTIC AND THERAPEUTIC ALGORITHM FOR CARDIAC ARREST DUE TO PULSELESS ELECTRICAL ACTIVITY (PEA) OR ASYSTOLE

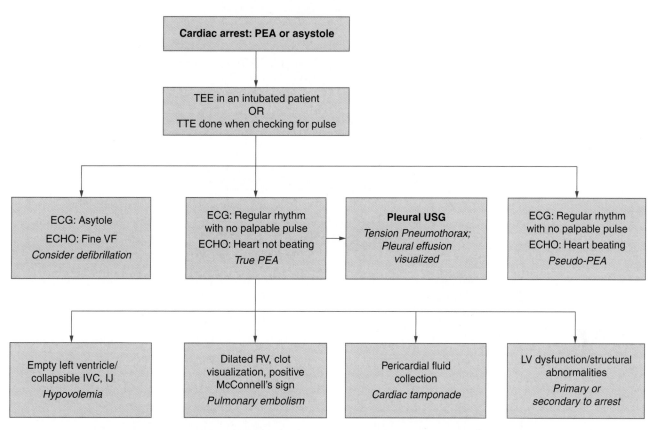

Note: PEA, pulseless electrical activity; TEE, transesophageal echocardiography; TTE, transthoracic echocardiography; ECG, electrocardiogram; ECHO, echocardiography; VF, ventricular fibrillation; USG, ultrasonographic; IVC, inferior vena cava; IJ, internal jugular; RV, right ventricle; LV, left ventricle

ALGORITHM FOR FEEL

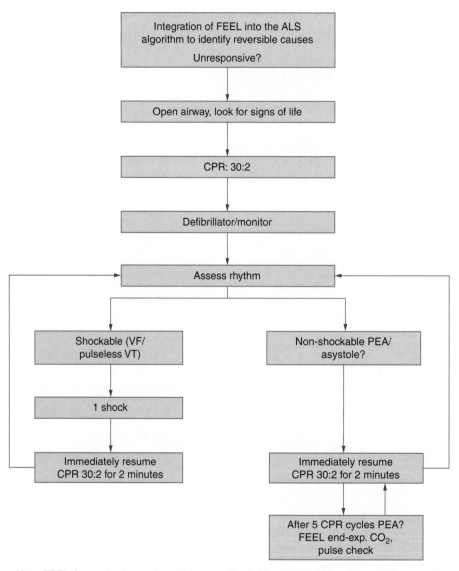

Note: FEEL, focused echocardiographic evaluation in life support; ALS, advanced life support; CPR, cardiopulmonary resuscitations; VF, ventricular fibrillation; VT, ventricular tachycardia; PEA, pulseless electrical activity

DIAGNOSTIC ALGORITHM FOR SHOCK

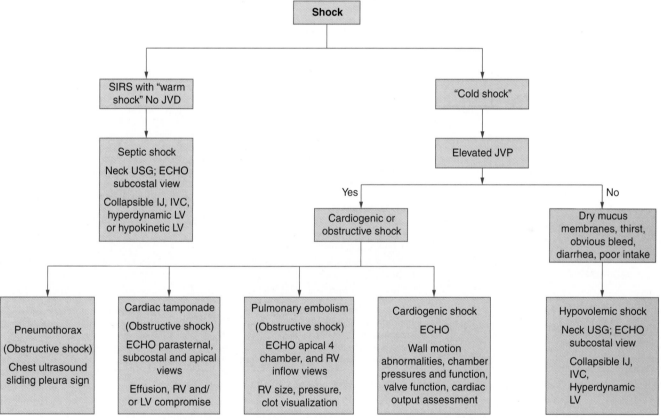

Note: SIRS, systemic inflammatory response syndrome; JVD, jugular venous distention; JVP, jugular venous pressure; USG, ultrasonography; ECHO, echocardiogram; IJ, internal jugular; IVC, inferior vene cava; LV, left ventricle; RV, right ventricle

DIAGNOSTIC ALGORITHM FOR TRAUMA (SEE ALSO CHAPTERS 7 AND 10)

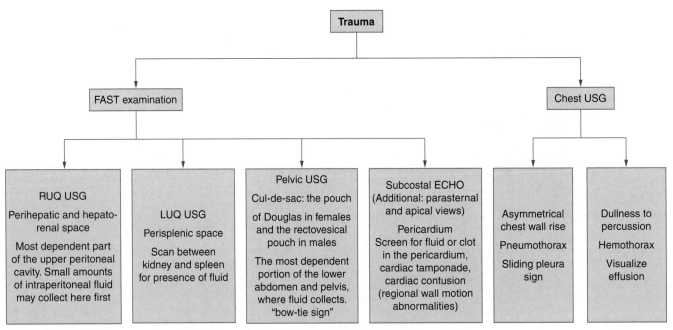

Note: USG, ultrasonographic; RUQ, right upper quadrant; LUQ, left upper quadrant; ECHO, echocardiography

DIAGNOSTIC ALGORITHM FOR ABDOMINAL PAIN (SEE ALSO CHAPTER 10)

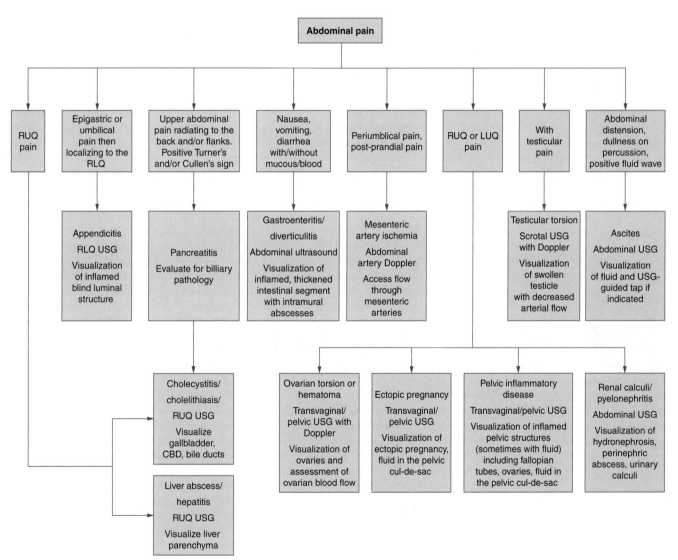

Note: RUQ, right upper quadrant; RLQ, right lower quadrant; LUQ, left upper quadrant; USG, ultrasonography; CBD, common bile duct

DIAGNOSTIC ALGORITHM FOR INCREASED ABDOMINAL GIRTH (SEE ALSO CHAPTER 10)

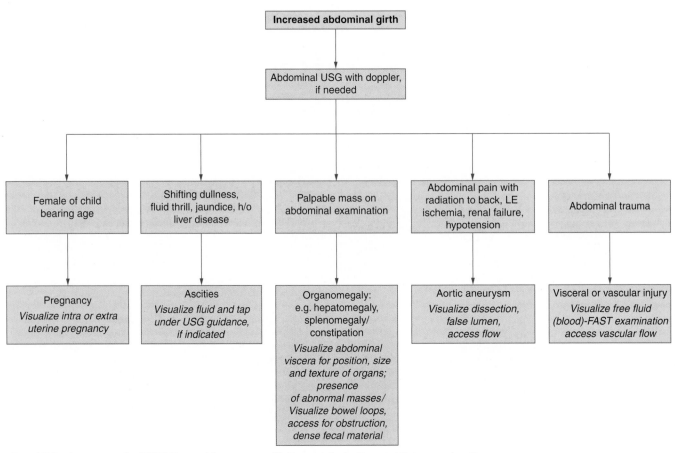

Note: USG, ultrasonography; FAST, Focused Assessment with Sonography for Trauma; LE, lower extremity

DIAGNOSTIC ULTRASOUND FINDINGS FOR FEMALE PATIENTS WITH ABDOMINAL PAIN (SEE ALSO CHAPTER 11)

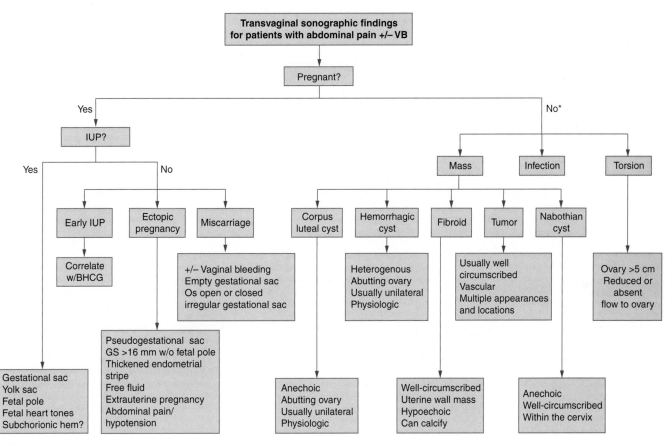

* Should obtain comprehensive scan

Note: IUP, intrauterine pregnancy; BHCG, beta human chorionic gonadotrophin; GS, gestational sac

DIAGNOSTIC ALGORITHM FOR RENAL INSUFFICIENCY

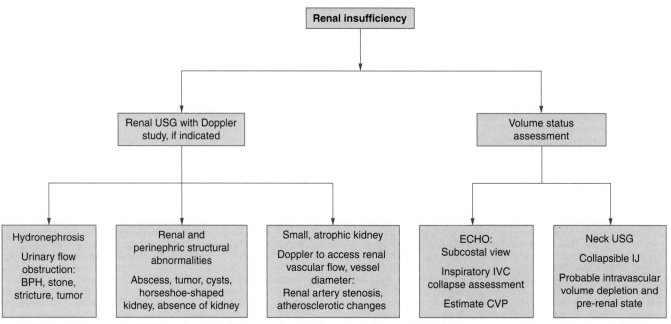

Note: USG, ultrasonography; BPH, benign prostatic hypertrophy; ECHO, echocardiogram; IVC, inferior vena cava; CVP, central venous pressure; IJ, internal jugular

DIAGNOSTIC ALGORITHM FOR LOWER EXTREMITY PAIN

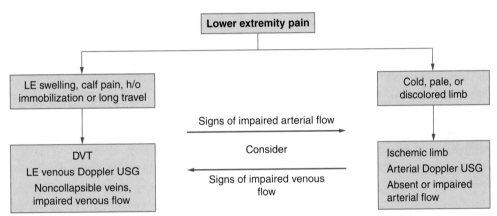

Note: LE, lower extremity; DVT, deep venous thrombosis; USG, ultrasonography

Table of Ultrasound Current Procedural Terminology (CPT)® Codes for Examinations and Procedures

- 2.76937—Ultrasonic guidance for vascular access
- 3.76942—Ultrasonic guidance for needle placement (i.e., aspiration injection)
- 4.76970—Follow-up for patency of established vascular access
- 5.76999—Other diagnostic procedures done at bedside
- 6.76775—Limited image of retroperitoneal space (e.g., abdominal aortic aneurysm rupture)
- 7.76705—Limited image of the abdomen (e.g., abscesses)
- 8.93308—Limited study of the heart (e.g., differential diagnosis of shock to assess left ventricular end-diastolic volume)
- 9.93321—Limited Doppler study of the heart (e.g., to assist with the bedside diagnosis of pulmonary embolism)
- 10.93307-08—Two-dimensional echocardiogram
- 11.93325—Echo color Doppler
- 12.93320—Echo Doppler
- 13.Q9957—Echo with intravenous contrast (same modifier for the stress echo)
- 14.93350—Stress echo
- 1.76930—Ultrasonic guidance for pericardiocentesis (in code situation)

Index

Numbers followed by "*f*" and "*t*" denote figures and tables, respectively.